Living and Dying with AIDS

Living and Dying with AIDS

Edited by
Paul I. Ahmed

National Center for Health Statistics
Centers for Disease Control
U.S. Department of Health and Human Services
Hyattsville, Maryland
and
Lecturer, Department of Health Education
University College
University of Maryland
College Park, Maryland

With the assistance of
Nancy Ahmed

Plenum Press • New York and London

Library of Congress Cataloging-in-Publication Data

Living and dying with AIDS / edited by Paul I. Ahmed.
       p.   cm.
    Includes bibliographical references and index.
    ISBN 0-306-43851-8
    1. AIDS (Disease)--Psychological aspects.   I. Ahmed, Paul I.
    [DNLM: 1. Acquired Immunodeficiency Syndrome--psychology.
  2. Adaptation, Psychological.   WD 308 L783]
  RC607.A26L58 1991
  362.1'969792--dc20
  DNLM/DLC
  for Library of Congress   ˙91-29060
                                                           CIP

Edited by Paul I. Ahmed in his private capacity. No official support or endorsement by the U.S. Department of Health and Human Services is intended or should be inferred.

ISBN 0-306-43851-8

© 1992 Plenum Press, New York
A Division of Plenum Publishing Corporation
233 Spring Street, New York, N.Y. 10013

Printed in the United States of America

To Irene

From her proud and loving father

Contributors

PAUL I. AHMED • Director, Special Foreign Currency Research Program, National Center for Health Statistics, Centers for Disease Control, U.S. Department of Health and Human Services, Hyattsville, Maryland 20782; and Lecturer, Department of Health Education, University College, University of Maryland, College Park, Maryland

MICHAEL H. ANTONI • Center for the Biopsychosocial Study of AIDS, Department of Psychology, University of Miami, Coral Gables, Florida 33124

DAVID D. CELENTANO • Professor and Chairman, Division of Behavioral Sciences and Health Education, Department of Health Policy and Management, The Johns Hopkins University, School of Hygiene and Public Health, Baltimore, Maryland 21205

ANNE J. DAVIS • Professor, Department of Mental Health, Community Health and Administrative Nursing, School of Nursing, University of California, San Francisco, San Francisco, California 94143-0608

JONELL EFANTIS • Department of Obstetrics and Gynecology, University of Miami School of Medicine, Jackson Memorial Hospital, Miami, Florida 33139

MARIA E. ESPOSITO • Assistant Professor, Department of Psychiatry, Uniformed Services University of the Health Sciences, Bethesda, Maryland 20814-4799

BARBARA G. FALTZ • Program Coordinator, CPC Belmont Hills Hospital, Belmont, California 94002

MARY ANN FLETCHER • Center for the Biopsychosocial Study of AIDS, Department of Medicine, University of Miami School of Medicine, Miami, Florida 33139

ROCHELLE GRIFFIN • Stichting Vuurulinder/Fire Butterfly Foundation for Conscious Living and Dying, 5328 AS Rossum, The Netherlands

HARRY C. HOLLOWAY • Deputy Dean and Professor, Department of Psychiatry, Uniformed Services University of the Health Sciences, Bethesda, Maryland 20814-4799

JOYCE HUNTER • HIV Center for Clinical and Behavioral Studies, New York, New York 10032

LARRY H. INGRAHAM • Department of Military Psychiatry, Walter Reed Army Institute of Research, Washington, D.C. 20307-5100

MARY ANNE JACKSON • University of Missouri, Kansas City, Children's Mercy Hospital, Kansas City, Missouri 64108

IRENE JILLSON-BOOSTROM • President, Policy Research, Inc., Clarksville, Maryland 21029

ARTHUR LAPERRIERE • Research Assistant Professor, Center for the Biopsychosocial Study of AIDS, Department of Psychiatry, University of Miami School of Medicine, Miami, Florida 33139

JENNIFER MARKS • Assistant Professor, Department of Medicine, University of Miami School of Medicine, Miami, Florida 33136

ANN E. NORWOOD • Assistant Professor, Department of Psychiatry, Uniformed Services University of the Health Sciences, Bethesda, Maryland 20814-4799

MARY JO O'SULLIVAN • Director, Department of Obstetrics and Gynecology, University of Miami School of Medicine, Jackson Memorial Hospital, Miami, Florida 33139

ANTHONY J. PUENTES • Public Health and Addiction Medicine Specialist, San Francisco, California 94131

JAMES R. RUNDELL • Department of Psychiatry, Uniformed Services University of the Health Sciences, Bethesda, Maryland 20814-4799

ROBERT SCHAECHER • The Calhoun School, New York, New York 10024

NEIL SCHNEIDERMAN • James L. Knight Professor of Psychology, Psychiatry, and Medicine, Center for the Biopsychosocial Study of AIDS, University of Miami, Coral Gables, Florida 33124

SANDRA C. SELLIN • Associate Clinical Instructor, City College of San Francisco, San Francisco, California 94112

SEANA HIRSCHFELD SHAW • Assistant Clinical Professor of Psychiatry, University of Miami, School of Medicine, Miami, Florida 33101

JAY SKYLER • Professor of Medicine, Psychology, and Pediatrics, Department of Medicine, University of Miami School of Medicine, Miami, Florida 33136

AMANDA BENEDICT SONNEGA • Division of Behavioral Sciences and Health Education, Department of Health Policy and Management, The Johns Hopkins University, School of Hygiene and Public Health, Baltimore, Maryland 21205

ALEXANDRA TEGUIS • Professor of Psychology, Manchester Community College, Manchester, Connecticut 06040

BRIAN M. WICKLUND • University of Missouri, Kansas City, Children's Mercy Hospital, Kansas City, Missouri 64108

Foreword

In this nation, in this decade, there is only one way to deal with an individual who is sick—with dignity, with compassion, care and confidentiality, and without discrimination.

> Statement made by President George
> Bush at the National Business Leadership
> Conference

This book is about the care of sick human beings. It is about the heroic struggle of individuals with AIDS. It is about their daily coping in the workplace and at home; about economic problems, the loss of friendship and family support, and physical and emotional pain. But it is also about empowering them to deal with their disease, viewing them not as victims but as warriors, vital and active participants in their battle against AIDS.

This book is also about the social context in which HIV-infected persons and people with AIDS live. It is about how we must learn to deal with sickness in more compassionate and humanitarian ways and what we yet need to learn. It touches on the health care system that confronts those who are ill, on programs of prevention and education, and on the personal implications of broader national and local policies.

Information about this epidemic must play an important role in determining the resources our nation will invest in dealing with this monstrous disease. The U.S. Centers for Disease Control (CDC) continue to play a key role in establishing and maintaining a system of surveillance so that the nature and extent of the HIV/AIDS epidemic can be tracked. As of July 1991, there had been 186,895 AIDS cases reported and 110,411 deaths among those. Current estimates of the number of HIV-infected persons in our country range from 650,000 to 1.4 million, depending on the method used. Granted, these numbers do not tell the stories of the lives and deaths they encompass, but they do indicate the breadth of the problem we face.

This disease has profoundly challenged those it has stricken, and likewise it has demanded thoughtful innovation of all who work in the health-care field. Our research scientists have faced the task of unraveling the workings of an extremely complex virus. Our treatment and care providers have instituted revolutionary procedures for drug testing and methods for delivery of services. The challenge of providing accurate information on an epidemic that has brought such profound grief to so many and has created such controversy over proper ways of protecting the privacy of individuals and preventing discrimination against them has been of particular interest to me.

We at CDC's National Center for Health Statistics were given the task of exploring the feasibility of developing better estimates of the extent of HIV infection through a survey of a national probability sample. In this work we discovered that success could be obtained only by establishing ways of developing survey plans in collaboration with the two communities selected as test sites. Development of a full partnership with the Allegheny County Health Department in Pittsburgh, Pennsylvania, and with the Dallas County Health Department in Texas was the first step toward building communication with the broader communities. Each health department then appointed a committee representing groups and constituencies greatly interested in AIDS/HIV issues. Through these bodies we provided information about intent and substance of a local household HIV survey and attempted to resolve concerns raised from many points of view. Some felt that a certain amount of "scientific rigor" was sacrificed to the compromises made in this collaborative planning, but our team did achieve the capacity to complete two respectable surveys. Through such collaborative processes we hope that in the future we will be able to communicate even more successfully the value of certain scientific survey methods and be able to intervene in the midst of "controversy" to develop invaluable information.

Like everyone who has contributed to this book, a number of my old assumptions have been challenged by the AIDS epidemic and new strategies have been learned. I recall something our survey planning team told me they had heard many times from old hands in AIDS work (something they were to learn very quickly when they started planning the "*usual*" survey), "with AIDS, nothing is '*as usual*'." This book prompts us to understand the unusual realities of AIDS and challenges us to take constructive action, which will eventually stimulate thinking about other outbreaks in the future. As a result we are indebted to the editor and authors of this stimulating work.

Manning Feinleib

Hyattsville, Maryland

Preface

HIV illness confronts a fundamental existential issue: the need to live and die with dignity, and to provide personal and societal mechanisms to deal with the needs of the patients. How society responds to this fundamental issue will determine whether this is a time of disaster or a time of growth and of building new capacities.

This book deals with one of the most important issues in public health of the 1980s and 1990s—the health and welfare of patients stricken with AIDS: mothers, children, the young, and the old. It deals with their emotional crises in work settings and at home and with relatives and friends. It addresses the major coping strategies that arise from the severe emotional and physical stress related to the actual disease processes. The life and family crises of those stricken with AIDS, and their friends, are presented in personal ways and adaptive tasks and skills are identified.

AIDS patients need a wide range of medications and, sometimes, procedures that raise issues of trauma, self-esteem, isolation, chronic pain, surgery, and hospitalization. To deal with these psychological issues, the book is divided into five parts.

Part I presents a general perspective on life and death issues for AIDS patients and discusses the importance of addressing psychosocial factors in coping with the patients' battle for survival. Also outlined in this section are medical, legal, and ethical issues facing AIDS care providers.

Part II deals with various personal issues of adolescents, mothers, and families regarding AIDS and discusses the role of peer groups and families in creating adaptive strategies for peer management and settlement of life issues. The chapter on adolescents recommends sensitivity to countertransference issues for adolescents prone to depression and suicide. It points out intervention models that will assist adolescents in translating the knowledge they have about AIDS into effective behavioral changes. The chapter on mothers emphasizes the effect individual differences in the number and type of psychosocial stressors, the level of coping, and the extent of immunological functioning can have on pregnancy complications, perinatal transmission, and GU infections among seropositive pregnant women. Another chapter deals with methods of psychotherapy, in this case an integrated approach, for HIV patients and their families. This chapter points out that, with every phase of illness, the patient and the family face a different set of psychological tasks and adaptive measures, such as open acknowledgment of feelings of sickness, loss, and general grieving.

Part III deals with issues of living with HIV infection and the onset of disease. Coping processes and strategies and personal resources among the HIV spectrum of diseases are discussed. In addition, issues relating to substance abuse among AIDS patients are discussed and coping strategies are provided. A chapter on coping processes and strategies points out the need for longitudinal investigations of the effects of coping and social support on psychological functioning. Also pointed out is the need for evaluations of active interventions affecting coping styles or altered social support networks. Innovative intervention strategies for bolstering coping efforts and new social support mechanisms are recommended. A chapter on workplace issues and strategies to deal with HIV infection is also included in this section.

Part IV deals with grief, sadness, and loss of those dying or soon to die. This is a touching section in which Alexandra Teguis and Rochelle Griffin reflect about their long involvement with the pain of those suffering and those dead from HIV infection. Their writings bring to life the extraordinary suffering and the lack of resources for HIV-infected patients in the latter stages of the disease. A chapter by a county medical director, who suffered the loss of a friend, poignantly describes the tremendous obstacles—legal, social, and governmental—facing patients trying to receive services.

Part V discusses special circumstances AIDS creates for minorities, army personnel, and hemophiliacs. Special programs and therapies dealing with each group's needs are discussed. In addition, the scope of the problem for each of the groups is identified.

The present volume was assembled to fill the need for more information on consultation techniques and coping practices for AIDS patients. It is meant to be pragmatic in focus—to feel the pain of the patients and to offer insights into how to operate as a consultant to AIDS patients in such varied demanding settings as schools, churches, and workplaces. The emphasis is on providing information, insights, and coping practices to the self-help groups, consultant practitioners, and advanced novices on what is current in coping with AIDS. It is a volume for "feelers" and "doers" and activists who want to function more effectively in self-chosen roles as mental health consultants for AIDS patients, and for those professionals who want to learn more about consultation practices with such patients.

This book has been broadly conceived in order to meet the needs of diverse audiences. The materials are relevant for policy planners and program managers and for incorporation into university courses in AIDS management in a variety of disciplines such as nursing, medicine, public health, social work, psychiatry, and behavioral science.

Like many books, this one has been a long time "aborning," but that labor has been one of love and affection. I am a firm believer in the role of community and self-help groups in coping with HIV infection, and I am pleased with the distinguished and creative group of authors who agreed to participate in this effort. My debt to them is great—for their patience and understanding throughout the long periods of telephone conversations, correspondence, and editing. I owe a special thanks to Alexandra Teguis, whose affection for AIDS patients and creative guidance and participation in the development of this book have been an inspiration. Thanks are also due to Nancy Ahmed, who took responsibility for the production of this book, and to Paul, Jr., Irene, and Rochelle, who tolerated my devotion to the book during evening hours though it caused slight neglect of their needs from a loving father. I hope this book will inspire them to develop their academic careers to the fullest and further their resolve to help the needy and the sick.

Paul Ahmed

Silver Spring, Maryland

Contents

PART II. AIDS, FAMILIES, AND ADOLESCENTS

Chapter 3

Adolescents and AIDS: Coping Issues

Joyce Hunter and Robert Schaecher

Chapter 4

Mothers with AIDS

Michael H. Antoni, Neil Schneiderman, Arthur LaPerriere,
Mary Jo O'Sullivan, Jennifer Marks, Jonell Efantis,
Jay Skyler, and Mary Ann Fletcher

Chapter 5
Psychotherapy of the HIV-Positive Patient and Family: An Integrated Approach
Seana Hirschfeld Shaw

PART III. LIVING WITH AIDS

Chapter 6
Coping Processes and Strategies and Personal Resources among Persons with HIV-Spectrum Disease
David D. Celentano and Amanda Benedict Sonnega

PART IV. DYING WITH AIDS

Chapter 9
Dying with AIDS
Alexandra Teguis

Chapter 10
Living with AIDS: Surviving Grief
Rochelle Griffin

Chapter 11

A Personal Perspective on Living and Dying with AIDS

Anthony J. Puentes

PART V. AIDS AND SPECIAL GROUPS

Chapter 12

Coping with HIV Disease in the Army

Ann E. Norwood, James R. Rundell, Maria E. Esposito,
Larry H. Ingraham, and Harry C. Holloway

Chapter 13
The Impact of HIV on Minority Populations
Irene Jillson-Boostrom

Chapter 14
Coping with AIDS in Hemophilia
Brian M. Wicklund and Mary Anne Jackson

Coping with AIDS

Living with AIDS
An Overview

ALEXANDRA TEGUIS and PAUL I. AHMED

AIDS has altered our entire conception of death as an event and our relationship to it as a force. As one teenager articulated, "our parents used condoms to prevent birth; now we use them to prevent death" (Klimek, 1988).

There is no precedent for AIDS. There are no precedents for coping with the spectrum of issues around AIDS; therefore, it is difficult to assess what might be defined as adaptive or maladaptive coping.

AIDS, like many other major world events, is full of paradoxes; among them are (1) that in our golden age of science and our extraordinary success at conquering much of both outer and inner space, a microscopic, mutable virus eludes us; (2) that the disease progresses more rapidly than most other diseases today, yet the incubation period may last up to 10 years and the window for developing antibodies also eludes us by 6 weeks to a year (Baumgartner, 1985); (3) that AIDS prompts the most brave and generous acts, yet provokes the most mean-spirited and nonrational behavior (Fineberg, 1988).

Indeed, although the morbidity/mortality statistics may seem too remote to us to be taken personally, we cannot even fathom the enormity of the problem or its relationship to us individually, even when it is put in clearer terms (see Figure 1). We know that a new case of AIDS is reported in the United States every 15 minutes and that someone in the world dies of AIDS every 30 minutes (Klimek, 1988). No part of the world is spared: 133 countries have reported at

ALEXANDRA TEGUIS • Manchester Community College, Manchester, Connecticut 06040.   PAUL I. AHMED • Foreign Currency Program, National Center for Health Statistics, Centers for Disease Control, U.S. Department of Health and Human Services, Hyattsville, Maryland 20782; and Department of Health Education, University College, University of Maryland, College Park, Maryland.

Living and Dying with AIDS, edited by Paul I. Ahmed, Plenum Press, New York, 1992.

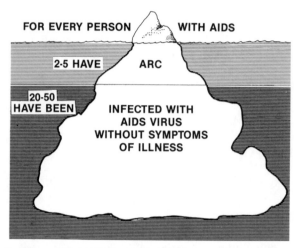

FIGURE 1. The iceberg model of AIDS illustrating that known incidence and prevalence of AIDS cases reflect merely a tiny proportion of the entire picture surrounding AIDS (ARC, AIDS-related complex).

least 81,433 cases, 74% of which are from the Americas, 12% from Africa, 13% from Europe, and 1% from Asia and Oceania (Fleming, Carballo, Fitzsimons, Bailey, & Mann, 1988).

Despite its precedence in other pandemics (e.g., Black Death, Dancing Manias, syphilis, smallpox, leprosy, influenza, TB, and polio; Altman, 1986; Durkee, 1859; Gregory, 1851; Gussow, 1989; Hecker, 1837; Sontag, 1978, 1989), it is our first *media* pandemic; that is, we can keep track of it daily via media, much as Vietnam was our first television war.

One outcome of viewing "AIDS" as the adversary is that we see people as "casualties" or "victims," exacerbating rather than altering a sense of impotency and helplessness. In addition, we tend to place victims along a continuum of "innocence" or "guilt" of worthiness of our compassion to a greater or lesser degree, and of deservedness or nondeservedness of the disease; thus, whites, heterosexuals, married people, babies, adolescents, hemophiliacs, middle-class individuals, professionals, and persons who acquired AIDS via transfusions would fall, clearly, in some minds, at various points to the right of center, whereas IV drug users, remote Third World inhabitants, gay and bisexual men, and lesbian women would fall at various marks to the left of center. Additionally, the concept of "victim" is disempowering and requires the concept of "perpetrators" to inflict suffering, as well as "rescuers" or "caretakers" (the distinction between caregivers and caretakers being that caretakers need to save the world and operate out of a needy framework where burnout is inevitable). Since some PWAs would be viewed, via this model, as perpetrating their *own* victimization, it would appear that psychosocial morbidity and subsequent maladaption would be guaranteed, and there would seem to be little hope of extricating oneself from this quagmire to develop more effective coping strategies.

A major effect of seeing people as statistical categories, particularly in the medical model, is to view them as victimized. Victimization frequently leads to blaming them for their condition.

Blaming the victim is not a phenomenon new to AIDS. William Ryan described it in detail almost two decades ago in a powerful polemic regarding middle-class ideology and bias. He suggested the logical outcome of analyzing social problems in terms of the deficiencies of victims is the creation of programs whose objectives are to change the victim. He further stated that victim blaming is an ideological process, deriving from motivated, but unintended, distortions of reality. Additionally, by objectifying or *remoting* those people so affected, we risk turning well-intentioned description into ideology and practice (Ryan, 1971). Although Ryan presented his arguments in the context of social inequities in the late 1960s and 1970s, the overrepresentation in the AIDS population of those very groups he describes—the poor, minorities, IV drug cultures, and prisoners—seems to underscore his findings (Murphy & Curran, 1988). Indeed, if we extend Ryan's views to the current AIDS situation, reactions range from offering ID cards as positive social incentive to those who test HIV negative (O'Leary, 1989) as well as ID cards to identify AIDS carriers (McCarroll, 1988); agreement with the concept of publicly isolating people with AIDS (Poling, Redman, & Burnette, 1990; D. Smith, 1986); differential views of *who* should practice safe sex (Fineberg, 1988); to the extreme solutions of offering active euthanasia (also termed "going to Amsterdam") to implement an "easy" death, (Hamerman *et al.,* 1986) developing isolation centers (Hamerman *et al.,* 1986) or reactivating death camps as warehouses (Kirby, 1988). It is interesting to speculate whether stimatization would have been diminished or even have existed if AIDS had been discovered first in children or in middle-class, white newborns. AIDS was first detected as GRID (gay-related immune deficiency) among users of recreational poppers (amyl and butyl nitrate) and simultaneously in sexually promiscuous gay men ("Patient Zero" being exemplary of this, having claimed 250 sexual partners annually; Shilts, 1988).

It should be obvious that massive educational efforts need to be made, not only to break through stereotypical assumptions, but also to dispel half-truths and misconceptions. One such false belief occurred about eight years ago when one company marketed a vaccine designed to be effective with a potentially fatal immune disorder in cats. Its posters depicted a rather sinister-looking cat and the large, bold print described the disorder, rather hysterically, as "CAT AIDS." Numerous cat owners, irrationally fearing that they could "catch" AIDS from their pets, sought to have their cats euthanized, some even wondering if their clothes had been contaminated.

Additionally, veterinarians also have described undue concern by many PWAs over acquiring toxoplasmosis from their cats. Though people fear contagion, vets say the disease is only problematic in the oocyte stage (within 4 hours of using a litter box). Proper disposal and hand washing eliminates the contamination (and more euthanized pets) (S. Beauchesne and D. Burnett, personal communication, 1991).

Another problem inherent in seeing PWAs as "victims" or mere statistics is that we fail to see the positive aspects of coping with AIDS and supplementary or alternative treatment efficacy (e.g., Fisher, 1987; Gavzer, 1988; Hay, 1988; Hinson, 1989; Jacobs & Serinus, 1987; Kübler-Ross, 1975, 1983a, 1987, 1989; Laventure, 1988; Levine, 1982, 1984; Lopez & Getzel, 1984; Melton & Garcia, 1988; Moffatt, 1987; Monette, 1989; Ruskin, 1988; Serinus, 1986; I. Smith, 1986; Spence, 1980; Tilleraas, 1988). These approaches may consist of psychological or other means such as biofeedback, hypnosis, autogenics, immune boosting, exercise regimens, meditation, and griefwork or regrieving, including Morita therapy.

We constantly read and hear about people being victimized, and we almost unconsciously place these individuals at some point along the victim continuum; thus, we hear about the "innocent" victims and place them at some point to the right of center; the "littlest" victims fall at the extreme right, or perhaps off the scale! James Hurley, a real estate attorney from Connecticut, articulated this statement about victimization a week before his death: "It galls me when I hear reporters say babies who contracted AIDS are the innocent victims of AIDS, as though the rest of us are somehow *guilty* victims. There's no such thing. Either you have AIDS or you don't. To have it is to have a disease that will end your life" (Hurley, 1987).

One month before his death, Mark Feldman addressed a candlelight march in San Francisco, and concluded with the words:

> On November 1, 1982, I was just a person, a human being. On November 23, my medical diagnosis and so much of the world *labelled me a "victim";* then it proceeded to call me "*a patient with* AIDS." Well, as many of you know, I'm in the process of defining myself. *I am a person with AIDS, a human* being, not a victim, and only a patient when I am in a hospital. L'Chayim. To life. (Altman, 1986, p. 24)

It was at a Denver conference of PWAs in 1983 that two survival guides for PWAs were conceived: *Surviving and Thriving with AIDS* and *Collected Wisdom.* At the end of *Collected Wisdom,* 17 rights and recommendations were set forth that formed a basis for empowerment, rather than victimization, of people with AIDS. It was here that they decided to call themselves PWAs rather than patients or victims (Cunningham, 1989). Indeed, many PWAs are now asserting that to instill an even more positive and hope-engendering image they be called PLWAs (people living with AIDS)!

A number of practitioners suggest that those PWAs who see themselves as "innocent" victims are more prone to anger (Runck, 1986). Although this anger is frequently directed at "victims" at the *other* end of the continuum, my experience has been that the will to live is inherent in virtually every human, and that anger has been an "equal opportunity emotion," expressed strongly at every point along the AIDS continuum. Although the targets may vary (e.g., individual people, the health care delivery system, or the virus itself), the *intensities* of the feelings are equally potent.

THE HUMAN SIDE OF AIDS

We all too often fail to consider the human dimension of AIDS because it is overshadowed by the specter of the virus. All too often we behave as if HTLV-III exists as a living, conscious entity on its own, amoebalike, an Andromeda strain, if you will, only remotely, if at all, connected to the suffering, vulnerable human host within which it resides. Tomes have been written, and endless conferences, seminars, and workshops have been given, dedicated to this one mysterious, almost godlike entity. This bias became very apparent with the long-anticipated release of the first lay, single-topic issue of *Scientific American.* On the cover loomed a gigantic micrograph of the virus against a bright red background. Although the issue was filled with state-of-the-art information on HIV, there was scant evidence that the *human* dimension was considered. Dr. Fineberg's sole article on psychosocial dimensions was brilliantly executed, but it was a whimper in the wilderness in contrast to the rest of the publication: of 152 pages, only 7 were devoted to the penultimate object of the virus's attack (Fineberg, 1988). Similarly, in the AIDS and Public Health special issue of the *American Journal of Public Health,* consisting of 115 pages, only three articles of a possible eighteen dealt with psychological or human issues—two concerning risk-reducing behaviors, and one regarding adolescents' condom use (Yankauer, 1988). It very much reminds me of the Hindu legend of the six blind men, each of whom stumbled upon a different part of an elephant, with which they had never before had an encounter. Each was positive that he had defined the entire elephant according to the part he had touched, and, since they could not concur, each went his separate ways, mumbling his superior reasoning. They were *all* correct, but they collectively missed the greater, more important context, that of its human dimensions.

No one would question for a moment the urgency of and benefits to tracking the course of the AIDS pandemic by way of statistical analysis of high-risk groups. It might be more efficacious to assess the effects of particular behavioral changes that occur as a result of educational efforts (or lack thereof) on prevalence. Indeed, it is by assessing *specific behavioral changes* that we are now beginning to comprehend how specific rates are changing. One instance reflecting this rate change concerns the reduced high-risk sexual behavior for the cohort of homosexual men in San Francisco, showing no new infections in 1987 (Murphy & Curran, 1988). Also, a phone survey in that same cohort from August 1984 to April 1985 indicated a 12% increase in monogamy or celibacy (Ulene, 1987). In another category, however, specifically the area of IV drug use, specific behaviors do not necessarily alter incidence or prevalence. A case in point is the inaccurate (or at the very least, incomplete) perception of the widely publicized educational message "Don't share needles!" Indeed, that admonition has been taken seriously but implemented with insufficient understanding. Numerous individuals, failing to comprehend the blood-borne nature of HIV, are now snorting heroin and other substances and transmitting AIDS via broken nasal capillaries by sharing snorting straws or rolled-up dollar bills (M. Magaz, personal communication, Dec., 1989; Mr. Magaz is a clinical social worker with the Hartford [CT] Dispensary, AIDS Unit). Only recently has risk education-oriented literature reflected the emphasis on *behavior* rather than on groupings or categories (American Red Cross, 1988). The overriding message presently conveys that it's not *who* you are (categorically speaking) but *what* you specifically *do* that puts you at greater risk. Adolescents are at special risk for extreme denial as a result of belief in a personal fable, that is, the illusion that they are impervious to any misfortune or demise as a result of their youth (category), vigor, or status (heterosexual, middle class, white, or affluent). Again, the *revised* literature at present admonishes teens about needle-sharing of steroids (common among athletes and bodybuilders), of hormones or vitamin shots, or of unsterile tattoo needles or ear-piercing equipment (American Red Cross, 1988).

Additionally, there are some categories in which specific behaviors are masked. In the transmission category of homosexual/bisexual males, for instance, is it possible that statistics don't adequately describe a group? How is "bisexual" defined? What proportion of homosexual behavior is bisexual? Is the bisexuality current? Simultaneous? Serial? Does one experience in the past constitute its definition? Given a possible 10-year incubation period, it appears these might be significant behaviors to determine. Where are the numbers for the bisexual males' women partners reflected? What about the "undetermined" category? Could it be that bisexual behavior is far more common than any of us imagine? There are numerous anecdotal accounts to suggest this is so, but hard data are still lacking. The state of Maryland has established a special outreach facility for high-risk special populations (gay and bisexual men, as well as male and female prostitutes) as part of an effort by the AIDS Health Services to target specific behaviors and increase risk reduction (P. Pasternak, personal communication, Sept., 1991. Mr. Pasternak is coordinator of Outreach to Special Populations, AIDS Health Services, Department of Health and Mental Hygiene, Maryland.) They hope to complete a behavioral study targeting such specifics in March of 1992, as extensive denial in dealing with such issues has prevented surveys like this from being conducted heretofore.

Mr. Pasternak also points out that the manner in which the interviewer poses the question determines the accuracy of the response. In some communities, for example, as with many people of color, persons would not acknowledge themselves as "gay" or "bisexual," as they do not classify themselves as such; they will, however, respond affirmatively when asked, "Do you have sex with other men?" or "Do you have sex with both men and women?"

This comment from a 16-year-old male prostitute underscores the need for documenting behaviors: "Many of my customers are married men who offer three times the going rate for sex without condoms" (Klimek, 1988).

One novel approach to changing specific sexual behaviors that has been shown to be effective is the use of cleverly designed tag lines on matchbooks and in condom packets. Use of such slogans appears to use an easy, nonthreatening approach to lowering risky behavior. Here are some that have been effective: "Stops transmission fluid leaks"; "Sleep with a lifeguard tonight"; "Smart sportswear for the active man"; "Don't go home without them"; "Have a lifesaver"; "Here's a ring for your next engagement" (McElhany & Foote, 1986). According to HERO (Health Education Resource Organization), distributors and developers of such material, the campaign, which uses the double entendre, has been well received in the gay community (K. Day, personal communication, Dec., 1989; Mr. Day is Chief of Material Distribution, HERO, Baltimore, Maryland). The AIDS outreach at the Maryland Department of Health has found the approach so efficacious that it has hired the same designer to create a series of condom posters all of which underscore the point that condoms provide "living" proof of stopping AIDS. These eye-catching signs read, "In 1984, we discovered the AIDS virus: In 1850, we discovered a way to stop it"; "Last night this woman slept with every one of her boyfriend's ex-lovers"; and a third poster, for IV users: "If you don't want to kick an old habit [needles], start a new one [condoms]" (McElhany, 1988). It is another telling aspect of the paradox, however, that the most glib and superficial of Madison Avenue ploys is being utilized as the vehicle to curtail one of the most serious and lethal agents known to man.

If one were to look at the leading causes of death today, one would find a contrasting picture to the one that existed at the turn of this century in the United States and most of the Western world. Indeed, you could go back a century or further and find that the leading causes of death were all of epidemic and infectious causes (Durkee, 1859; Gregory, 1851; Hecker, 1859; Kalish, 1981). Currently, the leading causes of death are all, in some form, stress involved; all major cardiovascular causes combined account for nearly half of all deaths, followed by cancers, cirrhosis of the liver, complications from diabetes, accidents (more than half of which involve alcohol or another addictive substance), and suicide. Pneumonia, influenza, and tuberculosis combined account for less than 3% (Kalish, 1981). In 1900, to contrast, influenza and pneumonia were leading causes of death, followed closely by tuberculosis (Kalish, 1981). One can only wonder how difficult it will be to deal with the double jeopardy of AIDS and stress-involved diseases in the next few decades. It will be a time of burgeoning interest, research, and application in the field of psychoneuroimmunology, where the interrelationships of thoughts, attitudes, beliefs, and expectations on neurotransmitters, hormonal functioning, and immunocompetence are examined. It will likely be a time of experimenting with all manner of strategies, from nutritional to psychical to self-empowering modalities, in order to cull the most effective approaches from the armamentarium available to fight the battles (and the war).

We would be well advised to be cognizant of the roles of denial and bargaining in all this search. Then, as now, in times of great uncertainty, such as have existed in numerous epidemics, desperate and open-minded people who have exhausted all conventional means of treatment may be "victimized" by illegitimate means. It is well to remember that there exists a fine line, propelled by desperation, between an open mind and gullibility, even by way of treatment by well-meaning, "scientifically respectable" sources.

The following case histories illustrate further evidence that we need to look beyond statistical groups and in more depth at individual behaviors (Melchreit, 1988).

AIDS Case History No. 1

When she was 6 months old, Stephanie Ernest (not her real name), the daughter of a prominent real estate developer and his wife, died of *Pneumocystis carinii* pneumonia and AIDS. She was a beautiful baby, bright and lively until the illness began. First there was a brief hospitalization for diarrhea, then a longer hospitalization at a large medical center when the diarrhea recurred and didn't respond to conventional treatments. Finally, at the age of 5 months, she was hospitalized for severe respiratory distress that required mechanical ventilator support to allow her to breathe. Her parents were at her bedside when she died one month later.

Her parents said this couldn't be AIDS, and extensive interviews of both parents uncovered no risk factors. The parents were in excellent health.

Two years later, Stephanie's mother was diagnosed with disseminated tuberculosis. Soon after, she also developed *Pneumocystis carinii* pneumonia and died. Until her death she said it was impossible for her to have AIDS. Again, an investigation revealed no risk factors.

Within 6 months of his wife's death, Stephanie's father was diagnosed with cytomegalovirus (CMV) infection and AIDS. Before dying he was finally able to tell doctors there was in fact a risk factor that even his wife was not aware of. Occasionally, on weekends, he shot heroin with his sister's husband, and they shared needles.

A 7-year-old daughter is the only survivor of this family.

AIDS Case History No. 2

Sandra Watson (not her real name) worked hard to escape a life of poverty. She excelled in college and decided to enhance her opportunities for a fulfilling and more prosperous life by enrolling in graduate school. In 1984, as a second-year graduate student, Sandra noticed that she tired easily and felt run down. She consulted the Student Health Service, which initially attributed her problem to "exam stress." However, Sandra's symptoms persisted and worsened even after final exams were over.

Within several months, Sandra developed *Pneumocystis carinii* pneumonia, and opportunistic disease commonly associated with AIDS. Tests confirmed that she had AIDS. Sandra, her family, and her physician were shocked and devastated. An investigation of potential risk factors for AIDS in Sandra's life revealed that two former boyfriends were at increased risk for AIDS. One of Sandra's boyfriends in college was bisexual, and another of her former lovers was from a country in central Africa where heterosexually transmitted AIDS rates are higher than in the United States. Both men had been healthy during their involvement with Sandra. Neither of the two men experienced any symptoms of AIDS at the time Sandra's diagnosis was confirmed.

Sandra's condition worsened at the hospital. She died 2 weeks after her AIDS diagnosis was confirmed.

PEOPLE, NOT STATISTICS

Toby McCarroll is a monk who, with three lay Catholic sisters, formed a community in northern California called Starcross. Although they had cared for foster children for years there, in 1986 they committed to caring for children with AIDS who would have otherwise spent their entire young lives since birth in hospital nurseries or pediatric units (described as "boarder" babies: children who would never touch grass, pet a cat, or play outdoors; e.g., Kübler-Ross, 1987; Whitmore, 1988b). He described how he was moved to adopt such children, having seen an article with an accompanying picture of a 10-month-old boy in a walker tied to a doorknob in a windowless hospital corridor. The back of the child's walker was labeled "17 North" and was numbered; his plastic bottle lay on the floor (McCarroll, 1988).

McCarroll goes on to describe Aaron, the first child who died of AIDS at the Community, at the tender age of one year, after local firefighters deliberately failed to respond to an emergency call via dispatch. After Aaron's death and a subsequent investigation, the volunteer firemen explained that they had made a clear prior decision not to respond because they felt inadequately trained for such circumstances. One fireman's rationale was that he thought the children didn't have long to live anyway (McCarroll, 1988). McCarroll points out the importance of viewing PWAs not as statistics, but as persons deserving of compassion and love. It is all too remote to cite the statistics, as alarming as they may be: that in New York City alone, AIDS is the leading killer of young women between the ages of 25 and 29 (McCarroll, 1988); that the risk of a newborn acquiring HIV from an infected mother is 20–50% (Klimek, 1988); that in New York City, 1 out of every 61 mothers giving birth at the end of 1987 tested HIV positive (McCarroll, 1988); that 40–50% of HIV-positive babies develop AIDS in 10–12 months (Klimek, 1988). McCarroll speaks of the high probability that at the time of Aaron's death, there likely was another child with AIDS who died somewhere else in the United States, after having lived all her life in a hospital ward and who, despite a concerned caregiver who made her last hours comfortable, died alone, anomic, a "statistic." He continues:

> Aaron was *not* a statistic. He was recognized and respected as a unique human being. In learning to live and to die, Aaron was encouraged by a loving, extended family. The death of the other little girl would have been an entry in some medical log. Aaron's passing was reported on the front page of the country's principal newspaper. Calls and cards came from all over. Church congregations offered prayers, I never understood how the word had spread. Aaron was not defined as a pitiful product of a dirty IV drug needle. He was a *person*. He lived, died, and will be remembered as a *person*. Until his death, we did not see clearly that our function, perhaps our assignment, in the war against AIDS is to see that as many babies as possible are given the *chance* to be people instead of statistics. (McCarroll, 1988, p. 144)

McCarroll asserts that many more babies could be helped to live as full a life as possible if one could only unclog the legal system and cut through the massive welfare and judicial red tape. Many infants die before being placed because the process is often held up for months (McCarroll, 1988). In New York City alone, currently 350 children await placement, and while authorities claim there are a dearth of suitable homes, Kübler-Ross claims she has 150 frustrated families awaiting children (Kübler-Ross, 1987, 1989; Whitmore, 1988b). Indeed, Kübler-Ross details quite extensively the role that fear of contagion and paranoia play in precluding appropriate care for these children in the course of attempting to establish an AIDS children's hospice on her 200-acre farm in Virginia. Her efforts were blocked by well-meaning but uninformed residents who believed that there were no cases of AIDS in their state and that their air and water supplies might be contaminated by these afflicted children (Kübler-Ross, 1987, 1989)! Indeed, one can readily comprehend why Kübler-Ross calls AIDS our "ultimate" challenge, separating "wheat" from "chaff" with regard to testing our compassion in light of our fears.

It is also well to consider that blaming the victim is not merely something that occurs in traditional, middle-class systems, but also has the capacity to inflict more guilt on PWAs utilizing more "new age" or popular cultural approaches to illness and health.

DISRUPTION OF PSYCHOSOCIAL STAGES

Let us look at some of the major issues and losses. Of persons with AIDS, 91% are in the prime of life between 20 and 49 years; 22% are in their 20s, 47% are in their 30s, and 22% are in their 40s.

Elsewhere, we are reminded of the fact that the grief model proposed by Kübler-Ross and others applys to *all losses,* whether they are death losses, symbolic losses, or even losses subjectively, rather than objectively, experienced (Baumgartner, 1985; Lopez & Getzel, 1984; Martin, 1988; Murphy & Curran, 1988).

It might be useful to review some of the major symbolic, psychological, and physical losses other than actual death losses that occur with persons with AIDS. Before we do this, perhaps it might be especially helpful if we go back to review the concept of developmental tasks expected to be accomplished at each life period, proposed by the model of Eric Erickson. He postulated that there were eight life stages from birth to death, beginning with the development of trust versus mistrust in infancy; through identity versus role confusion in adolescence; intimacy versus isolation in young adulthood; to ego integrity versus despair in the last stage of life. The two stages that encompass the majority of people with AIDS in the their 20s, 30s, and 40s are *intimacy* versus *isolation.* At a time when one normally develops a few intimate, soul-baring, vulnerable partnerships, perhaps preparing one for lifelong close companionship (either sexual or nonsexual, same or opposite gender), the PWA is thrust into a situation where out of fear of contagion (in either direction), he or she is isolated, or relegated back to adolescentlike confusion, awkwardness, or numbing of feelings completely. Although it is not impossible, it is far more difficult to recapture this skill later, and the reinforcement of lack of self-trust as well as lack of trust in others may make it difficult, at best, to reestablish trust later. In one's 30s and 40s, the task is generativity (to leave some legacy behind) versus self-absorption (Erickson, 1963).

At a time when people reach a peak in terms of career and life goals established in earlier years, many adult PWAs see this fulfillment as abruptly aborted. This is a time when many people have reached their zenith in terms of productivity; PWAs find themselves at their nadir, subject to forces external to themselves, beyond their ability to control. This pertains not only to white, middle-class gay males but to many people who've acquired AIDS through occasional, or recreational, drug use, or other risky behaviors.

In addition to the truncating effect AIDS has on these prior stages, AIDS by its chronic relapsing and progressive nature also forces PWAs to confront tasks usually relegated to one's aging final years, in one's 60s onward, when the dying trajectory is more expected and for which people are gradually prepared. There is generally more time and opportunity for anticipatory grieving. The rapid deterioration and mental effects often experienced as part of brain changes or dementia (which occur in about 75% of cases; Baumgartner, 1985) force the PWA and significant others to experience the process in a manner more consistent with sudden death. PWAs, then, are required to complete tasks not typically psychosocially experienced at their age. Fixation or perseveration is another possible coping style PWAs may utilize to insure task completion. Alternatively, as I have frequently witnessed, AIDS may also provide an opportunity to quickly prioritize tasks in such a manner as to enable the person to make the most of time remaining.

As risk behaviors and subsequent categories shift, and large numbers of people in various other psychosocial stages become affected, we should be more vigilant to the ways in which coping styles change in an effort to compensate for this change in homeostasis.

MAJOR LOSSES AND ISSUES SURROUNDING AIDS

The major losses associated with AIDS pervade every facet of a person's life. They include the following:

1. Loss of financial, job, or health care security. Many adults due to single or childless status have never taken on life insurance or adequate health insurance policies. One in five PWAs has no medical insurance (Fineberg, 1988).

2. Stigmatization and social ostracism. People are denied entrance to schools, restaurants and the like (McCarroll, 1988; Whitmore, 1988b).

3. Loss of pride and self-esteem. Employers force PWAs to stay home even though they are well enough to work; needs to create and to produce are blocked. Even after death there is secrecy—one-half to one-third of the names in the AIDS quilt book of names are first names only, or are "anonymous" (Names Project, 1989a,b).

4. Loss of innocence. Childhood, or childlike innocence ends when AIDS begins.

5. Aborted continuum of recovery for those who had finally conquered their addictions in treatment programs or alcohol or narcotic recovery and support groups such as AA or Narcotics Anonymous.

6. Loss of physical contact, touching, due to ill-informed fears regarding casual contagion. Some health professionals enforce unnecessary precautions and infection control practices, further isolating the patient (Lopez & Getzel, 1984); however, staff members, through open discussion, can learn to work through their fears and concerns (Baumgartner, 1985). Volunteer massage programs, such as "Service Through Touch," currently existing in several hospitals on the West coast address this need (I. Smith, 1986).

7. Isolation. Some dentists, physicians, and hospitals transfer PWAs out or refuse to treat them so that "real" patients will not be driven away (Ettelbrick, 1988; Fineberg, 1988; O'Leary, 1989; Whitmore, 1988a).

8. Loss of a sense of stability or concreteness. This is especially true of people with AIDS-related complex (ARC) or people in the "grey zone" called the "worried well" (Lopez & Getzel, 1984; Runck, 1986).

9. Loss of future hopes, dreams, and goals. Sometimes the pain of knowing one will never attain something is deeper than the pain of having attained something and lost it.

10. Loss of one's entire peer group. This loss is similarly felt by health professionals, where it is not uncommon to lose 20–30 patients a month; or as many friends in a year, one's cohort.

11. Loss of youth or vigor, energy, physical appearance, particularly with cytomegalovirus or Kaposi's sarcoma.

12. Multiple death losses and traumatic degenerative ones. Except for natural disasters and wars, this experience doesn't occur typically until *much* later in life (Lopez & Getzel, 1984). This loss is frequently magnified as well for many health and caring professionals who may have experienced the deaths of 30 to 50 patients over a period of a month to a few years.

13. Loss of feelings of control, especially for groups like hemophiliacs, mothers of infants with AIDS, transfusion patients, and the like.

14. Loss of privacy entailed in having to reveal one's most private life; also high visibility of the macules of Kaposi's sarcoma lesions reveal the secret—people avoid mirrors, as they are a reminder of the inevitable progression of AIDS. In a study by Coppola, four out of five urban gay men had not revealed their homosexuality to their families (Coppola & Zabarsky, 1983).

15. Dementia and CNS involvement blurs distinctions and creates confusion and distress.

16. Loss of "benefits" of the sick role, compassion (e.g., that cancer patients receive). PWAs now are treated stigmatically as were cancer patients in the past (Lopez & Getzel, 1984; D. Smith, 1986).

17. Loss of support of family of origin, in contrast to cancer patients where the family often rallies and becomes reinvolved. PWAs often need to lie and tell their family they have cancer (Lopez & Getzel, 1984). PWAs have also experienced rejection from their reconstituted gay families, due to homophobia or AIDS phobia.

18. Loss of former lifestyles. As problematic as some of this may have been, it served the person for as long as it occurred and enabled him to "survive."

It is important to note here that in relation to phases in the grief process (i.e., *one* model being denial and isolation followed often by anger and rage, then bargaining or atonement, depression, and ultimately a coming to terms with death), AIDS, unlike any other terminal illness experienced in our culture, involves shame as well as guilt. Shame, as opposed to guilt, involves one's entire being, one's worth as an entity. Guilt, by contrast, revolves around failures of doing or not doing—one's acts, or one's words. Excessive shame, by virtue of the stigma surrounding AIDS, causes one to believe he or she is "defective" in some deep, unchangeable, excessive way, a concept Potter-Efron and Potter-Efron have termed the "shame-based person" (Potter-Efron and Potter-Efron, 1989). Possessing such an identity leads one, paradoxically, not only to denial and nonrecognition of symptoms, but also to postponing help until the disease has progressed. This leaves one in a catch-22 position in terms of developing a sense of helplessness exacerbated by a shamed sense of self. The trivialization of this distress by professionals further focuses on problem-solving efforts as opposed to emotion-focused coping (Lazarus, 1985). Kübler-Ross also expresses that entire societies and subcultures experience the grief process as do individuals (Kübler-Ross, 1983b). If this is indeed so, we might well ask which stages we have already passed through and where we, as a nation, or as health professionals, now find ourselves. In describing AIDS as the ultimate challenge, Kübler-Ross illustrates that since AIDS potentially affects all of us, we cannot continue to judge others, for eventually we end up judging ourselves. Ultimately, the answer lies in unconditional and nonjudgmental love, and compassion for those suffering. Ultimately, our moral mandate is clear: that our solutions as well as our challenges, in AIDS, rest on creating a more caring community for others and for ourselves (Dunphy, 1987). It is to this end that this book dedicates its efforts.

Fineberg articulates the challenges that lie ahead for us: "AIDS throws new light on traditions of value, compels a fresh look at the performance of the institutions we depend on and brings society to a crossroads for collective action that may, with the passage of years, mark a key measure of our time mark" (Fineberg, 1988).

REFERENCES

Altman, D. (1986). *AIDS in the mind of America.* Garden City, NY: Anchor Press/Doubleday, *viii,* 228.

American Red Cross. (1988, November). *Teenagers and AIDS* (pamphlet publication, Stock #329536).

Baumgartner, G. H. (1985). *AIDS, psychosocial factors in the acquired immune deficiency syndrome.* Springfield, IL: Thomas.

Coppola, V., & Zabarsky, Z. (1983, August 9). Coming out of the closet. *Newsweek,* p. 34.

Cunningham, C. (Ed.). (1989, May/June). *The gay men's health crisis newsletter for volunteers and supporters.* New York: G.M.H.C.

Dunphy, R. (1987). Helping persons with AIDS find meaning and hope. *Health Progress, 68*(4), 58–63.

Durkee, S. (1859). *Gonorrhea and syphilis.* Cleveland, Ohio: J. P. Jewett and Co.

Erickson, E. (1963). *Childhood and society.* New York: W. W. Norton.

Ettelbrick, P. (Ed.). (1988, October/November). *Cooperating attorney report.* New York: Lambda Legal Defense and Education Fund.

Fineberg, H. V. (1988). The social dimensions of AIDS. *Scientific American, 259,* 128–134.

Fisher, S. (1987). *AIDS and anger* [Audiotape]. Los Angeles: Northern Lights Alternatives.

Fleming, A., Carballo, M., Fitzsimons, D., Bailey, M., & Mann, J. (Eds.). (1988). *The global impact of AIDS.* New York: Alan Liss.

Gavzer, B. (1988, September 18). Why do some people survive AIDS? *Parade Magazine,* pp. 2–7.

Gregory, G. (1851). *Lectures on the eruptive fevers; as now in the course of delivery at St. Thomas' Hospital, in London.* New York, S. S. & W. Wood.

Gussow, G. (1989). *Leprosy, racism & public health.* Boulder, CO: Westview Press.

Hamerman, W. J., Grauerholz, J., Tennenbaum, J., Freeman, D., Lillge, W., Rosinsky, N., Shapiro, E., Burdman, M., Pauls, R., Cleary, C., Spahn, J., & Kellogg, B. (Eds.). (1986). *An emergency war plan to fight AIDS and other pandemics prepared by the EIR Biological Holocaust Task Force.* Washington, DC (P.O. Box 17390, Washington 20041): Executive Intelligence Review.

Hay, L. (1988). *Heal your body.* Santa Monica, CA: Hay House.

Hecker, I. F. C. (1859). *The epidemics of the middle ages.* Philadelphia: Haswell, Barrington, and Haswell.

Hinson, P. (1989). *Creating love, healing, and miracles* (an audiotape series for children with catastrophic illnesses using attitudinal healing principles). Jacksonville, FL: Hinson Associates.

Hurley, J. (1987, August 10). "I'm dying—AIDS is your problem now." *Newsweek,* pp. 38–39.

Jacobs, S., & Serinus, J. (1987, August). Living with AIDS. *Yoga Journal, 75,* 30–36.

Kalish, R. (1981). *Death, grief, and caring relationships.* Monterey, CA: Brooks/Cole.

Kirby, M. (1988). AIDS—"Return to Sachsenhausen." In A. Fleming *et al.* (Eds.), *The global impact of AIDS* (pp. 1–6). New York: Alan Liss.

Klimek, J. (Ed). (1988, June). *HIV Update.* Hartford, CT: Hartford Hospital Department of Medicine.

Kübler-Ross, E. (1975). *Death: The final stage of growth.* Englewood Cliffs, NJ: Prentice-Hall.

Kübler-Ross, E. (1983a). *On children and death.* New York: Macmillan.

Kübler-Ross, E. (1983b). *Death, dying and transition,* from a transcription of a workshop lecture tape, San Juan Bautista, CA, March 26th. Headwaters, VA: Elisabeth Kübler-Ross Center.

Kübler-Ross, E. (1987). *AIDS: The ultimate challenge.* New York: Macmillan.

Kübler-Ross, E. (1989). *AIDS, life and love* [Videotape]. Headwaters, VA: E.K.R. Center.

Laventure, A. (Ed.). (1988, Autumn). *PWA Voice.* Vol. 1, no. 3, pp. 1–6.

Lazarus, R. S. (1985). The trivialization of distress. In P. Ahmed & N. Ahmed. (Eds.), *Coping with juvenile diabetes.* Springfield, IL: Thomas.

Levine, S. (1982). *Who dies?* New York: Doubleday.

Levine, S. (1984). *Meetings at the edge.* New York: Doubleday.

Lopez, D. J., & Getzel, G. S. (1984). Helping gay AIDS patients in crisis. Social casework. *The Journal of Contemporary Social Work, 65(7),* 387–394.

Martin, J. L. (1988). Psychological consequences of AIDS-related bereavement among gay men. *Journal of Consulting and Clinical Psychology 56*(6), 856–862.

McCarroll, T. (1988). *Morning glory babies.* New York: St. Martin's Press.

McElhany, J., & Foote, D. (1986). *Condom and matchbook tagline series.* Baltimore: HERO (Health Education Resource Organization).

McElhany, J. (1988). *Matchbook taglines.* Baltimore: Maryland Department of Public Health.

Melchreit, R., Hadler, J., & Weinstein, B. (Eds.). (1988, April). *Connecticut responds to AIDS, A report of the Department of Health Services AIDS Prevention Programs* (Connecticut Preventable Diseases Division, D.H.S. Publication). Hartford, CT.

Melton, G., & Garcia, W. (1988). *Beyond AIDS. A journey into healing.* Beverly Hills, CA: Brotherhood Press.

Moffatt, B. C. (Ed.). (1987). *AIDS: A self-care manual.* Los Angeles: AIDS Project Los Angeles.

Monette, P. (1989). *Borrowed time, an AIDS memoir.* New York: Caldmon.

Murphy, F., & Curran, J. (1988). *AIDS and human immunodeficiency virus infection in the United States, 1988 update.* Atlanta: Centers for Disease Control.

Names Project. (1989a). AIDS memorial quilt list of names 1989–1990. San Francisco: Names Project.

Names Project. (1989b). Keep the love alive—the names project AIDS memorial quilt. San Francisco: Names Project.

O'Leary, J. (Ed.). (1989, Spring). *National gay rights advocate newsletter.*

Poling, A., Redman, W., & Burnette, M. (1990). Stigmatization of AIDS patients by college students in lower division psychology classes. *Journal of College Student Development 31,* 64–70.

Potter-Efron, R., and Potter-Efron, P. (1989). *Letting go of shame.* Center City, MN: Hazelden.

Runck, B. (1986). *Coping with AIDS: Psychological and social considerations in helping people with HTLV-III infection* (DHHS NIMH Publication No. ADM 85-1432). Washington, DC: National Institute of Mental Health.

Ruskin, C. (1988). *The quilt: Stories from the names project.* New York: Simon & Schuster.

Ryan, W. (1971). *Blaming the victim.* New York: Random House.

Serinus, J. (Ed.). (1986). *Psychoimmunity and the healing process.* Los Angeles: Celestrial Arts.

Shilts, R. (1988). *And the band played on.* New York: Penguin.

Smith, D. R. (1986). Who will bear the burden when serious illness strikes? Unpublished senior thesis, Eastern Connecticut State University.

Smith, I. (1986). *Guidelines for the massage of AIDS patients.* San Francisco: Service Through Touch.

Sontag, S. (1978). *Illness as metaphor.* New York: Farrar, Straus & Giroux.

Sontag, S. (1989). *AIDS and its metaphors.* New York: Farrar.

Spence, C. (1980). A homecoming and the harvest—A counselor's view on death, dying and bereavement. *Lifestory,* pp. 1–12.

Tilleraas, P. (1988). *The color of light: Meditations for all of us living with AIDS.* Hazelden Foundation, New York: Harper & Row.

Ulene, A. (1987). *Safe sex in a dangerous world.* New York: Random House.

Whitmore, G. (1988a). *Someone was here: Profiles in the AIDS epidemic.* New York: New American Library.

Whitmore, G. (1988b, January 31). Bearing witness. *New York Times Magazine,* pp. 14–54.

Yankauer, A. (Ed.). (1988, April). AIDS and public health [Special topic issue]. *American Journal of Public Health, 78*(4).

2

AIDS Care Providers and the Medical Care System
Ethical and Legal Issues

SANDRA C. SELLIN, BARBARA G. FALTZ, and
ANNE J. DAVIS

INTRODUCTION

The AIDS epidemic raises important ethical and legal issues for health care providers. Ethics in the Western philosophical tradition places much emphasis on individual rights and the obligation of society and its institutions to see that those rights are upheld. At the same time, because we are a society, it also focuses on the common good or what is best for the community as a whole. Sometimes these two ethical principles come into conflict, resulting in an ethical dilemma.

AIDS is one of many stigmatized diseases that result in multiple problems with diagnosis. The first set of difficulties is the physical and emotional sequelae resulting from HIV infection. Additionally, trauma often strikes patients because of societal attitudes toward behaviors correlated with risk for HIV infection. These attitudes can result in discrimination in housing, employment, and access to health care.

This chapter discusses selected ethical issues found in the AIDS epidemic and offers a context in which to formulate sane and ethical solutions. Specifically, it will address the tension between the values of privacy and self-determination

SANDRA C. SELLIN • City College of San Francisco, San Francisco, California 94112.   BARBARA
G. FALTZ • CPC Belmont Hills Hospital, Belmont, California 94002.   ANNE J. DAVIS •
Department of Mental Health, Community Health and Administrative Nursing, School of Nursing,
University of California, San Francisco, San Francisco, California 94143-0608.

Living and Dying with AIDS, edited by Paul I. Ahmed, Plenum Press, New York, 1992.

and the need to protect the public's health, the responsibility of clinicians and researchers to protect confidentiality of patients, the just and fair distribution of scarce medical resources, and the ethical development and testing of new treatments.

Patients and their families often face legal problems in connection with these ethical issues. Issues surrounding patients' competency to make health care decisions, specifically, the right to refuse treatment, the legal ramifications of informed consent, and patients' ability to designate others as power of attorney, are issues we will address. Particular attention will be paid to patient concerns and health care workers' responsibilities.

ETHICAL PRINCIPLES AND AIDS

The ethical principles that are particularly applicable to the concerns and needs of people with AIDS are those involving individual rights to liberty, informed consent, confidentiality, and distributive justice. Each principle will be considered briefly within the context of the professional–patient relationship.

Individual rights to liberty, informed consent, and privacy are values grounded in the principle of autonomy. Generally, *autonomy* is a Greek term referring to self-governance, or self-rule, and is grounded in the broader principle of respect for persons. According to Beauchamp and Childress (1983), the principle of autonomy presumes competence, and exercising it means being one's own person without constraints from others or from physical or psychological limitations. An autonomous person determines his or her own course of action in accordance with a chosen plan. Included in the principle of autonomy are the rights to self-determination, the right to seek or refuse treatment, the right to informed consent, the right to freedom from coercion, the right to confidentiality, and the right to considerate and respectful care. For each right that an individual has there is a corresponding duty on the part of another person or society. Hospitalized patients, or their advocates, have all the rights listed above, among others. And health care professionals have corresponding duties to protect and respect the rights of patients.

Liberty is the constitutionally granted freedom to pursue one's life goals without restraints from others. Liberty may be restricted only if the individual represents a clear and present danger to self or others, or if the individual is gravely disabled. Under normal circumstances, the restriction of one's liberty without due process of law represents a gross infringement of one's civil rights and is rarely ethically justifiable.

The Doctrine of Informed Consent involves the voluntary consent of individuals to medical treatments or research protocols based on full disclosure of information about the medical treatment or research protocol in question. It grows out of the principle of autonomy and protects individuals' rights of self-determination. It also promotes the informed voluntariness of individuals' participation in medical treatment and research (Beauchamp & Childress, 1983).

The rules of confidentiality and privacy involve the duty of health care professionals to protect information about patients that is of a confidential nature. It is generally agreed that patients have a right to privacy and to the protection of confidential information based on the principle of autonomy. Respecting the confidential nature of patient information helps build trust in the professional–patient relationship and makes effective medical care possible. There are, however, circumstances under which a health care professional's duty to protect a patient's health status information may conflict with a broader social duty to protect the public's health. The strength and limits of the rules of confidentiality and privacy often are determined by the nature of the information in question and the degree of harm that might result if the information is not disclosed (Beauchamp & Childress, 1983). For example, if a man with much public contact has a highly contagious disease, more harm might be done to those he comes in contact with by their not knowing than would be done to him by the disclosure of his health status information. The rules of confidentiality and privacy are therefore not absolute. Many situations may exist in which confidentiality should not be maintained in order to protect others from harm.

The principle of distributive justice involves the relative treatment of individuals within a society. Generally, distributive justice is concerned with the distribution of the benefits and burdens, of goods and evils, in any society where resources are limited. Individual need is commonly used to justify the distribution of scarce health care resources. Health care professionals consider the harm that may result if an individual does not receive a given service, and they then distribute services to those most in need (Davis & Aroskar, 1983).

While this brief discussion of ethical principles is far from comprehensive, it does provide a loose framework from which to view cogent ethical issues faced by health care providers working in the AIDS epidemic.

HIV DISEASE AND STIGMA

Although AIDS can be transmitted by intimate sexual contact, which includes the exchange of semen, blood, or vaginal secretions between any two individuals, 59% of cases in the United States have been gay or bisexual men (Centers for Disease Control, 1991). Additionally, in 22% of cases, there is a history of injection drug use (Centers for Disease Control, 1989).

Homophobia, fear of homosexuals, has been identified in health care providers as well as in AIDS patients who may internalize societal views of homosexuality (Wirth, 1986). Attitudes of health care providers about homosexuality may affect the quality of care given to gay patients (Dunkel & Hatfield, 1986; Pogoncheff, 1979). Specific actions that result from negative attitudes toward homosexual patients with AIDS can range from "inadvertent" violations of confidentiality to dehumanizing and unnecessarily restrictive "isolation techniques" to outright neglect of patient care responsibilities.

Substance abuse may also be viewed as a moral issue. Providers may consequently lecture patients to control their drug use, or blame patients for their diagnosis of AIDS (Faltz & Madover, 1986). They may also expect substance abusers to be uncooperative patients, thereby influencing a negative outcome of staff–patient interactions (Biener, 1983). Caregivers may also fail to discuss substance abuse at all with patients thus ignoring the obvious (Faltz & Madover, 1986). They may feel that after an AIDS diagnosis it is futile to treat substance abuse or other mental health problems. This "why bother" mentality can lead to failure of treatment and/or discharge plans. Neglect of a central patient problem such as substance abuse or another mental health problem can sabotage the best plans.

Health care providers sometimes use their religious or other beliefs to justify a lack of caring. There may be the implication that somehow the gay patient or injection drug user deserves AIDS. The implication may be more subtle, but nonetheless damaging, if one calls children and transfusion recipients the "innocent victims of AIDS."

HEALTH CARE WORKERS' RESPONSIBILITY TO CARE FOR PATIENTS

Even though risk is low for HIV transmission to health care workers, emotional reactions rather than factual information often influence professionals' behavior. For example, the American Nurses' Association Code for Nurses (1985) is clear about nurses' responsibility to provide care to all patients. According to the Code, "the nurse provides services with respect for human dignity and the uniqueness of the client, unrestricted by considerations of social or economic status, personal attributes, or the nature of the health problems" (ANA, 1985, Sec. 1). Attributes of patients such as age, sex, race, color, personality, sexuality, ethnicity, individual differences in background, customs, beliefs, attitudes, and lifestyles influence care delivery only insofar as they represent factors that caregivers must consider, understand, and respect in tailoring care to meet patients' personal needs and in maintaining the individual's self-respect and dignity (ANA, 1985, Sec. 1.2; Sande, 1986). They do not constitute ethically justifiable reasons for refusing to provide care (Dunkel & Hatfield, 1986; Lewis, Freeman, Kaplan, & Corey, 1986; Ostrow & Gayle, 1986). Other professions' codes of ethics contain similar provisions (Beauchamp & Childress, 1983).

For some health care providers, perceptions of personal risk associated with providing care to AIDS patients have led to attempts to refuse or avoid giving care. They argue that so much is still not known about AIDS. Such perceptions of uncertainty create fears in health care providers and give some what they think are ethically justifiable reasons to refuse providing care. As uncertainty lessens, however, it becomes more difficult to use such reasons to ethically justify actions.

Blumenfield and colleagues (1987) report that a high percentage of nurses they surveyed said they would seek a transfer from their assigned unit if they were required to work with AIDS patients regularly. Fear of contagion can often persist long after AIDS in-service education. Therefore, additional classes may not be adequate to allay fears. Such findings raise questions about the nature of professional obligation and the general understanding of professional codes of ethics with regard to ethical obligations to all patients, including those with AIDS. Do health care providers have similar reactions to other patients with diseases known to be contagious through casual contact? If the answer is yes, then the nature of the provider's obligation requires extensive examination. If the answer is no, then the provider's attitudes toward AIDS patients is based on factors other than fear of contagion, which is the stated reason because it seems more reasonable, tolerant, and ethical.

Safety versus the Contagiousness of AIDS

Medical experts currently consider AIDS to be a generally fatal disease. The number of diagnosed AIDS cases in the United States doubles each year (Krim, 1986). As of February 1991, over 164,000 people had been diagnosed with AIDS (Centers for Disease Control, 1991).

Precautions that health care workers can take when caring for AIDS patients apply also to caring for most other patients. The AIDS virus is fragile and is easily killed with germicidal soaps. Therefore, careful handwashing with soap and water becomes of prime importance in preventing spread of the disease. The conscientious use of gloves when handling contaminated equipment or linen and the proper disposal of these items can go far to protect providers from the AIDS virus (Bennett, 1986). Such basic and simple precautions, once understood and used, can eradicate numerous ethical issues related to caring for AIDS patients. The best way to provide care to people with AIDS and simultaneously protect oneself is to approach patients thoughtfully, respectfully, carefully, and rationally. In this way, patients' rights are not violated and providers' ethical obligations to patients are met.

PRIVACY AND PUBLIC HEALTH ISSUES

The conflict between the right of an individual to privacy and society's need to safeguard the public's health revolves around the extent to which autonomy and confidentiality can be afforded an individual with an HIV-related diagnosis. An example of this ethical issue is the incident in which the wife of an injection drug user with an HIV infection was unaware of her husband's medical condition and was 3 months pregnant. He refused to tell her about his diagnosis, and the drug treatment counselor debated whether to reveal the HIV-related diagnosis or to respect the privileged information the client revealed. Legally, the counselor was bound not to reveal medical information about his client to others. Under these circumstances, however, he had ethical obligations that differed from his legal ones. The ethical obligations in this instance involved considering the harms that might be done by not disclosing relevant information to those others directly involved in the situation, namely, the wife and the unborn child.

Several factors about the AIDS epidemic are relevant to this discussion. First, since specific behaviors are associated with high risk for AIDS, individuals need to be encouraged to take responsibility for the prevention of AIDS. For teaching about AIDS prevention, community health education targets those who are sexually active and who use intravenous drugs. When little was known about AIDS and its transmission, it was not possible to speak of preventing it. However, once such knowledge becomes available, individuals have obligations as members of society to use the knowledge to help prevent further spread of the disease.

Mass distribution of condoms, along with information on their proper use, and information regarding methods of sterilizing hypodermic needles and syringes are controversial but essential if individuals are to be encouraged to assume responsibility for AIDS prevention. These activities do, however, raise ethical issues for some who equate providing such equipment and information with encouraging and condoning illicit sex and drug abuse.

Another way of thinking about the situation involves raising a question regarding the possible harm done by not providing equipment and information to individuals who may be at risk for AIDS. Raising the question of harm essentially recognizes that there are groups in our society who engage in behaviors that put them at high risk to contract AIDS. Raising the question of harm does not attempt to morally judge the behaviors in question. Rather, it focuses on the potential physical, psychological, social, and moral harms that may result from not having certain information and acting on it.

Mass screening of persons at risk for AIDS has been suggested as a way of safeguarding the public's health. This could lead to a false sense of security for communities as well as for those tested. Individuals with a negative HIV antibody status could still be virus positive because it often takes up to one year to develop HIV antibodies. Additionally, the validity of the test lasts only as long as the individual does not engage in HIV risk behavior.

The confidentiality of one's HIV antibody status as well as possible diagnosis of AIDS or AIDS-related complex (ARC) has been generally safeguarded. However, threats to this confidentiality often arise. The conflict between those opposed to the maintenance of confidentiality and those who defend it can involve not only differing ethical perspectives but also legal and political processes.

The Limits of Compulsion in Controlling AIDS

AIDS presents health care providers with numerous policy questions that have ethical dimensions. Because of several factors, including the lethal quality of the disease, the stigma of those who were first reported as having AIDS, and fear on the part of health care professionals and the general public, pressure has been mounting on public health officials to consider compulsory infection control strategies. Some see such compulsory controls as both necessary and desirable since they will counter the epidemic. Others, however, raise questions regarding the legal and ethical justification of these measures as well as their projected effectiveness in slowing or stopping the AIDS epidemic.

Some health care professionals suggest that all HIV carriers should be identified, tested, and warned to change their sexual and drug habits before they spread the epidemic further. Others, specifically, civil rights groups, fear that tracking them down could threaten their privacy, job security, and access to health insurance. The first group counterargues that such a focus on individual rights without consideration for the common good permits the continued spread of this lethal disease. Some ethicists have said that AIDS patients' self-interests have wrongly eclipsed the moral obligation to warn former sex partners and those with whom one has shared intravenous drug needles. This opinion has been supported by health professionals who say that any individual who is infected should think about the good of the community (Gostin & Curran, 1986).

Current policy regarding HIV testing is based on encouraging persons at high risk to voluntarily seek anonymous HIV antibody testing to determine their serological status and then to modify their behavior. Obviously, the cooperation of these individuals is critical to success. While society has the obligation to protect the rights and dignity of its members, citizens also have an obligation to act on behalf of the common good (Gostin & Curran, 1986).

Ethical issues also arise in policy discussions focused on the *isolation* and *quarantine* of individuals. While these terms sometimes are used interchangeably, they do have different meanings. Quarantine affects healthy individuals who may have been exposed to the infectious agent but are not yet known to be infected. Isolation applies only to those people already known to be infectious— whether carrying the infectious agent or suffering from the disease.

All states have authorized control measures for large numbers of common diseases. However, state statutes classify AIDS as a communicable disease and not as a venereal or sexually transmitted disease. Such a classification does not authorize isolation unless state regulations are amended. However, isolation has been advocated as the only effective public health measure society has to control the disease (Macklin, 1986).

Isolation is the most serious form of deprivation of liberty that can be used against a competent and unwilling person. It is based on what the person might do in the future rather than what she or he has already done. This ethical problem is compounded by the fact that there are no time limitations on isolation, and rigorous due process procedures are lacking. Therefore, general isolation of all those who test positive for HIV antibodies or all those with the disease would, in some judgments, be both unethical and unconstitutional (Gostin & Curran, 1986).

With the increasing spread of AIDS, society has begun to look to the law for control measures. When examined objectively, however, legal commentators indicate that most legal and regulatory proposals would have little or counterproductive effects on the spread of HIV infection. Such measures, so the argument goes, impose disproportionate restrictions on the liberty, autonomy, and privacy of persons vulnerable to HIV infection. There will continue to be policy discussions of the ethical dilemma posed by AIDS that pit individual rights against the common good. In this discussion, one factor must be remembered: To safeguard individual rights is part of the common good. In any evaluation of the relative interests of individual and community, however, the burden of proof is always upon the community to prove its case for restricting the liberty of individuals (Callahan, 1984).

DISTRIBUTION OF RESOURCES

The spreading AIDS crisis poses great challenges for all American institutions, including the health care system and the public and private financial institutions that support it. The estimated cost for AIDS/ARC medical care over the next 5 years, according to the CDC, could amount to $14 billion (Sedaka & O'Reilly, 1986). The average per person cost of treating people with AIDS is estimated at $140,000 (Volberding & Abrams, 1985).

To compound the ethical issues, the AIDS epidemic began during a time of belt-tightening and increased fiscal restraint by health care providers and health insurance carriers. Hospitals increasingly closed empty beds and reduced services and staff to save money. Health insurance carriers set firm limits on which services they would and would not cover. The prospects of AIDS relative to insurance coverage have further complicated health insurance carriers' decisions about who and what to cover (Oppenheimer & Padqug, 1986).

Because AIDS often causes protracted physical disability, people often lose their jobs, their job-related health insurance, their homes, and their savings. This leaves public assistance programs to cover the costs of their treatment and care.

This situation creates added financial strain on local assistance programs (Altman, 1987).

The current and projected incidence rates of AIDS in the population over the next 5 years indicate that existing hospitals and long-term care facilities will not have enough general and intensive care beds to accommodate the projected need. Questions also exist about whether or not the supply of nursing and medical personnel will be sufficient to meet the needs of those who will develop AIDS during the coming years. Given the current nursing shortage, it is entirely possible that nursing staffs will be stretched even further than they are at present.

Exponential increases in the number of AIDS cases further complicates the already complex issues of the ethical and equitable distribution of health care resources and raises a number of questions. How much of America's health care resources should AIDS research, treatment, and education receive? If health care resources are indeed scarce, what other health care services could be restricted in order to accommodate the financial and space needs of AIDS researchers and patients? How should expensive intensive care services be used with AIDS patients? Is an intensive care unit the most appropriate place to care for AIDS patients in their last days? The restrictive, high-technology atmosphere of an intensive care unit does not seem a likely place for a terminally ill patient to experience the caring concern and support that is so necessary at such a critical time. In these situations, perhaps home care or hospice care would be a more beneficial and appropriate use of resources, both for the individual patient and for society.

Much effort and money have already been provided for scientific research into the cause and characteristics of AIDS, its means of transmission, and the possibilities for treatment and cure of those already stricken. The message becomes clearer every day that the only sure cure for AIDS is specific knowledge about the disease and prevention of it through self-protection (Altman, 1987).

If the general public, in addition to those whose behavior puts them at risk for AIDS, can be educated about the specifics of AIDS, its transmission, and the general relevancy of this information to everyone's life, perhaps millions of people could be spared HIV infection (Slaff & Brubaker, 1985). Additionally, if people could be helped to see that needle exchange programs and the distribution of condoms and bleach to those at risk are public health issues rather than moral issues, perhaps many more people could be spared HIV infection and AIDS.

While the ethics and pragmatics of distributing safer sex information and devices to the general public and sterile needles to intravenous drug users has captured much media attention in recent times, the fact remains that personal and social responsibility and accountability are the most important factors in halting the further spread of AIDS. As members of society, individuals have both social and moral responsibilities to protect themselves, and others with whom they come in contact, from HIV infection. Society has a corresponding responsibility to protect its members by providing individuals who are at risk for HIV infection with the means to protect themselves and others. Sex, drugs, and AIDS are all current facts of American society. A comprehensive AIDS prevention program should provide, among other things, street outreach to injection drug users and their partners, and include distribution of bleach and condoms (Smith, 1988) and a needle exchange program (Stimson, 1989).

ETHICAL ISSUES IN AIDS RESEARCH

AIDS patients have been described as members of a special population with a life-threatening illness who may be willing to incur greater risk to themselves for the good of others. Due to the dynamics of AIDS, research has been conducted in a different way than is usually the case. Much of the dynamic in this situation is due to the public urgency that is tied to the possible scope and deadly quality of the condition. Several ethical problems emerge in this research environment and include the following.

Basically, it must be noted that informed consent, or the individual's right to know about the research, to agree or refuse to participate as a human subject, and the right to withdraw is basic to all research situations. In this urgent environment of AIDS research, patients who are asked to be in research proposals may be coerced to participate. This issue is made more difficult because therapies have not had time to be fully tested in the laboratory prior to involving humans. Institutional review boards that exist to protect the rights of human subjects in research, under these circumstances, are pressed to rapidly approve protocols, to approve compassionate use of unapproved drug therapies, and to expedite approvals for new drugs without controlled trials. One profoundly difficult issue in the research arena with AIDS patients is antibody testing where there has not been a clear distinction between epidemiological, diagnostic, and public policy purposes. The essential problem here stems from the fact that what might be ethically justified for one purpose may not be ethically justified for another (Panem, 1985).

Given that the public's and health care professionals' response to AIDS is grounded in urgency and fear, many are concerned that there is insufficient information to inform subjects about potential risks and that the incidence of central nervous system disease in AIDS patients makes consent difficult, and at times impossible. In addition, the question arises as to who may appropriately give proxy consent. At the baseline of concern is the difficulty conceiving of voluntary consent when the subjects are so vulnerable. Given the very real situation with AIDS, what sort of choices can patients make?

The numbers of women with AIDS is increasing, and some of these women are and will become pregnant. Therefore, ethical questions with this population include abortion, postponement of pregnancy, and sterilization. Should a woman at high risk for HIV infection and AIDS have a baby? What role should the state and health professionals play? Can coercion of the individual be ethically justified in the name of the common good?

Some patients with an AIDS diagnosis talk about suicide. If health professionals have this information, do they have an obligation to attempt to prevent a patient from committing suicide? Can we ethically justify suicide in these instances by thinking of such an action as rational suicide? Would it be ethical to give patients requested information regarding methods of suicide? For example, should a patient be told the drug dosage necessary to kill an individual?

LEGAL ISSUES

Competency to Make Health Care Decisions

Whenever a person has a life-threatening illness, questions arise regarding the ability of that person to make health care decisions. People who have illnesses associated with AIDS offer no exception.

According to the President's Commission Report on Ethical Problems in Medicine (1982), in order for patients to participate fully in health care decisions they must possess the mental, emotional, and legal capacity to do so. The person must be able to communicate, to understand information adequately, and to reason and deliberate sufficiently well about the choices. The person must also be able to understand the consequences that might follow from her or his health care decisions. The Doctrine of Informed Consent is based on the premise that a person's interests and well-being are best served when the person fully understands the situation and can participate in deciding on the course of treatment and care.

In situations where people with AIDS are concerned, consultations between physicians and competent patients to determine a plan of treatment and care should occur early in the course of the illness before any conditions develop that could compromise the patient's decision-making ability. Early health care planning is essential because people with AIDS frequently develop sudden cognitive impairment secondary to viral infections of the central nervous system and severe respiratory complications that render them unable to participate in treatment and care decisions (Jonsen, Cooke, & Koenig, 1986; Steinbrook, Lo, Tirpak, Dilley, & Volberding, 1985).

Many problems in decision making arise when people become incompetent to make their own health care decisions prior to making their wishes known and prior to the appointment of a surrogate decision maker. In the event that a patient does not legally appoint a surrogate decision maker prior to incapacity, the patient's next of kin would become, by law, the decision maker, even though this might prevent the patient's expressed wishes from being implemented (President's Commission, 1983).

The legal status of next of kin as default surrogate decision makers for incapacitated patients is a cause for concern to many homosexual AIDS patients. Situations occur in which gay men with AIDS must break the news of the illness and their homosexuality to their families at the same time. This situation can cause conflicts between the patients and their families. As a result, many gay or bisexual men who are not close to their families or who have conflicted family relationships choose a trusted friend or significant other to act as a surrogate decision maker in the event of mental incapacity.

Designation of Power of Attorney

In the State of California, the Durable Power of Attorney for Health Care allows competent persons to appoint others to act as surrogate decision makers for health care and terminal care in the event of mental incapacity. Use of the Durable Power of Attorney legalizes the power of the appointed friend or significant other to make the necessary health care decisions desired by the patient if and when the patient becomes unable to do so. The legal aspects of surrogate decision making are particularly important to gay couples because the law does not acknowledge or recognize their spousal relationship (Steinbrook *et al.*, 1985).

The main reason for confronting the issues of competency and informed consent early in the course of an illness is to get people thinking and talking about the future possibilities before problems arise. Use of the Durable Power of Attorney for Health Care can prevent troublesome and frustrating situations from developing when patients become unable to make their own decisions. By planning ahead, patients have the best chance of making their health care wishes become realities.

SUMMARY

This chapter has discussed selected ethical and legal issues that arise with people with HIV disease. During the early phase soon after diagnosis, the ethical issues tend to be those surrounding treatment decisions and fear of contamination. In the midstage of the disease process, the issues shift to pain control and the extent of treatment wanted by the patient. During the terminal phase, ethical issues become those having to do with dying and death issues such as withholding treatment, coping with pain and suffering, and who speaks in the best interests of the patients when they cannot speak for themselves (Dilley, Shelp, & Batki, 1986).

Throughout all three phases, ethical issues of allocation of resources and research must be addressed. The ethical principles of individual rights to liberty, informed consent, confidentiality, and distributive justice need to be understood fully by health professionals and used in ethically reasoning through dilemmas. Only in this way can AIDS patients benefit from our humane caring.

REFERENCES

Altman, D. (1987). *AIDS in the mind of America.* Garden City, NY: Anchor Press.

American Nurses' Association. (1985). *Code for nurses with interpretive statements.* Kansas City, Kansas: American Nurses' Association.

Beauchamp, T., & Childress, J. (1983). *Principles of biomedical ethics* (2nd ed.). New York: Oxford University Press.

Bennett, J. (1986). What precautions do you take in the hospital? *American Journal of Nursing, 86,* 952–953.

Biener, L. (1983). Perceptions of patients by emergency room staff: Substance abusers versus non-substance abusers. *Journal of Health and Social Behavior, 24,* 264–275.

Blumenfield, M., Smith, P. J., Milazzo, J., Seropian, S., & Wormser, G. P. (1987). Survey of attitudes of nurses working with AIDS patients. *General Hospital Psychiatry, 9,* 58–63.

Callahan, D. (1984). Autonomy: A moral good, not a moral obsession. *Hastings Center Report, 14,* 40–42.

Centers for Disease Control. (1991, February). *HIV/AIDS surveillance,* pp. 9.

Davis, A. J., & Aroskar, M. A. (1983). *Ethical dilemmas and nursing practice* (2nd ed.) Norwalk, CN: Appleton-Century-Crofts.

Dilley, J. W., Shelp, E. E., & Batki, S. L. (1986). Psychiatric and ethical issues in the care of patients with AIDS: An overview. *Psychosomatics, 27,* 562–566.

Dunkel, J., & Hatfield, S. (1986, March/April). Countertransference issues in working with persons with AIDS. *Social Work,* pp. 114–117.

Faltz, B. G., & Madover, S. (1986). Substance abuse as a cofactor for AIDS. In L. McKusick (Ed.), *What to do about AIDS: Physicians and health care professionals discuss the issues* (pp. 155–162). Los Angeles: University of California Press.

Gostin, L., & Curran, W. J. (1986). The limits of compulsion in controlling AIDS. *Hastings Center Report, 16,* 24–29.

Jonsen, A. R., Cooke, M., & Koenig, B. A. (1986). AIDS and ethics. *Issues in Science and Technology, 2*(2), 129–139.

Krim, M. (1986). AIDS: The challenge to science and medicine. *Hastings Center Report, 15,* 2–7.

Lewis, C. E., Freeman, H. E., Kaplan, S. H., & Corey, C. R. (1986). The impact of a program to enhance the competencies of primary care physicians in caring for patients with AIDS. *Journal of General Internal Medicine, 1,* 287–294.

Macklin, R. (1986). Predicting dangerousness and the public health response to AIDS. *Hastings Center Report, 16,* 16–23.

Oppenheimer, G. M., & Padqug, R. A. (1986). AIDS: The risks to insurers, the threat to equity. *Hastings Center Report, 16,* 18–22.

Ostrow, D. G., & Gayle, T. C. (1986). Psychosocial and ethical issues of AIDS health care programs. *Quarterly Review Bulletin, 8,* 284–294.

Panem, S. (1985). AIDS: Public policy and biomedical research. *Hastings Center Report, 15,* 23–26.

Pogoncheff, E. (1979). The gay patient: What not to do. *RN Magazine, 24,* 46–49.

President's Commission for the Study of Ethical Problems in Medicine and Biomedical and Behavioral Research. (1982). *Making health care decisions.* Washington DC: U.S. Government Printing Office.

President's Commission for the Study of Ethical Problems in Medicine and Biomedical and Behavioral Research. (1983). *Deciding to forego life-sustaining treatment.* Washington DC: U.S. Government Printing Office.

Sande, M. E. (1986). Transmission of AIDS: The case against casual contagion. *The New England Journal of Medicine, 314,* 380–382.

Sedaka, S., & O'Reilly, M. (1986). The financial implications of AIDS. *Caring, 6,* 38–46.

Slaff, J., & Brubaker, J. (1985). *The AIDS epidemic.* New York: Warner Books.

Smith, D. E. (1988). The role of substance abuse professionals in the AIDS epidemic. *Advances in Alcohol & Substance Abuse, 7*(2), 175–193.

Steinbrook, R., Lo, B., Tirpack, J., Dilley, J. W., & Volberding, P. A. (1985). Ethical dilemmas in caring for patients with the acquired immunodeficiency syndrome. *Annals of Internal Medicine, 103,* 787–790.

Stimson, G. V. (1989). Editorial review: Syringe exchange programmes for injection drug users. *AIDS, 3*(5), 253–260.

Volberding, P. A., & Abrams, D. (1985). Clinical care and research in AIDS. *Hastings Center Report, 15,* 16–18.

Wirth, S. (1986). Reflections on archetypal aspects of AIDS and a psychology of gay men. In L. McKusick (Ed.), *What to do about AIDS: Physicians and health care professionals discuss the issues* (pp. 95–102). Los Angeles: University of California Press.

II

AIDS, Families, and Adolescents

3

Adolescents and AIDS
Coping Issues

JOYCE HUNTER and ROBERT SCHAECHER

The AIDS epidemic has been with us for a decade. In that time a tremendous amount has been learned about HIV infection in terms of its etiology and epidemiology. Most recently, new treatments have been developed that prolong the lives of people with AIDS. Also, until recently, little attention has been given to the risks that the adolescent population might experience and the unique problems they face in reducing their risk of exposure to the infection or coping with an actual HIV infection. This chapter examines the problems and possibilities of HIV infection among adolescents in the United States as we enter the next decade.

RATES OF INFECTION AMONG ADOLESCENTS

As of January 1991, there have been 629 adolescent cases of AIDS reported to the Centers for Disease Control (Centers for Disease Control, 1991). Currently, less than 1% of the AIDS cases have occurred among 13- to 19-year-olds. However, 21% of AIDS cases are in the 20- to 29-year-old age group. With a possible incubation period of over 10 years, many young adults have been infected during the adolescent years. At this point in time we only have limited measures of the impact of HIV infection in the adolescent population because few adolescents have been tested for HIV infection. The infection rates we currently have may

JOYCE HUNTER • HIV Center for Clinical and Behavioral Studies, New York, New York 10032. ROBERT SCHAECHER • The Calhoun School, New York, New York 10024.

Living and Dying with AIDS, edited by Paul I. Ahmed, Plenum Press, New York, 1992.

underreport the incidence of HIV in adolescents because adolescents, particularly from minority groups and lower social classes, do not receive regular medical care (Lockhart & Wodarski, 1989). Among military recruits the rate of HIV infection has been 1.5/1000 at the national level (but 16/1000 for recruits from Bronx County in New York City). Testing of Job Corps applicants (ages 16–21) found an infection rate of 3.3/1000. In an HIV-seroprevalence study of runaway and homeless youth at Covenant House, New York City, an infection rate of 8% (15% among ages 19–20) was found (Hein, 1989). More recent blood studies conducted by the Centers for Disease Control found that 1% of 15- and 16-year-olds in areas like New York and Miami are already infected. Outside of large cities, 3 in 1000 adolescents were infected (Kolata, 1989).

In a risk profile of an average high school student in the United States, Dr. Elizabeth Alexander of the University of Kansas School of Medicine in Wichita asserts that before a 14-year-old graduates from high school there is a 17% chance that the student will experiment with cocaine, a 40% chance that the student will be a partner in pregnancy, a 65% chance that the student will use alcohol on a regular basis, and an 86% chance that the first 6–9 months of sexual intercourse will be unprotected by any form of contraception, including condoms ("Research Describes," 1989). Many adolescent behaviors serve as useful indicators for possible exposure to HIV. What forces operate to foster such a high level of risk taking?

RISK-TAKING BEHAVIOR IN ADOLESCENCE

The Health Belief Model identifies five factors in assessing a person's ability to engage in healthy behaviors (Rosenstock, 1974). First, the person must perceive some measure of susceptibility or vulnerability to illness. Second, the person must perceive the illness as severe. Third, the person must see the benefits of changing behavior to avoid the illness. Fourth, the person must understand and overcome the barriers of possible negative effects of change. Finally, there must be present sufficient cues or stimuli to change behavior, such as symptoms or health communications.

In reference to these beliefs, adolescents, and indeed many adults, have difficulty perceiving their personal vulnerability to illness. Adolescents in particular operate under the "personal fable" that they are immune to severe illness. Two factors contribute to this sense of invulnerability. One factor is that few adolescents are symptomatic for HIV infection. There are few peers ill with AIDS, so the belief that as a teenager one is immune is reinforced. The notion of being an asymptomatic carrier of a deadly disease is difficult to accept or even understand for oneself or others. The media has added to the problem by focusing on the incidence of AIDS among adult gay men and IV drug users, thus contributing even further to the adolescent denial. In addition, the effects of many diseases are only apparent later in life. Many teenagers smoke cigarettes, negating the long-term health consequences of this behavior. Lung disease will show up late in life, a future perspective difficult for a teenager to grasp. The adolescent can indeed say in the present time frame that "it can't happen to me"—largely true for the end stage of the disease, but certainly not for the asymptomatic infection stage (Melton, 1988). Many street youth (runaways and throwaways) can to some degree personalize their own vulnerability because of what they have seen. However, they will often say "What do I have to live for?" This sense of hopelessness about their life situation engenders an attitude that supports high-risk behaviors.

Other problems that interfere with an adolescent engaging in HIV risk reduction behaviors include the short-term rewards for unprotected sexual intercourse or IV drug use, which can be very strong—whether those be pleasure, peer approval, or behaviors perceived as markers for a sense of independence. Adolescents are in the process of changing from a family (parental) orientation to a peer orientation. Peer influence is an important factor for much of adolescent risk-taking behavior (Kandel, 1985; Lewis & Lewis, 1984; Norem-Hebeisen & Hedin, 1981).

ADOLESCENT KNOWLEDGE, ATTITUDES, AND BELIEFS

Several key surveys conducted with adolescents present a picture of their attitudes and beliefs (DiClemente, Zorn, & Temoshok, 1986; Helgerson, Petersen, & AIDS Education Study Group, 1988; Koopman, Rotheram-Borus, Henderson, Bradley, & Hunter, 1990; McGill, Smith, & Johnson, 1989; Price, Desmond, & Kukulka, 1985; Strunin & Hingson, 1987). The surveys indicate that in recent years adolescents have increased knowledge about how AIDS is transmitted, but they still lack sufficient understanding about effective precautions to lessen risk of infection. Substantial ethnic differences are also found in the surveys. A greater proportion of white adolescents are aware of AIDS and effective prevention measures than other racial groups. Sexually active adolescents know about condoms, but the reported use of condoms has not increased significantly (Kegeles, Adler, & Irwin, 1988; Rickert, Jay, Gottlieb, & Bridges, 1989). By age 20, over 80% of males and over 70% of females report engaging in sexual intercourse at least once, and the percentages continue to rise (Hayes, 1987). Meanwhile, the age of first intercourse is dropping and the number of sexual partners is increasing. One-fourth to one-third of the adolescents engaging in sexual intercourse do not use any form of contraception. Adolescent pregnancy and sexually transmitted disease rates support these findings. Over one million adolescent females become pregnant each year (Byrne, 1983; Hayes, 1987). Sexually transmitted diseases

(STDs) strike an estimated 20 million people in the United States each year, and about 85% of all STDs occur in teenagers and young adults (Yarber, 1985).

While IV drug use is not as common among adolescents as adults, adolescents do share needles in other contexts—ear piercing, tatooing, and steroid injections. Some youths are at greater risk because they drop out of school and live on the streets of urban centers. Many of these youths are exposed to drugs and high-risk sexual encounters. Cross-dressing youths will illegally obtain hormones to develop a more feminine appearance, and they often share these needles with each other.

So adolescents are increasingly well informed about the nature of HIV infection, but incorporating the necessary behavioral changes into their lifestyle is less forthcoming.

COPING WITH HIV INFECTION

The following two case studies illustrate how some adolescents struggle to cope with HIV disease.

Case Study 1: Felix

Felix was an 18-year-old Hispanic gay male who lived with his mother and sister. Occasionally his brother lived at home as well. Felix never knew his father. The family's socioeconomic status was working class.

At the time he came for help to the Hetrick–Martin Institute serving lesbian and gay youth in New York City, he was still living at home. He described his problem as one of having left school because he was being harassed due to his sexual orientation. He was very lonely because he had no friends his own age. He wanted help in getting a high school diploma and meeting friends his own age.

Felix went into an alternative high school program and received individual supportive counseling and joined a weekly socialization group. He was a very difficult person to engage in counseling. His attendance was erratic. His self-esteem was very low because of difficulties coping with being gay. He felt that his family never fully accepted his homosexuality. His social skills were woefully underdeveloped. He would push people away before he thought they could reject him. In counseling he revealed that he was engaging in anonymous sexual activities in local bathhouses.

His attendance at an alternative school was regular. School was very important to him because he believed that he could go on to college and have a career. He was highly motivated around schooling. It kept him engaged at the Hetrick–Martin Institute and he did manage to make a best friend.

The teachers noticed that he was appearing tired and beginning to miss classes. By this time he was living independently with a friend. His counselor recommended that he go to a local clinic for a health evaluation. He never followed through on the referral. As months passed, his health deteriorated further. He began to lose weight. Felix continued to deny that he was sick. Finally, he got a very bad cough and his counselor took him to see a doctor. After several medical checkups there was enough medical evidence to suspect that Felix had pneumonia. When it was suggested to him that he have a bronchoscopy, he refused. He became very depressed and anxious. Having received basic AIDS information from the beginning of his contact with the Hetrick–Martin Institute, he knew that the bronchoscopy meant that he might have AIDS. He talked about feeling alone again and hopeless and losing a reason for living. Suicidal ideation was expressed.

Felix finally relented and was tested for HIV infection and PCP, an AIDS-related pneumonia. He was positive on both tests. He went into total denial and refused to talk about his illness and what it meant to him. In counseling he focused exclusively on school.

Interventions were tried to connect him with other AIDS resource organizations such as the Gay Men's Health Crisis and the People With AIDS Coalition. Felix did not follow through with the referrals. He felt out of place because the other clients were all older than he was.

At one point he became very ill and was hospitalized again. The hospital workers avoided attending to him as much as possible, yet while there he passed all of his tests to qualify for a high school diploma. He was so upset at the poor treatment he received at the hospital that he pulled out his IV and walked out of the hospital. It took a week of telephone counseling to convince him to be admitted to a different hospital. The second hospital refused to admit him because he was not perceived to be sick enough. His counselor found a doctor who worked with AIDS patients in a clinic, and he accepted Felix for treatment as an outpatient. He was well enough to attend his graduation exercises. After graduation his health continued to deteriorate, and he returned home for care. Two months after graduation he died.

Felix's experiences illuminate several issues. First, one of the key developmental tasks for adolescents is the creation of a personal identity through socialization. Heterosexual youth accomplish this task by having available to them extensive adult role modeling, positive portrayals in the media, and experiences practicing social behaviors with same- and opposite-sex peers. Both the home and the school are settings for rehearsing these socialization behaviors. But young gay males commonly experience difficulty socializing with their peers. The stigma attached to a homosexual orientation is often borne as a "secret shame." Gay youth lack positive role models, witness negative portrayals of homosexuals in the media, and know that if they openly acknowledge their homosexual identity they are likely to suffer the consequence of harassment or violence. Hiding their homosexual orientation does not permit young gay males to discuss their feelings and concerns with anyone, even with family members. Searching for a way to connect with other gay males and lacking a repertoire of socialization skills, they may resort to anonymous sexual encounters in gay bars, bathhouses, and the streets. Looking for friendship, companionship, and love, they instead find sex (Hunter & Schaecher, 1987).

Felix had internalized the negative images of homosexuality in our culture. He saw no other choices for meeting gay people. Starting at the age of 15, he turned to the only places he had heard of—the bars, baths, and streets. Sex with men older than himself substituted for relationships with his peers. The context of these encounters was unsafe sex, and the consequence was HIV infection.

The second issue is the stigma attached to HIV infection. "Children and adolescents, like adults, must contend not only with the disease itself, but also with the public's fear—a reaction that promotes social isolation, rejection, and ostracism. Vulnerability and victimization have become central themes in the lives of these youngsters" (Lockhart & Wodarski, 1989). Felix's sense of the stigma attached to HIV disease was played out by his strong denial of the presence of the disease and its symptoms in his body. Even in the face of significant weight loss and persistent coughing, he attributed these symptoms to poor nutrition and catching a cold. Despite his declining health, he continued to perform his school work and employment as if business was usual. For Felix, employment was a measure of his independence. As Rando (1984) notes:

> This maturing teenager now becomes an individual in his own right for the very first time. At a point when the adolescent is tasting the pleasures of personal mastery and self-achievement, and is first experiencing his sexuality, the threat of death is enormously cruel. The rage and bitterness is profound. (p. 389)

Finally, Felix embodied the stigma that society places on people who are considered to be on the fringes of their community. Herek (1989) has characterized HIV disease as a "disease of communities." To be a member of one of these communities is to be identified as the "other." Felix belonged to three stigmatized communities—he was an Hispanic gay male with AIDS.

Case Study 2: John

> John is a 17-year-old white male from a divorced family. He lived with his father until removed by family court because of physical abuse from his father. He was placed with a foster family at the age of 11 and stayed with them for 5 years.
>
> At age 15 he went to live with his mother, who was a recovering alcoholic at that time. As he became more aware of his homosexual orientation he felt alone and isolated as a gay person. He was referred to a gay-identified agency with the recommendation that he join an afterschool socialization program for gay adolescent males. Up to this point John's efforts to connect with other gay people took place solely through sexual contacts in public places. At intake he expressed a desire to meet a person his own age with whom he could develop a relationship. His mother did not yet know that her son was gay; however, he eventually came out to her, and she accepted him with a great deal of ambivalence.
>
> When family problems developed, John dropped out of his school and was not seen by the agency for a year. Within that year he became HIV positive and

returned to the agency for support services. Initially, he denied the seriousness of his infection by avoiding clinic appointments and getting sufficient rest. He was already beginning to lose weight. John stated to his counselor that he was "putting his sexuality on hold." When he had sex he claimed to have safe sex, but he was not informing his sex partners about his health status. The agency was obtaining Medicaid and public assistance for John. The application for benefits was withdrawn by his mother, who wished to keep her address secret. At this point John decided he wanted to get a summer job. However, he began to develop more symptoms, and he was referred to a hospital's adolescent HIV center. He became involved with the hospital program (including a teen theater group), and he also entered an alternative high school program. As school was beginning, he left home because of family problems and got an apartment with a friend. But this arrangement was short lived. His roommate left and he had to support the apartment by himself. He began to come down with other infections and was put on AZT. John had a bad reaction to AZT that finally caused him to confront his fear of illness and death. His defenses were down, and he spoke about being afraid of losing everything he had worked so hard to obtain and the sense of helplessness that ensued. When AZT was discontinued, he rebounded and returned to school, work, and the theater group.

Many of the issues discussed in Case 1 (Felix) apply to the case of John. He, too, struggled with establishing a personal identity that incorporated a homosexual orientation. While John was more comfortable with his homosexuality than Felix, he followed the same socialization pattern of anonymous sexual encounters. Denied opportunities to develop open and positive peer relationships in a gay context within the school or community, he did not develop the interpersonal skills appropriate to the adolescent stage of development. Deficits in these interpersonal skills can result in a diminished sense of self, alienation, and isolation. Compounding all of this, this adolescent must face the possibility of dealing with a terminal illness.

> At no other point in time is the ego so busy, both reliving past conflicts and attending to new and stronger impulses and developmental tasks. Terminal illness ravages the body, threatening the adolescent's development and integration of a sexual identity. It creates emotional, cognitive, and physical changes that work against successful socialization and development of a secure sense of self-esteem that will facilitate the growth of important peer and sexual relationships. (Rando, 1984, p. 390)

The capacity to cope means dealing with reality—in this case, the reality of infection and possible terminal illness. Seeking out a physician, following up on the medical regimen prescribed for the infection, and keeping medical appointments are markers for successful coping. John had difficulty following through with his medical care. Adolescents still living with their families have adults to help them cope with their illness. The adult family members get them to medical appointments and monitor the medications. However, adolescents like John who have left home lack such a support system.

Adolescents are still largely in a concrete stage of cognitive development. As concrete thinkers they have difficulty understanding the implications of their infection. What does concrete thinking mean in this context? Adolescents have a here-and-now present-time orientation, a poor sense of delayed gratification, and the need to see immediate results. Unless they feel the physical symptoms of HIV infection, denial is very easy—no coughing, no night sweats, no weight loss, no headaches, no illness. It wasn't until John experienced a severe reaction to AZT that he could break through some of his denial. While it was a reaction to AZT, it still brought home the fact that he could become that ill.

On the other hand, denial could be a positive coping skill in the face of a serious illness. "Among patients confronted with a potentially fatal illness, denial can be a useful and necessary defense mechanism because it gives them some control over when and how they will confront the issue of their mortality" (Moynihan, Christ, & Silver, 1988). John attempts to exert control over his life situation by engaging in a wide range of activities that occupy his attention.

CONCLUSIONS

The difficulties of coping with AIDS have been tellingly described in the popular and professional literature. Yet little attention has been given to the plight of adolescents struggling with HIV infection or AIDS. Many of the issues faced by adolescents are similar to those faced by adults. However, given their developmental stage, adolescents have fewer coping strategies to handle life-threatening crises, and many adolescent circumstances are unique to their age.

We have noticed some similarities in adolescent responses to HIV infection:

- Fear, anxiety, and other issues related to death and dying. Adolescents typically believe that they are immortal. The personal threat of death is not within their cognitive and emotional frame of reference.
- Adolescents must learn and integrate risk reduction behaviors into their existing behaviors.
- Consequently, adolescents will often deny the seriousness of the disease until they become symptomatic.
- Depression and suicidal ideation can result from the restrictions that the disease places on the adolescent's normal activities of work, school, and socialization.
- The shame of the disease and the consequent "secret" about it results in social isolation from friends and family. The association of HIV infection with homosexual behavior or IV drug use places an additional stress of identification with stigmatized groups.
- Some adolescents with HIV infection have many other problems to deal with besides their illness, for example, dysfunctional families with parental

alcoholism and child abuse, and living in foster care, on the streets, or in temporary accommodations.

- Lesbian and gay adolescents have unique psychosocial stresses because of the stigma attached to homosexuality. Professionals who work with these adolescents must be particularly sensitive and nonjudgmental.
- Adolescents encounter many obstacles in negotiating the health care system. There are very few services for HIV-infected adolescents. Health care for minors involves issues of parental consent and confidentiality. Many HIV-infected youth fear their parents will be informed and will question their sexual or drug behaviors. Child welfare agencies may become involved if the person is under the age of 18. The emancipated minor poses another set of complicated legal issues. Adolescents from both minority groups and a lower socioeconomic class are the least likely to seek medical care. The inadequacy of medical and social service support systems in handling the unique problems of adolescents can result in adolescents avoiding treatment.

RECOMMENDATIONS

- Given the weight of the problems described above, extensive pre- and posttest counseling for HIV antibody is essential.
- Medical and social services need to examine the gaps in services for HIV-infected adolescents and develop more systematic and appropriate services for these youth—services sensitive to the problems specific to their developmental stage.
- Mental health workers need to help adolescents with their concrete problems (housing, medical care, etc.) and help them explore their feelings about HIV infection. The workers need to be particularly sensitive to signs of depression and suicide. HIV-infected youths elicit many feelings in mental health workers, and they must be able to manage any countertransference issues that arise.
- Effective interventions by medical and social services take into account the ethnic, racial, and cultural diversity of the clients.
- Adolescents need greater access to correct information to challenge the numerous myths and misconceptions about HIV infection and AIDS.
- In AIDS prevention education, more focus must be placed on developing intervention models that will assist adolescents in translating the knowledge they have about AIDS into effective behavioral change.
- All levels of government must be committed to financially supporting innovative and effective programs of primary, secondary, and tertiary

interventions with adolescents that include assurance of professional training on HIV infection and homophobia.

The conclusions and recommendations we have described are but a preliminary sketch of the issues confronting adolescents with HIV infection and AIDS. Adolescents as a group have very few advocates, and health care providers must be at the forefront in challenging our society to meet their physical and mental health needs.

REFERENCES

Byrne, D. (1983). Sex without contraception. In D. Byrne & W. A. Fisher, (Eds.), *Adolescents, Sex, and Contraception* (pp. 3–31). Hillsdale, NJ: Lawrence Erlbaum.

Centers for Disease Control (1991, January). *HIV/AIDS surveillance.*

DiClemente, R. J., Zorn, J., & Temoshok, L. (1986). Adolescents and AIDS: A survey of knowledge, attitudes and beliefs about AIDS in San Francisco. *American Journal of Public Health, 76,* 1443–1445.

Hayes, C. D. (1987). *Risking the future: Adolescent sexuality, pregnancy, and childbearing.* Washington, DC: National Academy Press.

Hein, K. (1989). Commentary on adolescent acquired immunodeficiency syndrome: The next wave of human immunodeficiency virus epidemic? *Journal of Pediatrics, 114,* 144–149.

Helgerson, S. D., Petersen, L. R., & AIDS Education Study Group. (1988). Acquired immunodeficiency syndrome and secondary school students: Their knowledge is limited and they want to learn more. *Pediatrics, 81,* 350–355.

Herek, G. (1989). Illness, stigma and AIDS. American Psychological Association Master Lecture. In S. Landers, AIDS stigma reaches epidemic proportions. *Monitor, 20*(11), 5.

Hunter, J., & Schaecher, R. (1987). Stresses on lesbian and gay adolescents in schools. *Social Work in Education, 9,* 180–190.

Kandel, D. B. (1985). On processes of peer influences in adolescent drug use: A developmental perspective. In J. S. Brook, D. J. Lettieri, D. W. Drook, & B. Stimmel (Eds.), *Alcohol and substance abuse in adolescence* (pp. 139–163). New York: The Haworth Press.

Kegeles, S. M., Adler, N. E., & Irwin, C. E. (1988). Sexually active adolescents and condoms: Changes over one year in knowledge, attitudes and use. *American Journal of Public Health, 78,* 460–461.

Koopman, C., Rotheram-Borus, M. J., Henderson, R., Bradley, J. S., & Hunter, J. (1990). Assessment of knowledge of AIDS and beliefs about AIDS prevention among adolescents. *AIDS Education and Prevention: An Interdisciplinary Journal, 2*(1), 58–70.

Lewis, C. E., & Lewis, M. A. (1984). Peer pressure and risk-taking behaviors in children. *American Journal of Public Health, 74,* 580–584.

Lockhart, L. L., & Wodarski, J. S. (1989). Facing the unknown: Children and adolescents with AIDS. *Social Work, 34,* 215–221.

McGill, L., Smith, P. B., & Johnson, T. C. (1989). AIDS: Knowledge, attitudes, and risk characteristics of teens. *Journal of Sex Education & Therapy, 15,* 30–35.

Melton, G. B. (1988). Adolescents and prevention of AIDS. *Professional Psychology: Research and Practice, 19,* 403–408.

Moynihan, R., Christ, G., & Silver, L. G. (1988). AIDS and terminal illness. *Social Work, 69,* 380–387.

Norem-Hebelsen, A., & Hedin, D. (1981). Influences on adolescent problem behavior: Causes, connections, and contexts. In *Adolescent peer pressure: Theory, correlates, and program implications for drug abuse prevention* (pp. 21–46). Washington, DC: National Institute on Drug Abuse, U.S. Department of Health and Human Services.

Price, J. H., Desmond, S., & Kukulka, G. (1985). High school students' perceptions and misconceptions of AIDS. *Journal of School Health, 55,* 107–109.

Rando, T. A. (1984). *Grief, dying and death: Clinical interventions for caregivers,* Champaign, IL: Research Press.

Research describes student risk levels. (1989, February/March). *Adolescent Counselor,* p. 57.

Rickert, V. I., Jay, M. S., Gottlieb, A., & Bridges, C. (1989). Females' attitudes and behaviors toward condom purchase and use. *Journal of Adolescent Health Care, 10,* 313–316.

Rosenstock, I. M. (1974). The health belief model and preventive health behavior. In M. H. Becker, (Ed.), *The health belief model and personal health behavior.* Thorofare, NJ: Charles B. Slack.

Strunin, L., & Hingson, R. (1987). Acquired immunodeficiency syndrome and adolescents: Knowledge, beliefs, attitudes and behaviors. *Pediatrics, 79,* 825–828.

Yarber, W. L. (1985). *STD: A guide for today's young adults.* Reston, VA: American Alliance for Health, Physical Education, Recreation and Dance.

4

Mothers with AIDS

Michael H. Antoni, Neil Schneiderman,
Arthur LaPerriere, Mary Jo O'Sullivan,
Jennifer Marks, Jonell Efantis, Jay Skyler, and
Mary Ann Fletcher

EPIDEMIOLOGICAL TRENDS IN HIV-1 SEROPREVALENCE AND AIDS

Over the past few years, reviewers have suggested that the phenomena of human immunodeficiency virus-Type I (HIV-1) infection and acquired immunodeficiency syndrome (AIDS) among heterosexuals, women, and ethnic minority groups have been largely understudied while at the same time accelerating in incidence (Mays & Cochran, 1988). National and regional epidemiological data collected since 1985 appear to support the latter point. While reported cases of AIDS among homosexual men leveled off in major metropolitan areas (Berkelman *et al.*, 1989) and actually declined in some cities (Lindan, Rutherford, Payne, Hearst, & Lemp, 1989) between 1985 and 1988, the proportion of cases attributable to heterosexual transmission has been increasing more rapidly than

Michael H. Antoni and Neil Schneiderman • Center for the Biopsychosocial Study of AIDS, Department of Psychology, University of Miami, Coral Gables, Florida 33124.   Arthur La Perriere • Center for the Biopsychosocial Study of AIDS, Department of Psychiatry, University of Miami School of Medicine, Miami, Florida 33139.   Mary Jo O'Sullivan and Jonell Efantis • Department of Obstetrics and Gynecology, University of Miami School of Medicine, Jackson Memorial Hospital, Miami, Florida 33139.   Jennifer Marks and Jay Skyler • Department of Medicine, University of Miami School of Medicine, Miami, Florida 33136.   Mary Ann Fletcher • Center for the Biopsychosocial Study of AIDS, Department of Medicine, University of Miami School of Medicine, Miami, Florida 33139.

Living and Dying with AIDS, edited by Paul I. Ahmed, Plenum Press, New York, 1992.

those due to any other risk category (Creenberg et al., 1989; Friedland & Klein, 1987). It has been projected that by the early 1990s, heterosexual transmission will account for 5% of all adult AIDS cases in the United States, and the majority of these will occur in New York and Florida (Friedland & Klein, 1987).

Among the hardest hit by the increasing incidence of heterosexually transmitted HIV-1 cases have been women, who outnumber men in this transmission category by 5:1 (Guinan & Hardy, 1987). Recent accounts report that the incidence of AIDS has increased at a faster pace for women than for any other subgroup of the U.S. population since 1986 (Carpenter, Mayer, Fisher, Desai, & Durand, 1989). Chin (1990) reports that in some countries, AIDS is the leading cause of death for women aged 20–40. In 1988 AIDS accounted for 3% of all deaths in U.S. women 15–44 years of age (Chu, Buehler, & Berkelman, 1990). According to recent figures, the number of women diagnosed with HIV-1 infections climbed by 45% during 1989 and the rate of HIV-1 seropositivity in teens is doubling each year (Boyer & Schafer, 1990). One study found that women with HIV infection progress in disease three times faster than sociodemographically similar men (Brown & Rundell, 1990). Moreover, the survival time (from time of AIDS diagnosis to death) for women is typically half that of men in general and 1/10 that of the population that has previously garnered the most research attention—white gay men. The shorter survival times among women may be due to the hesitation of physicians to diagnose them with AIDS, as little is known about the unique array of HIV-1-related signs and symptoms that may emerge in this group. In New York City AIDS is the leading cause of death in women aged 25–34 (Chu et al., 1990), and according to a Centers for Disease Control (CDC) report released in June, 1990 at the Sixth International Conference on AIDS, nationwide, over 31% of the 13,600 female AIDS cases appear to have contracted HIV-1 through heterosexual intercourse. In greater metropolitan Miami (Dade County) women comprise 15% of AIDS cases and most of these can be attributed to IV drug use (IVDU) or heterosexual transmission from IVDU or bisexual male partners. Female AIDS cases studied in the Miami area (as well as those in New York and Los Angeles) have a poorer prognosis than their male counterparts (Fischl et al., 1987), though these latter findings have not been supported at all centers (Carpenter et al., 1989). This disparity may be due, in part, to the varying sociodemographic profiles of the samples studied, with lower postdiagnosis survival times noted in the lower socioeconomic status (SES) populations sampled (Fischl et al., 1987). Overall, women comprise approximately 10% of all AIDS cases (Chu et al., 1990), and by 1991, AIDS is expected to be among the top five causes of death among child-bearing women with new cases numbering 7200 in that year (Peterman, Cates, & Curran, 1988), and cumulative figures set at 22,000–30,000 (Chu et al., 1990; Bell, 1989; Ellerbrock, Chamberland, Bush, & Rogers, 1989; Mays & Cochran, 1988). Women who acquired AIDS via heterosexual contact with risk-index men increased from

14.8% to 25.6% from 1983–1988 (Chamberland, Conley, & Buehler, 1989). As of January 1989, the majority of heterosexually transmitted cases of AIDS continued to be female (75%) and blacks or Hispanics (70%) (Chamberland *et al.,* 1989; Lehman, Smith, Mikl, & Morse, 1989). Moreover, female AIDS cases tend to be significantly younger than nonhomosexual male cases, with an especially high incidence in the 20- to 29-year-old age group (Guinan & Hardy, 1987). Analysis of CDC female AIDS cases greater than 13 years of age from 1981 to 1989 showed that 85% were of reproductive age (15–44 years old) and 52% were black (Ellerbrock *et al.,* 1989). Black women had a cumulative incidence 12 times that of white women (Ellerbrock *et al.,* 1989). The age-adjusted death rate for HIV/AIDS in black women increased from 4.4/100,000 in 1986 to 10.3/100,000 in 1988 alone (Chu *et al.,* 1990). In 1988, the death rate from AIDS in black women in the 15–44 year age range was nine times the death rate for comparably aged white women (Chu *et al.,* 1990). In New Jersey, from 1981 to 1988, the relative risk of AIDS was 12.4 in blacks versus whites (Williams, Coye, & Ryan, 1989). It is apparent that the greatest increases in AIDS cases among women will occur in geographical regions characterized by high densities of drug abusers and young, low-SES minority populations (Friedland & Klein, 1987). Florida appears to be one such geographical region—claiming the third highest number of female AIDS cases nationwide (Guinan & Hardy, 1987) and the fourth highest age-adjusted AIDS death rate in the U.S. (Chu *et al.,* 1990). Of the heterosexually transmitted AIDS cases in Florida, the percentage of U.S.-born cases increased from 0.6% to 3.5% overall and jumped from 6.0% to 18.0% among female cases attributable to heterosexual transmission from 1980 to 1988 (Withum *et al.,* 1989). The majority of these women (69%) were black Americans, and 61% of the cases involved partners of intravenous drug abusers (IVDAs) (Holzman, Brandenburg, Sims, & Witte, 1989). Of all Florida regions, the greater Miami area has reported, far and away, the greatest number of AIDS cases among women of childbearing age (Withum *et al.,* 1989).

Although a great deal of effort has been expended to document the incidence and prevalence of AIDS cases, it could be argued that the determination of HIV-1 seroprevalence rates may be more useful in predicting future AIDS cases and identifying groups that might benefit from primary (e.g., at-risk populations) and secondary prevention (e.g., infected populations) interventions. It is estimated that as many as 1.5 million people may be HIV-1 seropositive (HIV+) in the United States (Quinn *et al.,* 1988). Heterosexual transmission is the leading route of HIV infection worldwide and is rapidly increasing in the United States, the first case being reported as early as 1983 (Friedland & Klein, 1987). Although there is evidence for bidirectional transmission of HIV-1 between heterosexuals (Calabrese & Gopalakrishna, 1986; Redfield *et al.,* 1985), the proportion of women infected via heterosexual transmission (72%) is much higher than the

50 MICHAEL H. ANTONI *et al.*

proportion of heterosexually infected men (29%) (Redfield *et al.*, 1985). This finding is supported by more recent work (Padian, Shiboski, & Jewell, 1990).

One study at our center noted that among HIV+ pregnant women screened in an obstetrics clinic, 76% appear to have contracted the virus heterosexually (Gloeb, O'Sullivan, & Efantis, 1988). Between 1982 and 1986, the prevalence of female HIV+ cases attributable to heterosexual transmission more than doubled (12% to 26%) (Guinan & Hardy, 1987), and recent reports note that women now account for greater than 10% of cases in the United States (Carpenter *et al.*, 1989). Given the importance of IV drug abuse in viral transmission (Quinn *et al.*, 1988), directly and indirectly in the seroprevalence of women, it is not surprising that HIV+ women comprise a younger subset of the general population than HIV+ male homosexuals. Sexually transmitted disease (STD) clinic data showed that 62% of HIV+ female cases are less than 25 years of age (Quinn *et al.*, 1988).

In a study of opportunistic infections (OIs) among female AIDS cases, Carpenter *et al.* (1989) noted that viral infections were among the most common OIs (83.3%) and caused the more serious sequelae. The most commonly noted infections among these were genital herpes simplex virus (HSV) and human papillomavirus (HPV), each occurring in 33% of cases studied (Carpenter *et al.*, 1989). Sexually transmitted gynecological disease (gonorrhea, syphilis, genital herpes) and abnormal Pap smears are commonly noted in black, inner-city women attending HIV clinics (Anderson *et al.*, 1989). A history of HPV-associated genital warts, perhaps the most common STD in society at large, has been shown independently to predict seropositivity among females, giving rise to the speculation that genitourinary (GU) disorders that disrupt epithelial (e.g., cervical) surfaces may enhance the risk of HIV-1 transmission (Quinn *et al.*, 1988). HIV-1 positivity has also been associated with genital HSV as well as HPV infections (Carpenter *et al.*, 1989) and syphilis (Quinn *et al.*, 1990). Since HPV-associated genital warts regressed as a function of zidovudine therapy that increased T4 lymphocyte counts (Onorato, Peterson, Pappaioanou, & Dondero, 1989), it appears likely that the proliferation of HPV infection can occur as a function of the immunosuppressed state of the host. This suggests that GU-associated pathology may follow (i.e., as OIs) as well as precede (i.e., as cofactor) HIV-1 infection, an issue that deserves further study.

As in the case of AIDS, women at greatest risk for HIV-1 infection include poor urban minority members (Mays & Cochran, 1988). Across multiple sampling periods from 1986 to 1988, public STD clinics have reported reliable increases in HIV+ rates among heterosexual blacks (Handsfield, Sohlberg, Hopkins, & Harris, 1989). In a study of 10,161 women attending prenatal and family planning clinics across eight geographic areas, the highest seroprevalence rates were noted among blacks and for the 25- to 29-year-old age group (Sweeny, Allen, & Onorato, 1989). However one study of white middle-class women in

New York City found a seroprevalence rate of 22%, the primary route of infection being through heterosexual contact with IVDUs (Glaser, Strange, & Rosati, 1989). In the state of Florida for the period of July through December 1988, 306 new HIV+ cases were identified among women of childbearing age, of whom 225 were nonwhite. Dade County (including Miami) showed the highest seroprevalence in this study. Perhaps more importantly, in this study, it was estimated that 1,000 HIV+ women in Florida will give birth in 1989 (Withum *et al.,* 1989).

The significant rate (20–50%) of perinatal transmission noted among seropositive women in various studies has prompted a major seroprevalence study at our center. Based on data from the population of women served by our obstetrics and gynecology clinics, the incidence of AIDS cases in women has increased steadily since 1983; during the past 1.5 years, the majority of this increase has been accounted for by IV drug abuse and heterosexual transmission. Our seroprevalence data have also suggested that among pregnant women delivering in our obstetrics clinics, there is an overall prevalence of 2.1%, and 91.2% of these women are black, predominantly Americans or Haitians. In fact, black Americans showed a 3.2% seroprevalence rate—a proportion that was 8 times greater than the rate for white Americans (O'Sullivan *et al.,* 1989). Similar to national statistics (Quinn *et al.,* 1988), 66% of these seropositive black Americans were less than 25 years of age, with a large proportion of these women being cocaine and/or crack abusers. These data suggest that our Miami medical facility should be considered an epicenter that is especially relevant for heterosexually and perinatally transmitted cases of HIV-1 infection and AIDS due to the high density of young, low-SES, pregnant black American women served by our obstetrics clinic. Additionally, the large number of nonpregnant women at risk for being or actually seropositive served by our gynecology clinics (comprising a similar demographic profile as the pregnant at-risk or infected groups) emphasizes the need for studying these populations in such metropolitan areas.

There are several reasons to study the phenomenon of heterosexually transmitted HIV-1 infection among black American women in urban epicenters such as Miami, and some of these have been reviewed in the literature (Bell, 1989; Mays & Cochran, 1987, 1988). Among these reasons are:

1. The accelerating incidence of AIDS and HIV-1 infection among women who are members of ethnic minority groups including blacks and Hispanics, a substantial number of whom have multiple partners (Efantis *et al.,* 1989) or partners who are IVDAs, thereby facilitating multiple transmission routes and recipients.
2. The relatively unknown natural history of HIV-1 infection in women, including opportunistic infections (OIs) that may be unique to women, as well as the role of sexually transmitted GU infections as cofactors in HIV-1 disease progression.

3. The need to study female host factors that determine perinatal transmission and other pregnancy outcomes among pregnant minority women with documented high seroprevalence rates;

4. The potential role of unique female phenomena (e.g., pregnancy-related and postpartum changes in immunological and endocrine functioning) that may impact the rate and nature of HIV-1 disease progression. Some have speculated that the "gender-specific likelihood" of infection with potential OI pathogens may be related to certain anatomic, biochemical, or neuroendocrine differences that exist between men and women (Carpenter *et al.*, 1989). The latter two gender differences may become more or less pronounced during pregnancy and postpartum periods.

5. The unknown role of psychosocial stressors (which are prevalent in this population) on host physiological factors (immunological and endocrine functioning) that might affect disease progression and perinatal transmission.

6. The fact that the target population lacks organized support and information-providing networks (that other HIV-infected groups—e.g., homosexual males—have benefited from) to aid in necessary behavior change and coping skills acquisition mandated by knowledge of HIV-1 seropositivity.

Awareness of the alarming epidemiological shifts in seroprevalence along with multiple unknowns in the female AIDS picture have already begun to impact federal funding priorities. One avenue of research that is likely in this emerging trend is psychoneuroimmunology.

ROLE OF PSYCHONEUROIMMUNOLOGY IN HIV-1 INFECTION

A unique feature of HIV-1 infection is that it can have an asymptomatic phase that may last as long as 10–15 years (Munoz *et al.*, 1988). During the asymptomatic phase the individual is capable of transmitting this disease (Stevens, Taylor, & Zang, 1986), and immune functioning is compromised (Fletcher *et al.*, 1988). Because the individual infected with HIV-1 typically goes through several stages of progressive quantitative and qualitative decrements in immunological functioning that may be associated with disease progression over an extended period of time, the HIV-1 syndrome should be viewed as a chronic disease. As HIV-1 disease progresses, a loss in overall immunocompetence leaves infected individuals susceptible to OIs, which most commonly include *Pneumocystis carinii* pneumonia, cryptococcal meningitis, and toxoplasmosis-related meningoencephalitis, candidal esophagitis, and herpes simplex encephalitis (Kaplan, Wofsky, & Volberding, 1987).

The relationships among behavior, immunological functioning, and HIV-1 disease progression are not yet understood, but there is reason to believe that such relationships may exist. First, there is a substantial body of literature relating natural (Glaser *et al.*, 1987; Irwin, Daniels, & Bloom, 1987; Jemmott & Locke, 1984; Kiecolt-Glaser *et al.*, 1987; Kiecolt-Glaser & Glaser, 1988; Patterson, Grant, & McClurg, 1986) and experimentally induced stressors (Borysenko & Borysenko, 1982; Monjan & Collector, 1977; Shavit & Martin, 1987) to changes in immune function. Second, individual differences in psychological variables such as mental depression (Calabrese, Skwerer, & Barna, 1986; Kiecolt-Glaser, Garner, *et al.*, 1984; Schleifer, Keller, Siris, Davis, & Stein, 1985), perceived loss of control, and feelings of helplessness (Baum, McKinnon, & Silva, 1987; Rodin, 1988) have been associated with impaired immune functioning. Third, suggestive evidence is beginning to accumulate associating psychosocial stress with the progression of HIV-1 infection (Coates, Temoshok, & Mandel, 1984; Donlou, Wolcott, Gottlieb, & Landsverk, 1985; Solomon & Temoshok, 1987), and putative mechanisms have been suggested to explain these associations, including stressor-triggered activation of latent HIV-1—a process not unlike that described for stressor effects on other viruses such as HSV and Epstein–Barr virus (Glaser & Kiecolt-Glaser, 1987; Solomon, 1987). Fourth, we have observed that both the anticipation and the impact of being told their HIV-1 antibody status influences immune function in seronegative gay males (Ironson *et al.*, 1988). Fifth, we have seen evidence of immune enhancement in HIV-1 seronegative and seropositive individuals who have undergone either a 10-week aerobic exercise training program (LaPerriere *et al.*, 1990) or a psychosocial stress management (including relaxation training) protocol (Antoni, Fletcher, LaPerriere, Schneiderman, & Ironson, 1989). In view of the current status of psychoneuroimmunological research, there is reason to raise the possibility that behavioral factors may influence immune function in victims of HIV-1 disease and that behavioral interventions (e.g., aerobic exercise, relaxation training) may provide some benefit especially during the early stages of this chronic disease.

Stress Hormones, Immune Function, and HIV-1

What mechanisms might explain the relationship between psychosocial stressors and immune system changes? The exact functional relationships between behavior and immune function are as yet unknown. However, relationships between various neurohormones and immune function have been sufficiently established to permit the advancement of hypotheses relating psychosocial variables on the one hand and immunomodulation on the other. An individual's perception of a stressor and the availability or unavailability of a coping response to that stressor may trigger a series of physiological events leading to specific autonomic nervous system (ANS), neuroendocrine, and neuropeptide changes

(McCabe & Schneiderman, 1985). The sympathoadrenomedullary (SAM) system, activated during "active coping" responses, releases norepinephrine (NE) and epinephrine (E), which prepare the organism for stressor confrontation. Another physiological pattern appears to be dominant when coping responses are unavailable (hypervigilance, lack of adequate coping resources, and conservation–withdrawal), and may be characterized by behavioral inhibition and activation of the hypothalamic–pituitary adrenocortical system (HPAC). Activation of the HPAC system is associated with adrenocorticotropin hormone (ACTH) and cortisol release following signaling by corticotropin-releasing hormone (CRH) (McCabe & Schneiderman, 1985). Preliminary findings suggest that elevations in CRH, ACTH, cortisol, NE, and E may be accompanied by decrements in immune function. Corticotropin-releasing hormone has been shown to inhibit human natural killer (NK) cell cytotoxic activity and may do so by stimulating cyclic AMP (cAMP) in large granular lymphocytes (Pawlikowski, Zelazowski, Dohler, & Stepien, 1988). This finding is significant in that CRH release from the parvocellular subdivision of the paraventricular nucleus of the hypothalamus is the initiation step in HPAC activation (McCabe & Schneiderman, 1985). Downstream HPAC products (i.e., ACTH, cortisol) appear to be important as well.

Organisms subjected to uncontrollable stressors have displayed such immune system decrements as thymic involution (Selye, 1976), decreased helper/suppressor (T4/T8) cell ratios (Teshima *et al.,* 1987), suppressed lymphocyte proliferative responses (Laudenslager, Ryan, Drugan, Hyson, & Maier, 1983), and impairments in NK cell cytotoxicity (Shavit & Martin, 1987; Shavit, Lewis, Terman, Gale, & Liebeskind, 1984). Regarding physiological mediation of these findings, ACTH, plasma corticosteroid, and peripheral catecholamine elevations have been associated with both uncontrollable stressors (Mason, 1975; McCabe & Schneiderman, 1985) and immunomodulation (Antoni *et al.,* 1990a). Physiological doses of ACTH impair the responsiveness of T lymphocytes to antigenic (CD3 antibody) and mitogenic (concanavalin-A [Con-A]) stimuli and may do so via ACTH receptors on lymphocytes (Kavelaars, Ballieux, & Heijnen, 1988). Corticosteroids have been shown to decrease T-cell subpopulation number (Cupps & Fauci, 1982), production of several macrophage-regulating cytokines (Duncan, Sadlik, & Hadden, 1982), macrophage tumoricidal function (Pavlidis & Chirigos, 1980), NK cell cytotoxicity (Levy, Herberman, Lippman, & d'Angelo, 1987), cytokine production in response to phytohemagglutinin (PHA) (Hahn, Levin, & Handzel, 1976), and gamma interferon (γ-IFN) production (Stites, Stobo, Fudenberg, & Wells, 1982). Elevations in peripheral catecholamines have been associated with decreases in mouse and human NK cell cytotoxicity and decreased T-lymphocyte proliferative responses to mitogen—these effects potentially mediated by increases in intracellular cAMP levels (Plaut, 1987) secondary to activation of lymphocyte adrenergic receptors (Felten, Felten, Carlson, Olschawka,

& Livnat, 1985; Hadden, 1987; Livnat, Felten, Carlson, Bellinger, & Felten, 1985) by agents such as epinephrine. Human work has indicated that leukocyte number and lymphocyte proliferative responses are decreased following epinephrine infusion (Crary *et al.,* 1983; Livnat *et al.,* 1985). In sum, evidence exists for immunomodulatory effects of ANS and neuroendocrine elevations that may accompany periods of uncontrollable chronic stress.

Recent studies have related neurohormones as well as neuropeptides to HIV-1 disease. One study, for example, noted that the ability of HIV-1 to infect normal human lymphocytes is enhanced by supplementing the cell culture medium with corticosteroids (Markham, Salahuddin, Veren, Orndorff, & Gallo, 1986). This study suggests that adrenal stress hormones may affect the susceptibility of high-risk hosts to seroconversion following viral inoculation. Viral susceptibility may be related to the efficacy of lymphocyte or NK cell cytotoxic abilities, which may be compromised by glucocorticoid secretions during stress. In a second study, preliminary findings suggested that another stress-associated hormone, met-enkephalin, enhanced T-cell populations in AIDS patients with Kaposi's sarcoma (Plotnikoff, Wybran, Nimeh, & Miller, 1986). In a third study of seven AIDS-related complex (ARC) patients treated with met-enkephalin 3 times per week for 21 days, the following immunological changes occurred across the 3-week period: increases in OKT3, OKT4 (equivalent to CD4 or helper cell) number, NK cell cytotoxicity, interleukin-II (IL-II) production, and PHA mitogen response (Wybran *et al.,* 1987). These investigators have also noted impressive improvements in mitogen responses and regression of Kaposi's sarcoma lesions in AIDS patients treated with met-enkephalin (Wybran *et al.,* 1987). Many of these investigators have speculated that substances such as β-endorphin, β-lipotropin, and met-enkephalin may affect immune functioning (e.g., mitogen responsivity, NK cell activity) via changes in calcium uptake by immune cells (Sibinga & Goldstein, 1988), increases in IL-II receptor expression and production by lymphocytes (Plotnikoff *et al.,* 1986), and/or increases in other lymphokines such as γ-IFN (Brown & VanEpps, 1986) and leukocyte migration inhibitory factor (Sibinga & Goldstein, 1988). Further, increases in IL-II production, a noted effect of met-enkephalin administration, have been associated with increases in lymphocyte cGMP level, activation of protein kinase C, and consequent inhibition of adenylate cyclase, enhanced calcium mobilization, and facilitation of lymphocyte mitogen responsivity (Hadden, 1987). All of this work must be viewed, however, as preliminary, considering the small sample sizes and lack of replication across laboratories. These caveats notwithstanding, preliminary neuroimmunological findings do suggest several mechanisms by which psychosocial phenomena might impact immune status. Of course, any psychosocial phenomenon that is proposed as an immunomodulator would therefore need to be related to both neuroendocrine/neuropeptide as well as immunological alterations.

Psychosocial Stressors, Immune Function, and HIV-1

Several behavioral variables have been associated with both neuroendocrine changes and altered immune functioning. Animals subjected to uncontrollable stressors, for instance, have been noted to display elevated plasma corticosteroids and depleted brain NE levels (McCabe & Schneiderman, 1985; Pericic, Manev, Boranic, Poljak-Blazi, & Lakic, 1987) and increased peripheral catecholamine release (Mason, 1975), as well as the immune system decrements noted previously. Research involving naturally occurring uncontrollable stressors, in human subjects, has identified some parallels to the animal findings noted above. The experience of chronic environmental stressors characterized by a loss of personal control (e.g., being a resident of Three Mile Island during the nuclear reactor accident) among normal healthy subjects was accompanied by increased symptoms of psychological distress (e.g., anxiety, depression); elevations in urinary catecholamine levels; and decreases in total T-lymphocyte, macrophage, and CD4+ cell counts (Baum *et al.*, 1987).

Social stressors have been associated with elevations in stress hormone levels and impaired immune functioning in the animal and human literature. Social stressors most commonly associated with glucocorticoid elevations and cellular immunomodulation (NK cell activity and lymphocyte responses to PHA and/ or Con-A mitogens) in human work include loneliness (Kiecolt-Glaser, Ricker, *et al.*, 1984), marital disruption (Kiecolt-Glaser *et al.*, 1987), poor social support networks (Levy *et al.*, 1987; Levy, Herberman, Maluish, Schlien, & Lippmann, 1985), and bereavement (Irwin, Daniels, & Weiner, 1987; Calabrese, Kling, & Gold, 1987; Kosten, Jacobs, & Mason, 1984). Regarding physiological mediation, it is noteworthy that 24-hr urinary catecholamine excretions of NE and E are elevated in bereaved subjects and in subjects threatened with a loss as compared to normals (Jacobs *et al.*, 1986). Other recent work has noted that a high stress level, increased depressive symptoms, dissatisfaction with social support, and limited use of adaptive coping strategies predicted decreased CD4+ cell number and increased CD8+ cell number among elderly women (McNaughton, Patterson, & Grant, 1988).

Clinical depression or depressed affect have been linked with impaired cellular immune functioning in numerous studies. Patients with major depressive disorder showed decreased PHA and Con-A responses (Calabrese *et al.*, 1986; Kronfol, 1983; Schleifer *et al.*, 1985) as well as lowered percentages of helper T lymphocytes (Krueger, Levy, & Cathcart, 1984). Severity of depressive symptomatology has also been associated with diminished Con-A and PHA responses in HIV-infected males (Monjan, 1987) and decreased NK cell activity in medical students (Kiecolt-Glaser, Garner, *et al.*, 1984) and bereaved spouses (Irwin, Daniels, Bloom, & Weiner, 1986). Furthermore, depressive symptoms were predictive of decrements in NK cell activity among women when measured before and after the death of their husbands (Irwin, Daniels, Smith, Bloom, & Weiner, 1987).

The model for stressor-related immunomodulatory effects that is implicit in our studies of HIV-1 involves a synthesis of the findings outlined in the two preceding sections ("Stress Hormones, Immune Function, and HIV-1; Psychosocial Stressors, Immune Function, and HIV-1"). According to this framework, stressors that decrease the host's sense of control (e.g., learning of HIV-1 seropositivity in self or offspring, bereavement) may lead to a cascade of psychosocial, neuroendocrine, and immunological events that may accelerate HIV-1 disease progression. The specifics of this model have been outlined elsewhere (Antoni *et al.*, 1990a).

PSYCHOSOCIAL STRESSORS PREVALENT IN AT-RISK AND HIV-INFECTED WOMEN

As mentioned previously, at-risk and infected women are disproportionately represented among minority populations, especially blacks. Young, black American, low-SES women have been characterized as a group experiencing multiple *chronic* psychosocial stressors (Freudenberg, Lee, & Silver, 1989; Mays & Cochran, 1987, 1988). These include chronic financial hassles, drug and alcohol dependency, poor social networks, medical problems, and a general feeling of helplessness and powerlessness. These stressors may interact to aggravate a perceived loss of control resulting in the previously mentioned affective, neuroendocrine, and immunological changes (Antoni *et al.*, 1990a).

HIV-1 seropositive and at-risk seronegative pregnant and nonpregnant subjects are also likely to experience several *acute* stressors, some of which have been shown in our previous work to have effects on affective and immunological functioning (Ironson *et al.*, 1990). These acute stressors include (1) anticipation and initial impact of HIV-1 antibody test results, (2) adjustment to diagnosis and decision to continue pregnancy to term (among pregnant HIV+ women) and decision to alter risk behaviors, (3) pregnancy-associated stressors (psychological and physiological), (4) postpartum stressors (psychological and physiological), and (5) day-to-day interpersonal relationship issues.

Anticipation, Impact, and Adjustment to Serostatus

We have data that suggest that immunological and affective changes occur during the one-month periods preceding and following serostatus notification in gay males (Antoni *et al.*, 1990b; Ironson *et al.*, 1990). It is reasonable to propose that similar decrements in immunological and psychological functioning may occur in female populations, though environmental and constitutional factors unique to the samples are likely to influence these outcome variables as well. In the period following notification, for instance, seropositive pregnant women are faced with several stressors, including decisions to terminate pregnancy and to inform partners and significant others of serostatus. For seropositive nonpregnant subjects, the demand for reductions in sexual risk behaviors (which might compromise financial and social status) as well as addiction-related (e.g., immunosuppressive substance abuse) behaviors may present multiple, formidable stressors that must be dealt with at the same time as these individuals are adjusting to a life-threatening diagnosis and caring for a "fatherless" family. Seronegative subjects are also faced with a multitude of behavior-change demands for which they may lack the necessary coping skills or social support.

Pregnancy-Associated Stressors

Pregnancy-associated *psychological* stressors (following the decision to deliver) include the psychological/affective burden of pregnancy and labor *per se,* and the uncertainty of perinatal transmission outcome. Pregnancy-associated *physiological* stressors/changes include alterations in endocrine factors (e.g., increases in cortisol-binding globulin [CBG] and thyroid-binding globulin [TBG]), which partly explain the elevations in cortisol, triiodothyhyronine (T3), and thyroxine (T4) often found during pregnancy (Casey, MacDonald, & Simpson, 1985). The effects of endocrine function on HIV-1 disease course in pregnant and postpartum women may therefore be unique and at present are unknown. Since it has recently been documented that increases in TBG may be found early in the course of HIV-1 infection (Lopresti, Fried, Spencer, & Nicoloff, 1989), one might speculate that HIV-related increases in CBG, for example, may also occur and exaggerate the expected pregnancy-related increase in cortisol. If some subtle adrenal dysfunction occurs related to the HIV infection, there may be a greater increase in ACTH levels than is usually observed as well as lower-than-usual stimulated cortisol and aldosterone levels.

Immunological function is also impaired during pregnancy (e.g., decreased NK cell cytotoxicity to K562 tumor target cells [Bailey & Schacter, 1985; Okamura, Fuurukawa, Nakakuki, Yamadak, & Susuki, 1987] as well as to HSV-infected targets [Gonik, Lee, West, & Kohl, 1987]). Such physiological changes during pregnancy have also been hypothesized to account for the increased incidence and progression of viral infections, such as genital HSV (Brown *et cl.,* 1985; Young, Killam, & Green, 1976), cytomegalovirus (CMV) (Woodward, Thomlinson, & Hambling, 1987), and other GU infections (MacDonald *et al.,* 1983), as well as an increased progression rate of HIV-1 infection (Castelli *et al.,* 1989; Deschamps, Pape, Madharan, & Johnson, 1989; Romaquera *et al.,* 1989), all of which may increase the risk of birth complications (Brown, Berry, & Vontver, 1986; Bujko, Sulovic, & Dotlic, 1986; Minkoff, 1987; Robb, Benirescke, &

Barmeyer, 1986). Moreover, women who are chronically immunosuppressed (e.g., renal transplant recipients on immunosuppressive regimens) are believed to be at compounded risk for further immunodeficiency and GU viral infections such as CMV and HSV during pregnancy (Gaudier, Delpin, Rivera, & Gonzales, 1988). It could be reasoned that women who are HIV-1 seropositive, representing a chronically immunosuppressed population, might also be at heightened risk for such sequelae during pregnancy.

Recent work has noted that a majority of pregnant women who are HIV-1 seropositive experience decreases in helper cell (CD4+) counts of greater than 40% during pregnancy (Schafer, Friedman, & Schwarthlander, 1989). One study of seropositive and -negative pregnant women found that seronegatives displayed a decrease in CD4+ counts at 8 weeks before delivery but returned to normal levels in the postpartum period. In contrast, seropositive women in this study had a larger drop in CD4+ cell number during pregnancy and showed no recovery during a 12-month postpartum period (Biggar *et al.,* 1989). Some of the work in our medical center has revealed a high frequency (33–39.5%) of GU infections (e.g., urinary tract infections, HSV, syphilis), HPV and cervical intraepithelial neoplasia (CIN), and birth complications (e.g., preterm labor) among pregnant HIV+ women (Gloeb *et al.,* 1988; Gloeb *et al.,* 1989). GU infections have been associated with preterm labor either directly through chorioamparamitis or indirectly, by stimulation of contractions secondary to increased production of tumor necrosis factor and interleukins that stimulate prostaglandin production (Gloeb *et al.,* 1988).

In our ongoing natural history study as well as in a review of Pap smears at our clinical facility, it is clear that HPV is common in HIV-infected women as are abnormal Pap smears (Gloeb *et al.,* 1988). Consistent evidence for viral initiation of CIN has been found for HPV, which is commonly associated with the transformation to squamous cell carcinoma of the cervix (Crum, Ikenburg, Richart, & Gissman, 1984; Macnab, Walkinshaw, Cordiner, & Clementz, 1986). Interestingly, the number of cases of cervical dysplasia and carcinoma *in situ* has rapidly increased over the past 15 years (Kaufman & Adams, 1986). Oncologists attribute this increase primarily to the increased incidence of HPV, types 16 and 18. Several studies have demonstrated that condyloma of the cervix (HPV lesions) often coexist with dysplasia, and these lesions, many of which contain HPV subtype 16 or 18, have at least a 30% incidence of malignant transformation (Crum *et al.,* 1984; Kaufman & Adams, 1986; Macnab *et al.,* 1986; Nelson, Averette, & Richart, 1984). For instance, HPV particles, antigens, and nucleic acids have been demonstrated in cervical dysplasia, and papillomavirus DNA has been identified in cervical carcinomas as well (Crum *et al.,* 1984; Penn, 1982, 1986; Shelley & Wood, 1981).

Recent work has identified abnormalities in cellular immunity accompanying advancing levels of cervical neoplasia. One line of evidence that suggests that CIN may be an immune-mediated phenomenon is the often-noted increased incidence of cervical carcinoma among immunosuppressed populations (Penn, 1986). It is believed by some that various types of HPV may have been the oncogenic virus that predisposes renal transplant hosts to experience a field effect (i.e., cervical carcinoma) when they are immunosuppressed (Penn, 1982, 1986). Others have noted a higher likelihood of malignant transformation of HPV to CIN among immunosuppressed women (Shokri-Tobibzadeh, Koss, Molnar, & Romney, 1981; Sillman et al., 1984). Recent work suggests that promotion of HPV to CIN and cervical carcinoma may be at least partially dependent upon depression in specific T-cell subpopulations (e.g., decreased OKT4/OKT8 ratio) (Castello et al., 1986), changes in cell-mediated immunity (Levy et al., 1978), decreased T-lymphocyte number and reactivity (Bashford & Gough, 1983; Catalona, Sample, & Chretien, 1973; Sawanobori, Ashman, Nahmias, Benigno, & LaVia, 1977), and a significantly greater degree of leukocyte migration inhibition indicating changes in lymphokine (leukocyte migration inhibition factor) secretion by T cells (Goldstein, Shore, & Gusberg, 1971; Rivera et al., 1979).

Cervical intraepithelial neoplasia is defined by three phases: CIN I, CIN II, and CIN III. Mild and moderate phases (CIN I and II), involve undifferentiated cells limited to less than 75% of the cervical thickness, while severe dysplasia (CIN III) involves undifferentiated cells permeating from 75% to the entire cervical epithelium. The stepwise, well-defined progression of cervical dysplasia renders it amenable to research investigating the concomitant factors (i.e., psychosocial variables) associated with the initiation and promotion of HIV-1 disease. Lymphomas and Kaposi's sarcoma are part of the AIDS picture and represent traditional opportunistic neoplasias in this syndrome. Cervical neoplasias may join the list of such malignancies that identify those individuals infected with HIV-1 as having AIDS or as candidates for imminent progression to AIDS due to the documented immunosuppression and HPV infections (as potential co-factors of HIV progression) that are probable criteria for the manifestation of CIN. Cervical neoplasia may be an especially pertinent pathophysiological phenomenon from which to identify psychoimmunological influences because promotion from viral infection to early CIN, and finally to invasive carcinoma, appears to be associated with both immunosuppressed states and psychosocial stressors (Antoni & Goodkin, 1988, 1989). A key goal of our future work will be to determine how multiple factors (endocrine, immunological, psychosocial, and gynecologic) contribute and interact in predicting HIV-1 disease progression, perinatal transmission, and birth complications among pregnant seropositive women.

Postpartum-Associated Stressors

A final set of acute stressors that are relevant for HIV-infected and at-risk women comprise those associated with the postpartum period. These include decisions regarding changes in risk behavior, the impact of learning the HIV-1 serostatus of their offspring, and the added responsibilities of caring for a potentially ill child. All of these stressors will be experienced during a period (postpartum) associated with maternal affective instability/lability that might exacerbate stress responses, feelings of helplessness, and perceived loss of control. These subjects may be unable to muster coping strategies and social resources necessary to resolve these stressors and might instead turn to maladaptive strategies such as drug abuse and sexual acting-out that may consequently lead to abandonment of risk reduction attempts, increased likelihood of heterosexual transmission, and possible accelerated disease progression.

Interpersonal Relationship Issues

As Mays and Cochran (1988) have noted, those behaviors that are central to HIV-1 transmission are interpersonal ones. Consequently, reduction in risk behaviors associated with transmission requires consideration and alteration of interpersonal relationships among at-risk and infected mothers. At least four sets of maternal interpersonal relationships are salient in this regard, and these can be classified as mother–child, mother–sexual partner, mother–health care provider, and the mother's relationship to other members of society.

Among issues relevant to the mother–child relationship are the decision to abort or continue pregnancy to term, fears of becoming too ill to care or provide for offspring, and preparing the older children for life as orphans. For instance, HIV-1 seropositive pregnant women who decide to deliver must face a 20–35% risk of perinatal HIV-1 transmission if this is their first child since becoming infected and as high as a 50% risk if they have already delivered an infected child (Scott, 1989). Indeed, the prevalence of second pregnancies following the delivery of a seropositive child are higher than one might suspect, and this is likely tied to the sociocultural value of childbirth among ethnic minority members (Mays & Cochran, 1988). Understanding the perceived benefits of childbearing among disadvantaged adolescents and young women is critical in predicting decisions to terminate pregnancy and to engage in non-impregnation-focused "safer sex" behaviors. These perceived benefits range from escape from an abusive parental household, obtaining financial independence, and becoming part of a social support group consisting of other young mothers, to a more idealistic belief in increasing the survival of one's ethnic group. According to Mays & Cochran (1988), the desire to leave behind a legacy may play a role in the choices made by some pregnant seropositive women.

Regarding the interpersonal issues related to the mother–sexual partner relationship, the serostatus of the partner is an important consideration. Seropositive mothers with uninfected partners are likely to face rejection by the father of their children, resulting in emotional and financial isolation at a time when they are most in need of support and care. Others must also face the guilt of bringing their child into a fatherless world—blaming themselves for driving away the person who might someday be the child's only guardian. Seropositive mothers may react to an infected partner with self-isolation or attempts at retribution, both of which are likely to leave her and her offspring alone. If both mother and child are seropositive, the lack of emotional and financial support in this scenario would compound their plight.

The mother–health care provider relationship is critical and may be the only means of tangible emotional support that is available to the infected pregnant or postpartum mother. Some have commented, in fact, that the periods immediately preceding and following birth and delivery—in which the woman is dependent to a large degree on the health care system—is the window of opportunity within which providers can educate and intervene in behavior-change efforts (Mays & Cochran, 1988). Additional salient mother–provider issues focus on two questions with which the health care professional may be confronted. First, should physicians treat pregnant seropositive women with retroviral (e.g., AZT) or immunomodulatory (e.g., IL-II) regimens that may have toxic or lethal effects on the fetus? While slowing maternal disease progression, these agents may increase the likelihood of birth complications and infant mortality and play an unknown role in determining the probability of perinatal transmission. Second, can pediatric specialists ethically entrust the care of infected babies to poverty-stricken, drug-addicted, or physically ill mothers? Here the emotional needs of the mother must be weighted against the physical welfare of the child—a decision that health care providers may find themselves ill-equipped to handle.

Finally, the mother–societal relationship is imperative to our understanding of the milieu of women infected with HIV-1. From society's point of view, the mother is a key pathway in the heterosexual chain of HIV infection—providing a perinatal, sexual, and intravenous source of influence on the risk of infectivity in the general population. The role of ethnic, racial, cultural, and religious factors in influencing sexual behavior patterns is well known (Mays & Cochran, 1988), and hence sociocultural influences on risk behavior reduction cannot be ignored. Moreover, these same influences cut to the heart of perceptions of AIDS risk in those populations for whom such risk is highest—ethnic minorities. The risk of AIDS, while acknowledged by most, is only one risk in a hierarchy of multiple risks prevalent in the daily existance of black and Latin seropositive women (Mays & Cochran, 1988). The key to behavior change is where in this list they place the relatively longer-term consequences of AIDS-related risk behavior in relation to the shorter-term consequences of the risks of daily living (e.g., need for shelter, food, and safety). From this vantage point, behavior-change specialists need to be cognizant of more immediate survival needs, which if met, can provide the opportunity for professionals to educate and intervene effectively. Within this deeper understanding of the sociocultural milieu is the knowledge that the pervasive powerlessness experienced by disadvantaged women at risk may lead them to disengage from any attempts at behavioral coping once informed about risk behavior. Social scientists are well advised, then, to develop only the most pragmatic, immediate, and face valid of coping strategies in their education protocols.

To successfully reduce risk behaviors and aid seropositive and at-risk women in coping with infectivity or risk, psychologists will need to focus on the individual perceptions and identities, social support networks, and ethnic and cultural norms (Mays & Cochran, 1988), all of which are "transmitted" via the maternal–societal relationship.

Summary

In sum, there appear to be several roles for psychoneuroimmunologic (PNI) research as related to HIV-infected and at-risk women. First, it is important to document baseline values and longitudinal changes in psychological, neuroendocrine, and immunological functioning that occur among pregnant and non-pregnant women infected with HIV-1 in order to understand the role of pregnancy in the disease course. Second, PNI research should provide mechanistic explanations for how psychological, neuroendocrine, and immunological factors interact in predicting disease progression and future behavior. Third, this approach must incorporate a consideration of individual psychosocial differences among hosts in predicting the effects of environmental stressors (e.g., pregnancy and postpartum-related) on subsequent emotional responses, future behavior, and health outcomes. Fourth, it is important to understand the role of sexually transmitted GU viral infections (e.g., HSV, HPV, CMV) and associated changes (e.g., CIN) as early, covert OI manifestations, and/or as cofactors for HIV-1 disease progression and perinatal transmission, and the degree to which these associations are a function of host psychological, neuroendocrine, and immunological factors. Fifth, it is essential to determine the role of stress and coping processes in risk behavior change and then to design behavioral interventions that reduce both stress responses (i.e., stress management) and risk behavior. In terms of the HIV-1 infected and at-risk female target populations, there appears to be a clear set of behavioral goals and physiological/biomedical goals that might accomplish these mandates. *Behavioral goals* would comprise (1) stress management and attenuation of affective distress, (2) change in risk behavior and decreased future pregnancy rate, and (3) acquisition of coping strategies and social support networks to facilitate (1) and (2). *Physiological/biomedical goals* would include (1) enhancement of immune functioning, (2) normalization of endocrine functioning, (3) decreasing GU pathology, and (4) retardation of HIV-1 disease progression and reduction in perinatal transmission and birth complication rate as facilitated by (1), (2), and perhaps (3).

BEHAVIORAL INTERVENTIONS, RISK BEHAVIOR CHANGE, AND STRESS MANAGEMENT

Central to the accomplishment of the goals noted in the previous section is an understanding that risk behavior reduction and stress management are interdependent. Before providing evidence for this assertion, the theoretical framework and empirical data regarding behavioral interventions that focus on risk reduction or stress management will be reviewed. Most of these approaches appear to share three components: information provision, coping skills training, and enhancement of social/interpersonal functioning.

Risk Behavior Reduction

A key component of risk reduction interventions is the provision of information relating specific behaviors to subsequent health-compromising consequences. Although the bulk of the literature documenting AIDS-related risk behaviors has pertained to homosexual transmission of HIV-1, several sources have suggested that transmission between heterosexuals may be accomplished by similar pathways that share a common feature—exchange of bodily fluids capable of transporting live HIV-1 (Calabrese & Gopalakrishna, 1986; Castro, Lieb, Galisher, Witte, & Jaffe, 1987; Fischl et al., 1987; Kelly & St. Lawrence, 1988; Redfield et al., 1987). An awareness of these and other specific risk behaviors has prompted the assembly of well-defined targets (Kelly & St. Lawrence, 1988; Stall, McKusick, Wiley, Coates, & Ostrow, 1986) and the implementation of behavioral intervention strategies (Coates, Stall, et al., 1987; Kelly & St. Lawrence, 1987a) focusing on the reduction of AIDS-specific risk behaviors among homosexual males. One such program (Kelly & St. Lawrence, 1988) outlined the following targets: encouragement of exclusive relationships; promoting the adoption of safer sex (low-risk) practices; discouraging casual, anonymous, or promiscuous high-risk sexual behavior; and reducing the abuse of chemical substances/intoxicants known to be associated with disinhibition and irresponsible high-risk behavior (Kelly & St. Lawrence, 1988). It is reasonable to suggest that such aims would be relevant for infected and at-risk heterosexual women and that behavioral strategies might achieve these ends.

Empirical support for the efficacy of risk reduction interventions with AIDS populations has begun to accumulate (Coates, Stall, et al., 1987; Kelly & St. Lawrence, 1987b; Siegel, Grodsky, & Herman, 1986). Kelly and St. Lawrence (1988) suggest the following components of risk reduction information provision: (1) provision of information about HIV-1 infection and transmission, (2) identification of high-risk sexual practices, and (3) identification of lower-risk practices. However, these investigators have cautioned that information provision alone may not be sufficient to reliably reduce risk behaviors, especially when such behavior is immediately reinforcing and when aversive consequences of the activity are not immediate (Kelly, St. Lawrence, Brasfield, & Hood, 1987). Previous literature focusing on sexual attitudes and behaviors tends to support this caveat (Lance, 1975; Zuckerman, Tushup, & Finner, 1976). Understanding the limitation of information provision alone and observing the variability in reduction of high-risk sexual behaviors among homosexual men, several investigators have sought to identify host psychological factors that predict the adoption of reduced-risk behaviors (Bartlett, Rabin, Taggart, Bandemer, Bellonti, 1987; McKusick, Horstman, & Coates, 1985; Siegel, Mesagno, Chen, & Christ, 1987; Stall et al., 1986). Overall, these studies suggested that factors which favored the adoption of reduced-risk behaviors include perceived self-efficacy in successfully reducing risk behaviors, having coping strategies for controlling high-risk sexual impulses, and possessing skills for negotiating with interpersonal contacts and social networks (Kelly & St. Lawrence, 1988). Moreover, continued risk behavior was associated with denial of virulence of (and therefore personal susceptibility to) the HIV-1 virus and frequent drug and alcohol use preceding sex (Kelly & St. Lawrence, 1988).

All of the above-noted factors may be especially salient for infected and at-risk minority women (Mays & Cochran, 1988). It is known that black adolescents are poorly informed about contraceptives and use birth control methods inconsistently, even in cases where individuals are knowledgeable about the ability of condoms to reduce HIV-1 transmission risk (Mays & Cochran, 1988). One recent review generated several reasons to explain why ethnic minority women perceive their risk for AIDS to be low (Mays & Cochran, 1988). These reasons include the perception of AIDS risk as low on the hierarchy of other risks of daily living (e.g., shelter, personal safety, safety of children, loss of financial support), their incredulity of risk information provided by "white" and/or male sources, and the fact that denial and downplaying of susceptibility is easier than significant behavior and lifestyle changes. These authors recommend that behavior change in such populations may be enhanced by providing specific interpersonal skills required for change, tailoring interventions to the "cultural realities" of the target population, and utilizing a credible (e.g., female) source for delivery of such information (Mays & Cochran, 1988). Other authors suggest that to raise the priority of AIDS education on the list of daily survival issues facing minority group members, information-provision programs must be embedded in multi-benefit interventions that offer, perhaps, health and child care as well as stress management (Freudenberg et al., 1989).

One successful intervention program, "Project Aires," designed to reduce risk behaviors among homosexual men, has operated from the premise that behavior change can most effectively be realized through a combination of information provision and coping skills training (Kelly & St. Lawrence, 1988). These investigators reported significant decreases in sexual risk behavior and increases in AIDS-risk knowledge and assertiveness among intervention group members as compared to controls (Kelly & St. Lawrence, 1988). Although these findings are impressive, it is important to consider the demographics and socio-cultural milieu of these subjects before generalizing to other populations. Specifically, these subjects were middle-class gay men living in a metropolitan area known for its extensive, well-organized gay support network. In contrast, most at-risk and infected women (e.g., low SES, black American heterosexual females) experience different stressors (as mentioned previously) and possess fewer coping resources (e.g., social support) than the previously studied group. Indeed, others have highlighted the importance of tailoring intervention programs to ethno-graphic qualities and population-specific stressors of target groups (Bartlett *et al.*, 1987; Kelly & St. Lawrence, 1988).

One important issue that has not yet received adequate attention concerns the desirability of risk behavior reduction in women already infected with HIV-1. Although the desirability of having these infected women engage in "safer sex" behaviors is apparent from the standpoint of society, it is unlikely that this will occur unless the women become convinced of the benefit to them. In this respect, it is necessary for women infected with HIV-1 to understand (1) the likelihood of unprotected sex leading to STD infection, (2) the havoc that this is likely to play on an already-compromised immune system, and (3) the consequences that the STD is likely to have in terms of symptoms because of the damage that has already been done to the immune system.

In sum, behavior-change programs need to address the specific behaviors to be changed (i.e., information provision) and other factors as well. These other factors include relevant stressors, cognitive coping processes and pragmatic coping strategies, social/interpersonal resources/skills, and perceived benefits to the target group. Therefore, it is reasonable to posit that behavioral "stress management" interventions that reduce the *affective* impact of stressors (e.g., relaxation training for anxiety reduction), improve *cognitive* coping skills (e.g., cognitive restructuring to decrease irrational, maladaptive thoughts and reactions), and enhance *inter-personal* functioning (e.g., assertiveness training to negotiate safer sex) and *social* support might facilitate behavior change attempts at the same time as "managing" stressors. It is equally important that such interventions provide some tangible benefit to women infected with HIV-1 (e.g., reduced risk of STDs and their sequelae via modifications in risk behavior).

Stress Management

We have operated from a framework that considers the importance of af-fective, cognitive, and social functioning under the umbrella of stress management efforts (Antoni *et al.*, 1988). Accordingly, our previous work with HIV-1 sero-positive and HIV-1 seronegative gay males has incorporated a combination of *anxiety reduction, cognitive skills training, and social/interpersonal skill building* strategies to improve psychological and immune functioning preceding and following subjects' adjustment to serostatus notification.

There is reason to believe that anxiety and its reduction may be important issues to consider in this line of research. Anxiety has been shown to be one of the most common reactions to notification of HIV-1 seropositivity (Coates, Morin, & McKusick, 1987), with reactive adjustment disorders involving anxiety being observed in as many as 75% of those infected (Tross, Hirsch, Rabkin, Berry, & Holland, 1987). Although anxiety need not be destructive, it can be detrimental if it interferes with the individual's daily functioning and contributes to a sense of helplessness and hopelessness (Kelly & St. Lawrence, 1988). Such by-products may engender a perceived loss of control that may subsequently lead to a continuation of maladaptive high-risk behaviors (Kelly & St. Lawrence, 1988), sustained affective distress, and detrimental physiological changes. Anxiety reduction strategies may provide individuals infected with HIV-1 with effective coping skills, help in overcoming preoccupations that compromise daily living, and the opportunity to experience mastery—all of which may enhance a sense of control and self-efficacy (Bandura, 1989; Kelly & St. Lawrence, 1988).

One of the most commonly employed, well-researched, and easily reproduced anxiety reduction techniques is relaxation training, often taking the form of progressive muscle relaxation (Jacobsen, 1938) or relaxing imagery. These procedures are often included in cafeteria-style stress management interventions (Meichenbaum & Jaremko, 1983) and have been useful in several health-related conditions in which anxiety plays a role, such as anticipatory nausea in chemotherapy patients (Burish, Carey, Krozely, & Greco, 1987), essential hypertension (Hoelscher, Lichstein, Fischer, & Hegarty, 1987) and postpartum distress (Halonen & Passman, 1985). The impetus for such investigations has been an increasing knowledge base regarding the effects that psychosocial stressors can have on the physiological mechanisms underlying these problems (McCabe & Schneiderman, 1985; McGrady, Woerner, Bernal, & Higgins, 1987). For example, relaxation training has been associated with significant decreases in urinary and plasma cortisol levels among hypertensives (McGrady *et al.,* 1987). Some work suggests that this form of training may also affect immune functioning.

Anxiety Reduction Techniques

There are two arguments to support the hypothesis that relaxation may have beneficial effects on immune function. First is the evidence that certain stressors can lead to declines in immune markers (Kiecolt-Glaser *et al.,* 1985). If relaxation training leads to a decrease in the perception of stressors and subsequent stress responses, then immune function might be enhanced by such a regimen. Second, plasma catecholamines and corticosteroids, which are released through the activation of the SAM and HPAC systems, may inhibit some immune functions (McCabe & Schneiderman, 1985); thus, relaxation training may indirectly benefit the immune system by decreasing sympathetic nervous system arousal and concommitant release of stress hormones.

In a field study of psychosocial immunomodulators in a geriatric population, residents of independent living facilities were assigned to either relaxation-training, social contact, or no-contact groups (Kiecolt-Glaser *et al.,* 1985). Results indicated that subjects in the relaxation group demonstrated a significant increase in NK cell activity and a significant decrease in HSV antibody titers at the end of the intervention; changes in these factors did not vary for the other groups. Kiecolt-Glaser and her colleagues (1986) also looked at the effects of relaxation training on immune function in a younger population, a group of medical students. This was actually a more rigorous test of the effectiveness of this treatment since outcome measures were collected during a stressful period, final exams. The first blood draw was one month before final exams, and the second was on the final day of exams. Results indicated that, while *group membership* did not affect percentage of helper cells (CD4+), suppressor cells (CD8+), or NK cells, *frequency of relaxation practice* was significantly correlated with percentage of helper cells during the exam period, when baseline levels were controlled. Thus, relaxation training prior to a stressful period does appear to moderate levels of helper cells, and this effect may be proportional to the frequency of relaxation-induced states achieved by practicing subjects. In sum, there appears to be some evidence that relaxation training can affect some enumerative and functional immune markers. This effect is more apparent when several sessions of training in the relaxation technique have been provided.

Another aspect of this initial work that may be of importance, as suggested by Kiecolt-Glaser *et al.* (1986), is the clinical relevance of immune changes to the study participants. To demonstrate, Kiecolt-Glaser's geriatric and medical student populations were not receiving the training for any immune-related clinical disorder. Therefore, they may not have been motivated to practice the relaxation exercises to a degree that would improve immune function significantly. Also, since their immune systems were relatively intact, compared to some clinical populations, there may not have been much room for improvement; that is, a ceiling effect may have been at play. Support for this latter suggestion comes from a study of cancer patients who received relaxation, biofeedback, and guided imagery training (Gruber, Hall, Hersch, & Dubois, 1988). This population represents a group for whom immunoenhancing interventions may have health implications. Compared to pretreatment levels, these patients showed significantly increased responses on a variety of cellular and humoral functional measures, as well as an increased number of NK cells, by the end of the relaxation intervention (Gruber *et al.,* 1988). Our work suggests that relaxation training may enhance certain aspects of cell-mediated immunity (e.g., CD4+ number) among asymptomatic seropositive and seronegative gay males who have recently learned of their serostatus and that such effects are related to the frequency of relaxation practice (Antoni, Baggett, Ironson, *et al.*, 1991; Baggett *et al.*, 1989). It is reasonable to suggest that such interventions may enhance immunological as well as affective functioning among HIV-1 infected and at-risk females.

Cognitive Coping Skills

Following HIV-1 serostatus notification, the infected individual is likely to harbor dysfunctional beliefs that may aggravate a perceived loss of control as well as anxiety and depression levels (Kelly & St. Lawrence, 1988). Recent accounts suggest that relevant cognitive factors here include the individual's perceptions, self-statements, attributions, and appraisals of seropositivity, HIV-1 exposure, and future health and life changes (Kelly & St. Lawrence, 1988). Although such processes can motivate the individual to reevaluate values and make "positive behavior changes," they may also fuel protracted periods of rumination and catastrophic thinking that lead to affective disturbances and interference with daily functioning (Kelly & St. Lawrence, 1988). Our own work suggests that during the weeks following serostatus notification, seropositive individuals experience marked increases in intrusive thoughts as well as heightened anxiety, depression, and confusion (Ironson *et al.*, 1990). It has been suggested that cognitive therapy to improve coping skills may be beneficial for such individuals (Kelly & St. Lawrence, 1988).

Cognitive therapeutic techniques have been utilized in a number of ways in the health field, including the areas of health promotion and disease prevention, detection, and treatment. Specific applications of cognitive stress management interventions have been developed for chronic illnesses such as asthma (Bartlett, 1983), rheumatoid arthritis (Parker *et al.*, 1987), and peptic ulcer (Brooks & Richardson, 1980). Additionally, cognitive strategies have been targeted at the reduction of postoperative cesarean-section pain (Baumstark & Beck, 1988), pain associated with cancer (Fishman & Loscalzo, 1987), and control of acute and chronic pain (Weisenberg, 1987). Although cognitive techniques have been widely researched in terms of general health outcomes, rarely have investigations focused upon hormonal or immunological changes following the implementation of these strategies.

Cognitive-behavioral stress management techniques include strategies such as cognitive reappraisal of stressors; cognitive restructuring of maladaptive thoughts and affective responses; and active problem-solving behaviors. These techniques are designed to change individuals' perceptions of environmental events and their ability to control the situation. The rationale for cognitive-behavioral techniques stems from the assumption that individuals can be taught new patterns of thinking, feeling, and behaving to help them achieve a sense of control over emotional states and maladaptive behaviors, thereby functioning as active contributors to their lives and not "helpless victims" (Turk, Holzman, & Kerns, 1986). According to this perspective, an individual's appraisals, beliefs, attitudes, cognitive coping strategies, and expectancies are important mediators in all realms of health, disease, and responses to treatment (Turk et al., 1986).

The effects of cognitive therapies on depression and anxiety have been investigated in several studies. This work is relevant in that these two affective processes appear to be related to both the individual's appraisal of environmental stimuli and immune functioning. Linn, Linn, and Jensen (1981) found that individuals experiencing psychological states of perceived stress and anxiety had impaired lymphocyte mitogen responsiveness. Similarly, depression has been linked to compromised immunological functioning and with the course of some immune-related disease processes. For example, Kemeny, Zegans, and Cohen (1987) found depressed mood to be associated with decreases in cytotoxic T-cell number and with increases in the rate of HSV-2 outbreaks.

Although depressive illness is often referred to as an affective disorder, it presents as a disturbance of psychological and physiological functioning. Recent studies have concentrated on two aspects of depression—changes in cognitions and alterations in HPAC activity. The thought content of depressed patients has been found to contain a negative bias with specific processing errors and excessively rigid idiosyncratic beliefs (Blackburn, Jones, & Lewin, 1986; Kovacs & Beck, 1978). These cognitive distortions are highly correlated with depressed mood, and maintenance of distorted thinking is associated with poor response to treatment among depressed patients (Simons, Garfield, & Murphy, 1984). Conversely, improvements in dysfunctional thinking often accompany recovery from depressive illness regardless of whether the treatment is pharmacotherapy or cognitive based, and greater cognitive enhancement and less relapse is seen with cognitive interventions (Blackburn & Bishop, 1983; Covi & Lipman, 1987; Murphy, Simons, Wetzel, & Lustman, 1984; Stavynski & Greenberg, 1987). Others have noted that compared with imipramine, cognitive therapy resulted in significantly greater decreases in hopelessness and more improvement in self-concept among nonpsychotic depressed outpatients (Rush, Beck, Kovacs, Weisenburger, & Holon, 1982).

Increased HPAC activity in depression has been consistently reported (Christie et al., 1986), and failure to suppress cortisol secretion after dexamethasone administration (dexamethasone suppression test) has been used to diagnose endogenous depression (Carroll et al., 1981). Moreover, elevated plasma concentrations of cortisol have been shown to return to normal in patients successfully treated with antidepressants (Carroll, Curtis, & Mendels, 1976) or electroconvulsive therapy (Christie, Whalley, Brown, & Dick, 1982). Depressed inpatients successfully treated with cognitive therapy also show a parallel fall in plasma cortisol (Christie et al., 1982). These findings, taken together with those of Rush *et al.,* (1982), suggest that cognitive-based interventions may alter psychological and physiological functioning among depressed patients. Despite these impressive findings supporting the efficacy of cognitive therapy among psychiatric patients, less is known regarding the psychological and physiological effects of cognitive interventions in nonpsychiatric groups experiencing a traumatic event, such as HIV-1 serostatus notification.

Some have suggested that cognitive techniques can be used to improve coping skills as well as general appraisals of self-efficacy (Bradley *et al.,* 1984). A limited number of studies have related cognitive coping styles and appraisals to immune functioning. In a study of coping styles, cellular immune functioning, and HSV-2 outbreaks, problem-focused coping was associated with greater cytotoxic T-cell activity and a longer period of dormancy between outbreaks, whereas emotion-focused coping was associated with lower cytotoxic T-cell activity and shorter latency periods (Kemeny, 1986). In a study of males in the early stages of HIV-1 infection, the amount of problem-focused coping strategies utilized was positively correlated with T helper cell number (Day, Patterson, & Grant, 1988). These findings suggest that specific coping strategies may modulate cellular immune functioning in certain individuals. Little is known, however, regarding immunomodulatory effects for cognitive-based coping skills training programs in such populations.

In addition to modulating affective and immune functioning, cognitive factors may also predict risk behavior reduction. It is well documented that attributions influence perceived control and predictability, which may then motivate risk behavior change and maintenance (Kelly & St. Lawrence, 1988). This phenomenon has been demonstrated among cardiac patients involved in behavior-change programs (Affleck, Tennen, Croog, & Levine, 1987). It is plausible that cognitive interventions might be helpful in motivating reduced-risk behavior. A synthesis of the empirical and theoretical literature suggests that changing cognitive processing of environmental stressors may have multiple effects that are relevant with HIV-1 infected and at-risk females. Specifically, cognitive strategies that alter causal attributions and enhance coping skills may increase perceptions of control. Such increases in perceived control may attenuate affective distress with consequent normalization of endocrine functioning and immunoenhancement on the one hand, and increased motivation for risk behavior change (secondary to improved self-efficacy) on the other.

Social Functioning

A final component of stress management involves the enhancement of social and interpersonal functioning. A common reaction to HIV-1 seropositivity is social withdrawal and isolation (Kelly & St. Lawrence, 1988). Some have noted that improving individuals' social support network can help them cope more successfully with a seropositive diagnosis (Zones, Beeson, Echenberg, Rutherford, & O'Malley, 1987), and several programs have emerged for just this purpose (Kelly & St. Lawrence, 1988). In addition to offering a sense of universality, such groups may also allow the individual infected with HIV-1 to express feelings and learn specialized styles of coping successfully employed by other group members.

Social interventions that include an active engagement in group activities may have the most potent role in stress reduction. Relatively few studies have been completed that evaluate social support group interventions as stress reducing and/or immunoenhancing agents. In one investigation of the effect of support group attendance on immunity, Kiecolt-Glaser and her colleagues noted that among family caregivers of Alzheimer's disease victims, those who attended such groups rated themselves as less lonely and had higher NK cell percentages than nonmembers (Kiecolt-Glaser, Glaser, Shuttleworth, et al., 1987). Other recent findings suggest that adequate social support resources may be associated with NK cell and lymphocyte functioning (Levy & Herberman, 1988), which may be mediated by increases in active coping (Sarason, 1979), and changes in physiological stress response systems (Cobb, 1974). Specifically, Sarason (1979) holds that social support may insulate stressed humans from self-preoccupying helplessness, thereby favoring the employment of active coping strategies.

Regarding physiological effects of social support, unemployed men receiving high levels of emotional support from their wives and families showed lower catecholamine levels than their lower-support counterparts (Cobb, 1974). Further, low social support states (e.g., loneliness) have been associated with elevated urinary cortisol levels as well as impaired NK cell activity and lymphocyte responsivity (Kiecolt-Glaser, Ricker, et al., 1984). Among female breast cancer patients, seeking social support as a primary coping strategy and receiving high levels of spousal support predicted better NK cell cytotoxic function (Levy & Herberman, 1988). In an ongoing longitudinal study of long-surviving AIDS patients, investigators noted that one important social support variable associated with survival was "problem-solving help used" (Solomon, Temoshok, O'Leary, & Zich, 1987).

These findings suggest that it may be the more active components of social support that possess protective effects. It seems especially important to investigate the efficacy of social support interventions in populations that are at high risk for social isolation and exposure to other social stressors (e.g., women who are HIV-1 seropositive). In addition to reducing distress, a new social support network may help the individual to adopt and maintain reduced-risk behaviors that would not be possible in previous social networks (e.g., IV drug abusers). In our stress management program designed for gay males, subjects first learn of the health benefits of social supports followed by individualized assessment of several parameters of their social network. Finally, subjects are sensitized to local community organizations and encouraged to initiate new relationships within these organizations and through contacts made in therapy groups (Antoni *et al.,* 1988).

In addition to enhancing social supports, stress management interventions should provide individuals with the skills needed to deal with stressful interpersonal encounters and to maintain reduced-risk behaviors in the face of sexual enticement and, possibly, coercion. Assertiveness training (Hersen, Eisler, Miller, Johnson, & Pinkston, 1973; Kelly, 1982) is an appropriate intervention for accomplishing these ends and has been suggested as a crucial component of interventions designed to reduce risk behavior among individuals who are HIV-1 seropositive (Kelly & St. Lawrence, 1988).

Summary

It is apparent that multimodal stress management interventions targeting affective, cognitive, and social/interpersonal functioning may be especially useful in attenuating stress responses and adopting (and maintaining) reduced-risk behaviors in HIV-1 infected and at-risk populations. Although recent work suggests that such interventions may be successful in decreasing distress (Baggett *et al.,* 1989; Coates & McKusick, 1987), enhancing immune functioning (Baggett *et al.,* 1989; Antoni *et al.,* 1991), and reducing the frequency of high-risk sexual behavior (Coates & McKusick, 1987; Kelly, St. Lawrence, Hood, & Brasfield, 1989) among seropositive and at-risk seronegative homosexual males, no such work has been conducted with infected and at-risk heterosexual females. However, by integrating information on prevalent psychosocial stressors, known barriers to risk reduction, and common maladaptive responses employed by low-SES minority women with available behavioral interventions, the benefits of a multifaceted stress management approach appear to be plentiful (see Table 1).

CONCLUSION

In summary, we hold that future work needs to focus on the following research agendas:

1. Immunological and psychological (affective) effects of serostatus notification among seropositive pregnant and nonpregnant minority women.
2. The natural history of HIV-1 infection in pregnant versus nonpregnant women.
3. Factors affecting seroconversion rate in at-risk seronegative women.
4. The incidence of GU viral infections (HSV, HPV, CMV) and cervical dysplasia (CIN) among seropositive pregnant and nonpregnant women as compared to seronegative (pregnant vs. nonpregnant) women.

TABLE 1
Factors, Targets, and Intervention Strategies That Affect High-Risk Behaviors
in Populations at Risk for HIV-1

Likely issues in population	Intervention strategy
Lack of information on risk behavior and transmission	Education in safer sex techniques
Denial of personal vulnerability to HIV-1	Confrontation of denial coping strategies in supportive environment
Difficulty in management of high-risk behaviors	Identification of high- and low-risk practices and employment of behavior change strategies (e.g., self-management training)
Inability to resist sexual coercion	Assertion training
Substance abuse as alternative coping strategy leading to disinhibition of behavioral impulses	Coping skills training stress management techniques
Lack of social supports conducive to self-pride and self-esteem	Social support sensitization, enrichment, and engagement
Financial stressors	Problem-solving strategies
Unmanageable anger and sexual acting out	Anger control strategies
Hopelessness and loss of sense of control	Self-efficacy training
Affective distress	Cognitive therapy for anxiety and depression

5. Psychoimmunological, immunological, and endocrine aspects/changes during pregnancy, labor, and the early postpartum period among seronegative and seropositive women.
6. The role of individual differences in psychosocial stressors, coping and immunological functioning on pregnancy complications, perinatal transmission, GU infections and disease progression to OIs among seropositive pregnant women.

This information should lead to the formulation of behavioral interventions. *Short-term goals* of such behavioral stress management interventions should include: (1) risk behavior change and future pregnancy reduction, (2) reduction of perceived stressors and affective distress responses (e.g., anxiety, depression) as well as enhancement of perceived control, (3) acquisition of coping skills, (4) enhancement of immunological functioning, (5) reduction in the incidence of GU viral infections and cervical dysplasia (CIN), and (6) decreasing seroconversion rates (among initially seronegative subjects). *Longer-term goals* should include: (1) maintenance of reduced-risk behavior changes and future pregnancy incidence, (2) decreased perceived stressors and distress responses as well as enhanced perceptions of personal control, (3) fortified social support networks, (4) optimal immunological functioning, (5) decreased incidence of GU viral infections, cervical dysplasia, and traditional AIDS-related OIs and neoplasia, and (6) continued reductions in seroconversion rate.

With the ominous projections for seropositive cases among women in coming years, and the potential for multiple pathways of transmission (heterosexually, perinatally, and intravenously) from each of these cases, mothers with AIDS are likely to become the focus of increased media and research attention. To achieve the goals suggested in this chapter, much of the information learned from the study of infected homosexual men can be integrated, yet tempered, with the knowledge of the unique psychological and physiological stressors that pregnant and postpartum seropositive women experience. It is encouraging that the realization of these goals might be achieved by behavioral means—a controllable aspect of a phenomenon (HIV-1 infection) that is more commonly associated with hopelessness and fatalism.

REFERENCES

Affleck, G., Tennen, H., Croog, S., & Levine, S. (1987). Causal attribution, perceived benefits, and morbidity after a heart attack: An 8-year study. *Journal of Consulting and Clinical Psychology, 55,* 29–35.

Anderson, J., Horn, J., King, R., Keller, J., Herbert, B., & Barbacci, M. (1989, June). *Selected gynecologic issues in women with HIV infection.* Paper presented at the V International Conference on AIDS, Montreal.

Antoni, M. H., & Goodkin, K. (1989). Host moderator variables in the promotion of cervical neoplasia. II. Dimensions of life stress. *Journal of Psychosomatic Research, 33*(4), 457–467.

Antoni, M. H., & Goodkin, K. (1988). Host moderator variables in the promotion of cervical neoplasia. I. Personality facets. *Journal of Psychosomatic Research, 32*(3), 327–338.

Antoni, M. H., Baggett, L., Ironson, G., LaPerriere, A., August, S., Klimas, N., Schneiderman, N., & Fletcher, M. A. (1991). Cognitive behavioral stress management intervention buffers distress responses and immunologic changes following notification of HIV-1 seropositivity. *Journal of Consulting and Clinical Psychology,* in press.

Antoni, M. H., Schneiderman, N., Fletcher, M. A., Goldstein, D., Ironson, G., & LaPerriere, A. (1990a). Psychoneuroimmunology and HIV-1. *Journal of Consulting and Clinical Psychology, 58*(1), 38–49.

Antoni, M. H., August, S., LaPerriere, A., Baggett, H. L., Klimas, N., Ironson, G., Schneiderman, N., & Fletcher, M. A. (1990b). Psychological and neuroendocrine measures related to functional immune changes in anticipation of HIV-1 serostatus notification. *Psychosomatic Medicine, 52,* 496–510.

Antoni, M. H., Fletcher, M., LaPerriere, A., Schneiderman, N., & Ironson, G. (1989, January). *Stress management, psychological, and immune functioning among asymptomatic HIV+ and HIV– gay males.* Paper presented at the scientific meetings of the American Association for the Advancement of Science, San Francisco, CA.

Antoni, M. H., August, S., Baggett, L., Saab, P., Ironson, G., Schneiderman, N., & Fletcher, M. (1988). *Cognitive/behavioral stress management intervention manual for HIV high risk groups.* Unpublished manuscript, University of Miami, Department of Psychology.

Baggett, L., Antoni, M. H., August, S., LaPerriere, A., Schneiderman, N., Ironson, G., & Fletcher, M. (1989, April). *Frequency of relaxation practice, state anxiety and immune markers in an HIV-1 high risk group.* Paper presented at the tenth annual scientific meeting of the Society of Behavioral Medicine, San Francisco, CA.

Baley, J., & Schacter, B. (1985). Mechanisms of diminished natural killer cell activity in pregnant women and neonates. *Journal of Immunology, 134,* 3042–3047.

Bandura, A. (1989). Human agency in social cognitive theory. *American Psychologist, 44*(9), 1175–1184.

Bartlett, E. (1983). Educational self-help approaches in childhood asthma. *Journal of Allergy and Clinical Immunology, 72*(5), 545–554.

Bartlett, E., Rabin, D., Taggart, V., Bandemer, C., & Bellonti, J. (1987, June). *Behavioral diagnosis for effective education of HIV-seropositive patients.* Paper presented at the III International Conference on AIDS, Washington, DC.

Bashford, J., & Gough, R. (1983). High-affinity erythrocyte rosette formation and inhibition in pre-malignant disease of the uterine cervix. *Cancer Research, 43,* 3955–3958.

Baum, A., McKinnon, Q., & Silvia, C. (1987, March). *Chronic stress and the immune system.* Paper presented at the eighth annual scientific meeting of the Society of Behavioral Medicine, Washington, DC.

Baumstark, K., & Beck, N. (1988, March). *A cognitive-behavioral treatment package for management of postoperative cesarean-section pain.* Paper presented at the 9th annual scientific meeting of the Society of Behavioral Medicine, Boston, MA.

Bell, N. (1989). AIDS and women: Remaining ethical issues. *AIDS Education and Prevention, 1*(1), 22–30.

Berkleman, R., Karon, J., Thomas, P., Kerndt, P., Rutherford, G., & Stehr-Green, J. (1989, June). *Are AIDS cases among homosexual males leveling?* Paper presented at the V International Conference on AIDS, Montreal.

Biggar, B., Minkoff, H., Gail, M., Willoughby, A., Mendez, H., Goedert, J., & Landesman, S. (1989, February). *The effect of pregnancy on immune status in HIV(+) and HIV(−) women.* Paper presented at the ninth annual meeting of the Society of Perinatal Obstetricians, New Orleans, LA.

Blackburn, I., & Bishop, S. (1983). Changes in cognition with pharmacotherapy and cognitive therapy. *British Journal of Psychiatry, 143,* 609–617.

Blackburn, I., Jones, S., & Lewin, R. (1986). Cognitive style in depression. *Clinical Psychology, 25,* 241–251.

Borysenko, M., & Borysenko, J. (1982). Stress, behavior, and immunity: Animal models and mediating mechanisms. *General Hospital Psychiatry, 4,* 56–67.

Boyer, C., & Schafer, F. (1990, 2 August). Adolescent risk behaviors, sexually transmitted diseases and AIDS. Paper presented at the annual scientific meeting of the American Psychological Association. Boston, MA.

Bradley, L., Young, L., Anderson, K., McDaniel, L., Turner, R., & Agudelo, C. (1984). Psychological approaches to the management of arthritis pain. *Social Science and Medicine, 19,* 1353–1360.

Brooks, G. R., & Richardson, F. C. (1980). Emotional skills training: A treatment program for duodenal ulcer. *Behavior Therapy, 11,* 198–207.

Brown, G., & Rundell, J. (1990). Prospective study of psychiatric morbidity in HIV-seropositive women without AIDS. *General Hospital Psychiatry, 12,* 30–35.

Brown, S., & VanEpps, D. (1986). Opioid peptides modulate production of interferon-γ by human mononuclear cells. *Cellular Immunology, 103,* 19.

Brown, Z., Berry, S., & Vontver, L. (1986). Genital herpes simplex virus infections complicating pregnancy. *Journal of Reproductive Medicine, 31*(5), 420–425.

Brown, Z., Vontver, L., Bendetti, J., Critchlow, C., Hickok, D., Sells, C., Berry, S., & Corey, L.

(1985). Genital herpes in pregnancy: Risk factors associated with recurrences and asymptomatic viral shedding. *American Journal of Obstetrics & Gynecology, 153,* 24–30.

Bujko, M., Sulovic, V., & Dotlic, R. (1986). Herpes virus hominis (HVH) infection in women with preterm labor. *Journal of Perinatal Medicine, 14,* 319–324.

Burish, T., Carey, M., Krozely, M., & Greco, F. (1987). Conditioned side effects induced by cancer chemotherapy: Prevention through behavioral treatment. *Journal of Consulting and Clinical Psychology, 55,* 42–48.

Calabrese, J., Kling, M., & Gold, P. (1987). Alterations in immunocompetence during stress, bereavement, and depression: Focus on neuroendocrine regulation. *American Journal of Psychiatry, 144*(9), 1123–1134.

Calabrese, J., Skwerer, R., & Barna, B. (1986). Depression, immunocompetence, and prostaglandins of the E series. *Psychiatric Research, 17,* 41–47.

Calabrese, L., & Gopalakrishna, K. (1986). Transmission of HTLV-III infection from man to woman to man. *New England Journal of Medicine, 314,* 987.

Carpenter, C., Mayer, K., Fisher, A., Desai, M., & Durand, L. (1989). Natural history of acquired immunodeficiency syndrome in women in Rhode Island. *American Journal of Medicine, 86,* 771–775.

Carroll, B., Curtis, G., & Mendels, J. (1976). Neuroendocrine regulation in depression. I. Limbic system-adrenocortical dysfunction. *Archives of General Psychiatry, 33,* 1034–1044.

Carroll, B., Feinberg, M., Greden, J., Tarika, J., Albala, A., Hasket, R., James, N., Kronfel, Z., Lohr, N., Steiner, M., De Vigne, J., & Young, E. (1981). A specific laboratory test for the diagnosis of melancholia. *Archives of General Psychiatry, 38,* 15–22.

Casey, M., MacDonald, P., & Simpson, E. (1985). Endocrinological changes of pregnancy. In D. Wilson, & D. Foster (Eds.), *William's textbook of endocrinology* (pp. 422–437). Philadelphia, PA: Saunders.

Castelli, F., Chiodera, A., Tarantini, M., Prati, E., Bianchi, U., & Carosi, G. (1989, June). *Pregnancy and HIV infection: An experience about 15 cases.* Paper presented at the V International Conference on AIDS, Montreal.

Castello, G., Esposito, G., Stellato, G., Mora, L., Abate, G., & Germano, A. (1986). Immunological abnormalities in patients with cervical carcinoma. *Gynecologic Oncology, 25,* 61–64.

Castro, K., Lieb, S., Galisher, C., Witte, J., & Jaffe, H. (1987, June). *AIDS and HIV infection.* Paper presented at the III International Conference on AIDS, Washington, DC.

Catalona, W., Sample, W., & Chretien, P. (1973). Lymphocyte reactivity in cancer patients: Correlation with tumor histology and clinical stage. *Cancer, 31,* 65.

Cecchi, R. L. (1984). Stress: Prodrome to immune deficiency. *Annals of the New York Academy of Sciences, 437,* 286–289.

Chamberland, M., Conley, L., & Buehler, J. (1989, June). *Surveillance of heterosexually acquired AIDS, U.S.A.* Paper presented at the V International Conference on AIDS, Montreal.

Chin, J. (1990). Current and future dimensions of HIV/AIDS pandemic in women and children. *Lancet, 336,* 221–224.

Chu, S., Buehler, J., & Berkelman, R. (1990). Impact of the human immunodeficiency virus epidemic on mortality in women of reproductive age, United States. *Journal of the American Medical Association, 264*(2), 225–229.

Christie, J., Whalley, L., Brown, N., & Dick, H. (1982). Effects of ECT on the neuroendocrine response to apomorphine in severely depressed patients. *British Journal of Psychiatry, 148,* 58–65.

Christie, J., Whalley, L., Dick, H., Blackwood, D., Blackburn, I., & Fink, G. (1986). Raised plasma cortisol concentrations a feature of drug-free psychotics and not specific for depression. *British Journal of Psychiatry, 148,* 58–65.

Coates, T., & McKusick, L. (1987, June). *The efficacy of stress management in reducing high risk* behavior and improving immune function in HIV antibody positive men. Paper presented at the III International Conference on AIDS, Washington, DC.

Coates, T., Morin, S., & McKusick, L. (1987, June). Consequences of AIDS antibody testing among gay men: The AIDS behavioral research project. Paper presented at the III International Conference on AIDS, Washington, DC.

Coates, T., Stall, R., Mandel, J., Bocellari, A., Sorensen, J., Morales, E., Morin, S., Wiley, J., & McKusick, L. (1987). AIDS: A psychosocial research agenda. Annals of Behavioral Medicine, 9(2), 21–28.

Coates, T. J., Temoshok, L., & Mandel, J. (1984). Psychosocial research is essential to understanding and treating AIDS. American Psychologist, 39(11), 1309–1314.

Cobb, S. (1974). Physiological changes in men whose jobs are abolished. Journal of Psychosomatic Research, 18, 245–258.

Covi, L., & Lipman, R. (1987). Cognitive behavioral group psychotherapy combined with imipramine in major depression. Psychopharmacology Bulletin, 23(1), 173–176.

Crary, B., Borysenko, M., Sutherland, D., Kutz, I., Borysenko, J., & Benson, H. (1983). Decrease in mitogen responsiveness of mononuclear cells from peripheral blood after epinephrine administration in humans. Journal of Immunology, 130, 694–697.

Creenberg, A., Thomas, P., Hindin, R., Greene, A., Rautenberg, E., & Schultz, S. (1989, June). The evolving epidemiology of AIDS in New York City: Trends in AIDS case surveillance data. Paper presented at the V International Conference on AIDS, Montreal.

Crum, C., Ikenburg, H., Richart, R., & Gissman, L. (1984). Human papillomavirus type 16 and early cervical neoplasia. New England Journal of Medicine, 310(14), 880–883.

Cupps, T., & Fauci, A. (1982). Corticosteroid-mediated immunoregulation in man. Immunology Review, 65, 133–155.

Day, J., Patterson, T., & Grant, I. (1988, March). A pilot study on the relationship between psychosocial variables and immune status in HIV-infected individuals. Paper presented at the 9th annual scientific meetings of the Society of Behavioral Medicine, Boston, MA.

Deschamps, M., Pape, J., Madhavan, S., & Johnson, W. (1989, June). Pregnancy and acceleration of HIV-related illness. Paper presented at the V International Conference on AIDS, Montreal.

Donlou, J. N., Wolcott, M. S., Gottlieb, M. S., & Landsverk, J. (1985). Psychosocial aspects of AIDS and AIDS-related complex: A pilot study. Journal of Psychosocial Oncology, 3(2), 39–55.

Duncan, M., Sadlik, J., & Hadden, J. (1982). Glucocorticoid modulation of lymphokine-induced macrophage proliferation. Cellular Immunology, 67, 23–36.

Efantis, J., Garcia, A., Potter, S., Johnson, B., O'Sullivan, M., Scott, G., Lowrance, B., & Plummer, P. (1989, September). Cross cultural case management: A medical and social service demonstration model for HIV positive women and their children. Paper presented at the V National Pediatric AIDS meeting, Los Angeles, CA.

Ellerbrock, T., Chamberland, M., Bush, T., & Rogers, M. (1989, June). National surveillance of AIDS in women, 1981–1988: A report from the centers for disease control. Paper presented at the V International Conference on AIDS, Montreal.

Felten, D., Felten, S., Carlson, S., Olschawka, J., & Livnat, S. (1985). Noradrenergic and peptidergic innervation of lymphoid tissue. Journal of Immunology, 135(2 Suppl.), 755s–765s.

Fischl, M., Dickinson, G., Scott, G., Klimas, N., Fletcher, M., & Parks, W. (1987). Evaluation of heterosexual partners, children, and household contacts of adults with AIDS. Journal of the American Medical Association, 257, 640–644.

Fishman, B., & Loscalzo, M. (1987). Cognitive-behavioral interventions in management of cancer pain: Principles and applications. Medical Clinics of North America, 71(2), 271–287.

Fletcher, M. A., Caralis, P., Laperriere, A. R., Ironson, G., Klimas, N. G., Perry, A., Ashman, M., & Schneiderman, N. (1988, June). Immune function and aerobic training as a function of anti-HIV status in healthy gay males. Paper presented at the meeting of the International Conference on AIDS, Stockholm, Sweden.

Freudenberg, N., Lee, J., & Silver, D. (1989). How Black and Latino community organizations respond to the AIDS epidemic: A case study in one New York City neighborhood. *AIDS Education and Prevention, 1*(1), 12–21.

Friedland, G., & Klein, R. (1987). Transmission of human immunodeficiency virus. *New England Journal of Medicine, 317*(18), 1125–1135.

Gaudier, F., Delpin, E., Rivera, J., & Gonzales, Z. (1988). Pregnancy after renal transplantation. *Surgery, Gynecology, & Obstetrics, 167,* 533–543.

Glaser, R., & Kiecolt-Glaser, J. (1987). Stress-associated depression in cellular immunity: Implications for Acquired Immune Deficiency Syndrome (AIDS). *Brain, Behavior, and Immunity, 1,* 107–112.

Glaser, R., Rice, J., Sheridan, J., Fertel, R., Stout, J., Speicher, C., Pinsky, D., Kotur, M., Post, A., Beck, M., & Kiecolt-Glaser, J. (1987). Stress-related immune suppression: Health implications. *Brain, Behavior, and Immunity, 1*(1), 7–20.

Gloeb, D., Efantis, J., Ricci, J., & O'Sullivan, M. (1989, February). *HIV infection in pregnancy.* Paper presented at the ninth annual meeting of the Society of Perinatal Obstetricians, New Orleans, LA.

Gloeb, D., O'Sullivan, M., & Efantis, J. (1988). Human immunodeficiency virus infection in women: I. The effects of human immunodeficiency virus on pregnancy. *American Journal of Obstetrics and Gynecology, 159,* 756–761.

Glaser, J., Strange, T., & Rosati, D. (1989). Heterosexual human immunodeficiency virus transmission among the middle class. *Archives of Internal Medicine, 149,* 645–649.

Goldstein, M., Shore, B., & Gusberg, S. (1971). Cellular immunity as a host response to squamous carcinoma of the cervix. *American Journal of Obstetrics & Gynecology, 111,* 751–755.

Gonik, B., Lee, L., West, S., & Kohl, S. (1987). Natural killer cell cytotoxicity and antibody-dependent cellular cytotoxicity to herpes simplex virus-infected cells in human pregnancy. *American Journal of Reproductive Immunology & Microbiology, 13,* 23–26.

Gruber, B., Hall, N., Hersh, S., & Dubois, P. (1988). Immune system and psychologic changes in metastatic cancer patients while using ritualized relaxation and guided imagery. *Scandinavian Journal of Behavior Therapy.*

Guinan, M., & Hardy, A. (1987). Epidemiology of AIDS in women in the United States: 1981–1986. *Journal of the American Medical Association, 257*(15), 2039–2042.

Hadden, J. (1987). Neuroendocrine modulation of the thymus-dependent immune system. *Annals of the New York Academy of Sciences, 496,* 39–48.

Hahn, T., Levin, S., & Handzel, Z. (1976). Leukocyte migration inhibition factor (LIF) production by lymphocytes of normal children, newborns, and children with immune deficiency. *Clinical Experimental Immunology, 24,* 448–454.

Halonen, J., & Passman, R. (1985). Relaxation and expectation in the treatment of postpartum distress. *Journal of Consulting and Clinical Psychology, 53,* 839–845.

Handsfield, H., Sohlberg, E., Hopkins, S., & Harris, N. (1989, June). *Trends in HIV seroprevalence in an urban sexually-transmitted disease clinic.* Paper presented at the V International Conference on AIDS, Montreal.

Hersen, M., Eisler, R., Miller, P., Johnson, M., & Pinkston, S. (1973). Effects of practice, instructions, and modeling on components of assertive behavior. *Behavior Research and Therapy, 11,* 443–451.

Hoelscher, T., Lichstein, K., Fischer, S., & Hegarty, T. (1987). Relaxation treatment of hypertension: Do home relaxation tapes enhance treatment outcome? *Behavior Therapy, 18,* 33–37.

Holzman, D., Brandenberg, N., Sims, J., & Witte, J. (1989, June). *Changing patterns of heterosexually acquired AIDS in Florida.* Paper presented at the V International Conference on AIDS, Montreal.

Ironson, G., LaPerriere, A., Antoni, M. H., O'Hearn, P., Schneiderman, N., Klimas, N., & Fletcher, M. (1990). Changes in immune and psychological measures as a function of anticipation and reaction to news of HIV-1 antibody status. *Psychosomatic Medicine, 52,* 247–270.

Ironson, G., O'Hearn, P., Laperriere, A., Antoni, M., Ashman, M., Schneiderman, N., & Fletcher, M. (1988, April). *News of HIV-1 antibody status and immune function in healthy gay males.* Paper presented at the ninth annual scientific meeting of the Society of Behavioral Medicine, Boston, MA.

Irwin, M., Daniels, M., & Bloom, E. (1987). Life events, depressive symptoms, and immune function. *American Journal of Psychiatry, 144,* 437–441.

Irwin, M., Daniels, M., Bloom, E., & Weiner, H. (1986). Life events and natural killer cell activity. *Psychopharmacology Bulletin, 22,* 1093–1096.

Irwin, M., Daniels, M., Smith, T., Bloom, E., & Weiner, H. (1987). Impaired natural killer cell activity during bereavement. *Brain, Behavior, and Immunity, 1*(1), 98–104.

Irwin, M., Daniels, M., & Weiner, H. (1987). Immune and neuroendocrine changes during bereavement. *Psychiatric Clinics of North America, 10*(3), 449–465.

Jacobs, S., Mason, J., Kosten, T., Wahby, V., Kasl, S., & Ostfeld, A. (1986). Bereavement and catecholamines. *Journal of Psychosomatic Research, 30,* 489–496.

Jacobsen, E. (1938). *Progressive relaxation.* Chicago: University of Chicago Press.

Jemmott, J., & Locke, S. (1984). Psychosocial factors, immunologic mediation, and human susceptibility to infectious diseases: How much do we know? *Psychological Bulletin, 95,* 79–108.

Kaplan, L. D., Wofsky, C. B., & Volberding, P. A. (1987). Treatment of patients with acquired immunodeficiency syndrome and associated manifestations. *Journal of the American Medical Association, 257*(10), 1367–1376.

Kaufman, R., & Adams, E. (1986). Herpes simplex virus and human papillomavirus in the development of cervical carcinoma. *Clinical Obstetrics & Gynecology, 29*(3), 353–360.

Kavelaars, A., Ballieux, R. E., & Heijnen, C. (1988). Modulation of the immune response by proopiomelanocortin derived peptides II. *Brain, Behavior, and Immunity, 2,* 57–66.

Kelly, J. (1982). *Social skills training: A practical guide for interventions.* New York: Springer.

Kelly, J., & St. Lawrence, J. (1987a). Cautions about condoms in prevention of AIDS. *Lancet, 1*(8528), 323.

Kelly, J., & St. Lawrence, J. (1987b). The prevention of AIDS: Roles for behavioral intervention. *Scandinavian Journal of Behaviour Therapy, 16,* 5–19.

Kelly, J., & St. Lawrence, J. (1988). *The AIDS health crisis: Psychosocial and social interventions.* New York: Plenum.

Kelly, J., St. Lawrence, J., Brasfield, T., & Hood, H. (1987, June). *Relationships between knowledge about AIDS risk and actual risk behavior in a sample of homosexual men: Some implications for prevention.* Paper presented at the III International Conference on AIDS, Washington, DC.

Kelly, J., St. Lawrence, J., Hood, H., & Brasfield, T. (1989). Behavioral intervention to reduce AIDS risk activities. *Journal of Consulting and Clinical Psychology, 57*(1), 60–67.

Kemeny, M. (1986, April). *Stress and coping in genital herpes simplex.* Paper presented at the seventh annual scientific meeting of the Society of Behavioral Medicine, New York.

Kemeny, M., Zegans, L., & Cohen, F. (1987). Stress, mood, immunity, and recurrence of genital herpes. *Annals of New York Academy of Sciences, 496,* 735–736.

Kiecolt-Glaser, J., Fisher, L., Ogrocki, P., Stout, J., Speicher, C., & Glaser, R. (1987). Marital quality, marital disruption, and immune function. *Psychosomatic Medicine, 49,* 13–34.

Kiecolt-Glaser, J., Garner, W., Speicher, C., Penn, G. M., Holliday, J., & Glaser, R. (1984). Psychosocial modifiers of immunocompetence in medical students. *Psychosomatic Medicine, 46,* 7–14.

Kiecolt-Glaser, J., & Glaser, R. (1988). Psychological influences in immunity: Implications for AIDS. *American Psychologist, 43,* 892–898.

Kiecolt-Glaser, J., Glaser, R., Strain, E., Stout, J. C., Tarr, K. L., Holliday, J. E., & Speicher, C. E. (1986). Modulation of cellular immunity in medical students. *Journal of Behavioral Medicine, 9,* 311–320.

Kiecolt-Glaser, J., Glaser, R., Shuttleworth, E. C., Dyer, S. C., Ogrocki, P., & Speicher, C. E. (1987). Chronic stress and immunity in family caregivers of Alzheimer's disease victims. *Psychosomatic Medicine, 49,* 523–535.

Kiecolt-Glaser, J., Glaser, R., Williger, D., Stout, J., Messick, G., Sheppard, S., Ricker, D., Romisher, S. C., Briner, W., Bonnell, G., & Donnerberg, R. (1985). Psychosocial enhancement of immunocompetence in a geriatric population. *Health Psychology, 4,* 25–41.

Kiecolt-Glaser, J., Ricker, D., George, J., Messick, G., Speicher, C., Garner, W., & Glaser, R. (1984). Urinary cortisol levels, cellular immunocompetency, and loneliness in psychiatric inpatients. *Psychosomatic Medicine, 46*(1), 15–23.

Kosten, T., Jacobs, S., & Mason, J. (1984). The dexamethasone suppression test during bereavement. *Journal of Nervous and Mental Disorders, 172,* 359–360.

Kovacs, M., & Beck, A. (1978). Maladaptive cognitive structures in depression. *American Journal of Psychiatry, 135,* 525–535.

Kronfol, Z., Silva, J., Greden, J., Dembinski, S., Gardener, R., & Carroll, B. (1983). Impaired lymphocyte function in depressive illness. *Life Science, 33,* 241–247.

Krueger, R., Levy, E., & Cathcart, E. (1984). Lymphocyte subsets in patients with major depression: Preliminary findings. *Advances, 1,* 5–9.

Lance, L. (1975). Human sexuality course socialization: An analysis of changes in sexual attitudes and sexual behavior. *Journal of Sex Education and Therapy, 2,* 8–14.

LaPerriere, A., O'Hearn, P., Ironson, G., Caralis, P., Ingram, F., Perry, A., Klimas, N., Schneiderman, N., & Fletcher, M. (1988, April). *Exercise and immune function in healthy HIV-1 antibody negative and positive gay males.* Paper presented at the ninth annual scientific meeting of the Society of Behavioral Medicine, Boston, MA.

Laudenslager, M., Ryan, S., Drugan, R., Hyson, R., & Maier, S. (1983). Coping and immunosuppression: Inescapable but not escapable shock suppresses lymphocyte proliferation. *Science, 221,* 568–570.

Lehman, S., Smith, P., Mikl, J., & Morse, D. (1989, June). *Heterosexually transmitted AIDS in New York State.* Paper presented at the V International Conference on AIDS, Montreal.

Levy, S., & Herberman, R. (1988, April). *Behavior, immunity, and breast cancer: Mechanistic analyses of cellular immunocompetence in patient subgroups.* Paper presented at the ninth annual scientific meeting of the Society of Behavioral Medicine, Boston, MA.

Levy, S., Herberman, R., Lippman, M., & d'Angelo, T. (1987). Correlation of stress factors with sustained depression of natural killer cell activity and predicted prognosis in patients with breast cancer. *Journal of Clinical Oncology, 5*(3), 348–353.

Levy, S., Herberman, R., Maluish, A., Schlien, B., & Lippman, M. (1985). Prognostic risk assessment in primary breast cancer by behavioral and immunological parameters. *Health Psychology, 4*(2), 99–113.

Levy, S., Kopersztych, S., Musatti, C., Souen, J., Salvatore, C., & Mendes, N. (1978). Cellular-immunity in squamous cell carcinoma of the uterine cervix. *American Journal of Obstetrics & Gynecology, 130,* 160–164.

Lindan, C., Rutherford, G., Payne, S., Hearst, N., & Lemp, G. (1989, June). *Decline in rate of new AIDS cases among homosexual and bisexual men in San Francisco.* Paper presented at the V International Conference on AIDS, Montreal.

Linn, M., Linn, B., & Jensen, J. (1984). Stressful events, dysphoric mood, and immune responsiveness. *Psychological Reports, 54,* 219–222.

Livnat, S., Felten, S., Carlson, S., Bellinger, D., & Felten, D. (1985). Involvement of peripheral and central catecholamine systems in neural immune interactions. *Journal of Neuroimmunology, 10,* 5–30.

Lopresti, J. S., Fried, J. C., Spencer, C. A., & Nicoloff, J. T. (1989). Unique alterations of thyroid hormone indices in the acquired immune deficiency syndrome (AIDS). *Annals of Internal Medicine, 110,* 970–975.

MacDonald, P., Alexander, D., Alexander, R., & participants in NIH workshop (1983). Summary of a workshop on maternal genitourinary infections and the outcome of pregnancy. *Journal of Infectious Diseases, 147*(3), 596–605.

Macnab, J., Walkinshaw, S., Cordiner, J., & Clementz, J. (1986). Human papillomavirus in clinically and histologically normal tissue of patients with genital cancer. *New England Journal of Medicine, 315*(7), 1052–1058.

Markham, P., Salahuddin, S., Veren, K., Orndorff, S., & Gallo, R. (1986). Hydrocortisone and some other hormones enhance the expression of HTLV-III. *International Journal of Cancer, 37,* 67–72.

Mason, J. (1975). A historical view of the stress field. I. *Journal of Human Stress, 1,* 6–12.

Mays, V., & Cochran, S. (1987). Acquired immunodeficiency syndrome and Black Americans: Special psychosocial issues. *Public Health Reports, 102*(2), 224–231.

Mays, V., & Cochran, S. (1988). Issues in the perception of AIDS risk and risk reduction activities by Black and Hispanic/Latina women. *American Psychologist, 43*(11), 949–957.

McCabe, P. M., & Schneiderman, N. (1985). Psychophysiologic reactions to stress. In N. Schneiderman & J. T. Tapp (Eds.), *Behavioral medicine: The biopsychosocial approach* (pp 99–131). Hillsdale, NJ: Lawrence Erlbaum.

McGrady, A., Woerner, M., Bernal, G. A. A., & Higgins, J. T. (1987). Effect of biofeedback-assisted relaxation on blood pressure and cortisol levels in normotensives and hypertensives. *Journal of Behavioral Medicine, 10,* 301–310.

McKusick, L., Horstman, W., & Coates, T. (1985). AIDS and sexual behavior reported by gay men in San Francisco. *American Journal of Public Health, 75*(15), 493–496.

McNaughton, M., Patterson, T., & Grant, I. (1988, April). *Psychosocial factors, depression, and immune status in a group of elderly women.* Paper presented at the ninth annual scientific meeting of the Society of Behavioral Medicine, Boston, MA.

Meichenbaum, D., & Jaremko, M. (Eds.). (1983). *Stress reduction and prevention.* New York: Plenum.

Minkoff, H. (1987). Care of pregnant women infected with human immunodeficiency virus. *Journal of the American Medical Association, 258,* 2714–2717.

Monjan, A. (1987, March). *Behavioral modulation of immune functioning.* Paper presented at the eighth annual scientific meeting of the Society of Behavioral Medicine, Washington, DC.

Monjan, A., & Collector, M. (1977). Stress-induced modulation of the immune response. *Science, 196,* 308–308.

Munoz, A., Wang, M. C., Good, R., Detels, H., Ginsberg, L., Kingsley, J., Phair, J., & Polk, B. F. (1988, June). *Estimation of the AIDS-free times after HIV-1 seroconversion.* Paper presented at the meeting of the International Conference on AIDS, Stockholm, Sweden.

Murphy, G., Simons, A., Wetzel, R., & Lustman, P. (1984). Cognitive therapy and pharmacotherapy: Singly and together in the treatment of depression. *Archives of General Psychiatry, 41,* 33–41.

Nelson, J., Averette, H., & Richart, R. (1984). Dysplasia, carcinoma-*in-situ* and early invasive cervical carcinoma. *CA-A Cancer Journal Clinic, 34*(6), 5–26.

Okamura, K., Fuurukawa, K., Nakakuki, M., Yamadak, & Susuki, M. (1984). Natural killer cell activity during pregnancy. *American Journal of Obstetrics & Gynecology, 149,* 396–399.

Onorato, I., Peterson, L., Pappaioanou, M., & Dondero, T. (1989, June). *Prevalence of HIV infection in heterosexual persons in the United States, 1988–89.* Paper presented at the V International Conference on AIDS, Montreal.

O'Sullivan, M., Fajardo, A., Ferron, P., Efantis, J., Senk, C., & Duthely, M. (1989). *Seroprevalence in a pregnant multiethnic population.* Paper presented at the V International Conference on AIDS, Montreal.

Padian, N., Shiboski, S., & Jewell, N. (1990, June). The relative efficiency of female-to-male HIV sexual transmission. Paper presented at the sixth International Conference on AIDS, San Francisco, CA.

Parker, J., Frank, R., Beck, N., Smarr, K., Bevscher, K., Phillips, L., Smith, E., & Anderson, S. (1987). *Pain management in rheumatoid arthritis: A cognitive-behavioral approach.* Unpublished manuscript.

Patterson, T., Grant, I., & McClurg, J. (1986, April). *Relationship between immune status and stressful events in an elderly population.* Paper presented at the seventh annual scientific meeting of the Society of Behavioral Medicine, New York.

Pavlidis, N., & Chirigos, M. (1980). Stress-induced impairment of macrophage tumoricidal function. *Psychosomatic Medicine, 42,* 47–54.

Pawlikowski, M., Zelazowski, P., Dohler, K., & Stepien, H. (1988). Effects of two neuropeptides, somatoliberin (GRF) and corticoliberin (CRF), on human lymphocyte natural killer activity. *Brain, Behavior, and Immunity, 2,* 50–56.

Penn, I. (1982). The occurrence of cancer in immune deficiencies. *Current Problems in Cancer, 6,* 1–64.

Penn, I. (1986). Cancers of the anogenital region in renal transplant recipients. *Cancer, 58,* 6111–6116.

Pericic, D., Manev, H., Boranic, M., Poljak-Blazi, M. & Lakic, N. (1987). Effect of diazepam on brain neurotransmitters, plasma cortisol, and the immune system of stressed rats. *Annals of the New York Academy of Sciences, 496,* 450–458.

Peterman, T., Cates, W., & Curran, J. (1988). The challenge of human immunodeficiency virus (HIV) and acquired immunodeficiency syndrome (AIDS) in women and children. *Fertility and Sterility, 49,* 571–581.

Plaut, M. (1987). Lymphocyte hormone receptors. *Annual Review of Immunology, 5,* 621–669.

Plotnikoff, N., Wybran, J., Nimeh, N., & Miller, G. (1986). Methionine enkephalin: Enhancement of T-cells in patients with Kaposi's Sarcoma (AIDS). *Psychopharmacology Bulletin, 22,* 695.

Quinn, T., Cannon, R., Glasser, D., Groseclose, S., Brathwaite, W., Fauci, A., & Hook, E. (1990). The association of syphilis with risk of human immunodeficiency virus infection in patients attending sexually transmitted disease clinics. *Archives of Internal Medicine, 150,* 1297–1302.

Quinn, T., Glasser, D., Cannon, R., Matuszak, D., Dunning, R., Kline, R., Campbell, C., Israel, E., Fauci, A., & Hook, E. (1988). Human immunodeficiency virus infection among patients attending clinics for sexually-transmitted diseases. *New England Journal of Medicine, 318*(4), 197–203.

Redfield, R., Markham, P., Salahuddin, S., Wright, D., Sarnagadharan, M., & Gallo, R. (1985). Heterosexually acquired HTLV-III/LAV disease (AIDS-related complex and AIDS): Epidemiologic evidence for female-to-male transmission. *Journal of the American Medical Association, 254,* 2094–2096.

Rivera, E., Hersh, E., Bowen, J., Barnett, J., Wharton, T., & Murphy, S. (1979). Leukocyte migration inhibition assay of tumor immunity in patients with cervical squamous cell carcinoma. *Cancer, 43,* 2297–2305.

Robb, J., Benirescke, K., & Barmeyer, R. (1986). Intrauterine latent herpes simplex virus infection: I. Spontaneous abortion. *Human Pathology, 17,* 1196–1209.

Rodin, J. (1988, April). *Aging, control, and health.* Paper presented at the ninth annual scientific meeting of the Society of Behavioral Medicine, Boston, MA.

Romaquera, J., Zorilla, C., Diaz, C., Moscoso, R., De La Vega, A., & Carrodeguas, J. (1989, June). *Pregnancy outcome in women. HIV infection in Puerto Rico in a population of predominant heterosexual transmission.* Paper presented at the V International Conference on AIDS, Montreal.

Rush, A., Beck, A., Kovacs, M., Weisenburger, J., & Holon, S. (1982). Comparison of the effects of cognitive therapy and pharmacotherapy on hopelessness and self-concept. *American Journal of Psychiatry, 139*(7), 862–866.

Sarason, I. (1979, 2 August). *Life stress, self-preoccupation, and social supports.* Paper presented at the annual meeting of the Western Psychological Association, Washington, D.C.

Sawanobori, S., Ashman, R., Nahmias, A., Benigno, B., & La Via, M. (1977). Rosette formation and abilities in cervical dysplasia and carcinoma *in-situ. Cancer Research, 37,* 4332–4335.

Schafer, A., Friedman, W., & Schwarthlander, B. (1989, June). *Differences in immunosuppression during pregnancy in HIV-infected women.* Paper presented at the V International Conference on AIDS, Montreal.

Schleifer, S., Keller, S., Siris, S., Davis, K., & Stein, M. (1985). Depression and immunity: Lymphocyte function in ambulatory depressed patients, hospitalized schizophrenic patients, and patients hospitalized for herniorrhaphy. *Archives of General Psychiatry, 42*(2), 129–133.

Scott, G. (1989). Perinatal HIV-1 infection: Diagnosis and management. *Clinical Obstetrics & Gynecology, 32*(3), 477–484.

Selye, H. (1976). *Stress in health and disease.* Reading, MA: Butterworths.

Shavit, Y., & Martin, F. (1987). Opiates, stress, and immunity: Animal studies. *Annals of Behavioral Medicine, 9*(2), 11–15.

Shavit, Y., Lewis, J., Terman, G., Gale, R., & Liebeskind, J. (1984). Opioid peptides mediate the suppressive effect of stress on natural killer cell cytotoxicity. *Science, 223,* 188–190.

Shelley, W., & Wood, M. (1981). Transformation of the common wart into squamous cell carcinoma in a patient with primary lymphedema. *Cancer, 48,* 820–824.

Shokri-Tabibzadeh, S., Koss, L., Molnar, J., & Romney, S. (1981). Association of human papillomavirus with neoplastic processes in the genital tract of four women with impaired immunity. *Gynecologic Oncology, 12,* S129–S140.

Sibinga, N., & Goldstein, A. (1988). Opioid peptides and opioid receptors in cells of the immune system. *Annual Review of Immunology, 6,* 219–249.

Siegel, K., Grodsky, P., & Herman, A. (1986). AIDS risk-reduction guidelines: A review and analysis. *Journal of Community Health, 11*(4), 233–243.

Siegel, K., Mesagno, F., Chen, J., & Christ, G. (1987, June). *Factors distinguishing homosexual males practicing safe and risky sex.* Paper presented at the III International Conference of AIDS, Washington, DC.

Sillman, F., Stanek, A., Sedis, A., Rosenthal, J., Lanks, K., Buchhagen, D., Nicastri, A., & Boyce, J. (1984). The relationship between human papillomavirus and lower genital intraepithelial neoplasia in immunosuppressed women. *American Journal of Obstetrics & Gynecology, 150,* 300–308.

Simons, A., Garfield, S., & Murphy, G. (1984). The process of change in cognitive therapy and pharmacotherapy: Changes in mood and cognition. *Archives of General Psychiatry, 41,* 45–51.

Solomon, G. F. (1987). Psychoneuroimmunologic approaches to research on AIDS. *Annals of the New York Academy of Sciences, 496,* 628–636.

Solomon, G. F., & Temoshok, L. (1987). A psychoneuroimmunologic perspective on AIDS research: Questions, preliminary findings and suggestions. *Journal of Applied Social Psychology, 17*(3), 286–308.

Solomon, G., Temoshok, L., O'Leary, A., & Zich, J. (1987). An intensive psychoimmunologic study of long-surviving persons with AIDS. *Annals of the New York Academy of Sciences, 496,* 647–655.

Stall, R., McKusick, L., Wiley, J., Coates, T., & Ostrow, D. (1986). Alcohol and drug use during sexual activity and compliance with safe sex guidelines for AIDS: The AIDS behavioral research project. *Health Education Quarterly, 13*(4).

Stevens, C. E., Taylor, P. E., & Zang, E. A. (1986). Human T-cell lymphotropic virus Type III in a cohort of homosexual men in New York City. *Journal of the American Medical Association, 225,* 2167–2171.

Stites, D., Stobo, J., Fudenberg, H., & Wells, J. (1982). *Basic and clinical immunology* (4th ed.). Los Altos, CA: Lange.

Stravynski, A., & Greenberg, D. (1987). Cognitive therapies with neurotic disorders: Clinical utility and related issues. *Comprehensive Psychiatry, 28*(2), 141–150.

Sweeney, R., Allen, D., & Onorato, I. (1989, June). *HIV infection among women attending women's health clinics in the United States, 1988–89.* Paper presented at the V International Conference on AIDS, Montreal.

Teshima, H., Sogawa, H., Kihara, S., Nagata, S., Ago, Y., & Nakagawa, T. (1987). Changes in populations of T cell subsets due to stress. *Annals of the New York Academy of Sciences, 496,* 459–466.

Tross, S., Hirsch, D., Rabkin, B., Berry, C., & Holland, J. (1987, June). *Determinants of current psychiatric disorder in AIDS spectrum patients.* Paper presented at the III International Conference on AIDS, Washington, DC.

Turk, D., Holzman, A., & Kerns, R. (1986). Chronic pain. In K. Holroyd, & T. Creer (Eds.), *Self-management of chronic disease: Handbook of clinical interventions and research.* Orlando, FL: Academic Press.

Weisenberg, M. (1987). Psychological intervention for the control of pain. *Behavioral Research & Therapy, 25*(4), 301–312.

Williams, N., Coyne, M., & Ryan, J. (1989, June). *The relative risk of AIDS for the Black and Hispanic communities in New Jersey.* Paper presented at the V International Conference on AIDS, Montreal.

Withum, D., LaLota, M., Holtzman, D., Buff, F., Chan, M., & Lieb, S. (1989, June). *Prevalence of HIV antibodies in childbearing women in Florida.* Paper presented at the V International Conference on AIDS, Montreal.

Woodward, C., Thomlinson, J., & Hambling, M. (1987). Immunity to cytomegalovirus amongst pregnant women with differing racial backgrounds. *Public Health, 101,* 329–332.

Wybran, J., Schandene, L., Van Vooren, J., Vandermoten, G., Latinne, D., Sonnet, T., deBruyere, M., Toelman, H., & Plotnikoff, N. (1987). Immunologic properties of methionine-enkephalin, and therapeutic implications in AIDS, ARC, and cancer. *Annals of the New York Academy of Science, 496,* 108–113.

Young, E., Killam, A., & Green, J. (1976). Disseminated herpes virus infection: Association with primary genital herpes in pregnancy. *Journal of the American Medical Association, 235,* 2731–2733.

Zones, J., Beeson, D., Echenberg, D., Rutherford, G., & O'Malley, P. (1987, June). *Management of confidentiality by a cohort of gay and bisexual men who have learned their antibody status.* Paper presented at the III International Conference on AIDS, Washington, DC.

Zuckerman, M., Tushup, R., & Finner, S. (1976). Sexual attitudes and experience: Attitude and personality correlates and changes produced by a course on sexuality. *Journal of Consulting and Clinical Psychology, 144,* 7–19.

5

Psychotherapy of the HIV-Positive Patient and Family
An Integrated Approach

SEANA HIRSCHFELD SHAW

INTRODUCTION

HIV infection is a catastrophic event for the individual and family members. The diagnosis of HIV infection can be regarded as a traumatic event. In addition to the awareness of being infected by an infectious virus, there is fear of loss of financial security and social status. Social isolation and the stigma of being HIV positive lead to feelings of alienation and despair. An integrated and comprehensive psychotherapy approach can address the multifaceted issues.

Health care providers are faced with the challenge of learning the nuances of treatment of the HIV infection and the acquired immunodeficiency syndrome. A biopsychosocial approach is most useful. It will be necessary to become knowledgeable about the advances in diagnosis and treatment of HIV infection as well as the natural history of the infection and the special characteristics of HIV. There is resistance to acquiring such information due to the shroud of stigma and societal rejection that surrounds the HIV situation. HIV infection can be devastating to the individual and family. Death and dying issues in young persons are especially hard for professionals to deal with. Public health policy, confidentiality, and privacy issues may be formidable obstacles in communicating and acquiring information about the HIV status of patients and those at risk for being infected by HIV. The professional may avoid the patient rather than become involved in a situation that is fraught with ambivalence and complexity. High-

SEANA HIRSCHFELD SHAW • University of Miami, School of Medicine, Miami, Florida 33101.

Living and Dying with AIDS, edited by Paul I. Ahmed, Plenum Press, New York, 1992.

risk populations may be particularly difficult to treat because of characterological problems and countertransference issues.

The health care professional is usually the initial provider of mental health care. The initial contact with the HIV-positive person, usually at the time of pretest counseling or when notifying the person of his or her HIV test status, is crucial in preparing the person for the psychological traumata that will be part of the HIV infection. Notifying parents of HIV positivity of their child is particularly stressful for the health care professional.

Preparing the patient for the stress of the initial adjustment to the diagnosis can modify and often prevent severe depressive and adjustment problems. In addition, there are underground treatments and several research treatments that the HIV-positive patient will consider in the course of the illness. The HIV-positive patient experiences the HIV infection as a psychic trauma and is caught in a tragic situation. Shame and stigma are part of the psychological and social experience. Depression and suicidal ideation are common consequences. The trauma, tragedy, shame, and stigma need to be worked through as part of the psychotherapeutic treatment.

REVIEW OF LITERATURE

There are numerous articles on psychosocial treatment issues involving special patient populations. Lomax and Sandler (1988) summarize the psychological issues and propose a goal-oriented approach. Morin, Charles, and Malyon (1984), describe the psychosocial reaction accompanying the AIDS diagnosis in gay men. Dilley (1984) describes the psychological issues and treatment approaches in the three stages in the progression of the illness. Nichols (1983, 1985) discusses the four phases of the HIV condition and uses a supportive and cognitive behavioral approach. Knowledge of the psychodynamics of the dying patient is useful. Death and dying issues as explicated in the work of Kübler-Ross (1969) and Becker (1973) can readily be applied to AIDS patients. Psychological stress on the family is outlined by Frierson, Lippmann, and Johnson (1987). They highlight the frequent sources of stress as being the revelation of homosexuality or bisexual activity, the unremitting nature of the condition, loss of privacy, grief, and a sense of helplessness. Of benefit is the provision of information, nonjudgmental attitude, grief counseling and peer support groups. Volberding (1988) describes an integrated approach to the treatment of the patient with AIDS, drawing from early experience with the world's first inpatient unit at San Francisco General Hospital.

BACKGROUND OF HIV EPIDEMIC

In June of 1981, the Centers for Disease Control first reported that two unusual and seemingly dissimilar outbreaks of Kaposi's sarcoma and *Pneumo-*

cystis carinii pneumonia were occurring in gay men and intravenous drug abusers (CDC, 1981). In 1983, the etiologic agent was identified. The acquired immunodeficiency syndrome (AIDS) is caused by the human immunodeficiency virus (HIV), which renders the host profoundly immunoincompetent. Patients with AIDS are susceptible to a plethora of bacterial, protozoal, fungal, viral, and helminthic opportunistic infections, as well as unusual malignancies. AIDS has already killed hundreds of thousands of people in over 100 countries. In addition to illness, disability, and death, AIDS has brought fear to the hearts of many—fear of disease and fear of the unknown.

At the beginning of the AIDS pandemic, many people had little sympathy for patients with AIDS. The feeling was that somehow people from certain groups deserved their illness. The traditional dread of homosexuality has become part of the irrational reaction to AIDS.

The epidemic of AIDS is without parallel in the history of medicine. Victims are stripped of their immunity, develop unusual malignancies, and succumb to recurrent and progressive opportunistic infections. As of January 1991, AIDS has afflicted more than 100,000 people in the United States and is stressing our medical resources, with the total number of AIDS patients doubling every 14 months.

SPECIAL CLINICAL ISSUES IN THE MILITARY

In October 1985, the U.S. Armed Services began testing all active duty personnel for evidence of infection with the HIV virus. Mandatory testing is essential, as active duty soldiers are given attenuated-live virus vaccinations. This procedure can be life threatening to an immunocompromised individual. In addition, soldiers in combat zones may be needed as blood donors, and the HIV status is required to be a blood donor. The mandatory-testing situation created a unique clinical situation in that otherwise healthy individuals were involuntarily tested for their HIV status. Those who were found to be positive faced the stigma and shock of diagnosis. In 1984 and 1985, there was considerable stigma and hysteria.

The testing procedure involved an educational briefing about the HIV virus, including how it was transmitted and the common risk factors for infection, that is, sexual transmission, IV drug use, or blood transfusion. Blood samples for HIV antibody testing were obtained, and the soldier was told that he or she would be notified if the test was positive. Shortly after the start of this testing it was discovered that soldiers, on learning that they tested positive, were experiencing severe psychological reactions including a high frequency of suicidal behavior. These soldiers had been informed that they tested positive and had been counseled, as required by Department of Defense policy, regarding the progressive and infectious nature of their infection (Herbold, 1986).

Stress Reactions and Suicidal Behaviors

In January 1986, a soldier who was at the Walter Reed Army Medical Center (WRAMC) for staging and evaluation of his HIV infection killed himself. Pfc AA was a 27-year-old Caucasian, active duty new recruit whose basic training was interrupted when the testing results became known. He was transferred to WRAMC for medical evaluation. In the medical hold barracks (an open-bed facility for soldiers), he displayed sexually provocative behaviors with peers and superiors. Information obtained from several sources indicated that he had a history of emotional distress prior to his military service. Pfc AA committed suicide a few weeks after returning from Christmas leave to visit his family. Investigation subsequent to his suicide revealed that, on the night of his death, he had been distressed after a telephone call to his family, had suffered a "rejection" by his barracks' mates, and had been drinking heavily.

This case brought to the awareness of the hospital authorities the severity of the emotional stress that these soldiers experience in the process of adjusting to the diagnosis of HIV infection. Psychiatric intervention is directed at suicide prevention, psychological support, and appropriate treatment for the HIV-seropositive soldier. An important finding was derived from experience during World War II—that a soldier's relationship to his group was the determining factor as to how well he would function in battle. Thus, the supports and comforting aspects of HIV-positive patients' immediate environment are important and significantly influence their fate.

Pfc AA had several risk factors. He was HIV positive (in 1985 this factor alone carried an estimated 100-fold increased risk for completed suicide compared to the overall military suicide rate). Additional factors that increased this soldier's risk of suicidal behavior were deviant sexual behavior, peer rejection, risk-taking behavior, alcohol abuse, and threat of administrative action terminating his army career.

Empirical Findings

During the period of January 1986 to September 1988, approximately 550 patients were evaluated on a multidisciplinary unit at WRAMC (Shaw, 1988). These were active duty or retired soldiers and their families. Patients received a psychosocial evaluation and educational program while undergoing evaluation of their HIV status. Of the group of patients seen initially, approximately 50% have been recommended for a medical board. Of those that are retired, there is a sense of relief and a reorganization of their lives. For those with supportive families, there is a return to their family of origin. For those still on active duty, there is a wish to remain healthy and productive. Many are casualties of demoralization and a sense of alienation and isolation. Fear of disability, dependence, and disfigurement is paramount in some individuals.

Career and promotion-oriented soldiers experience loss of stature and prestige and gradual deterioration in morale and self-confidence. The soldier feels insecure and unsupported. There is a loss of identity as a competent, effective soldier. The level of performance falls under this pressure. The soldier is left with the new identity of a damaged person who must accept the illness label. The bar to deployment overseas and the loss of identification with a combat-ready unit is mourned. The symptoms of anxiety and depression usually can no longer be denied, and they take their toll in somatic symptoms such as headaches, chronic fatigue, and sleep disturbance (Rothberg et al., 1990).

The risk factors associated with suicide and suicidal behaviors in the HIV seropositive patient are (1) deviant sexual behavior causing rejection by peers and family; (2) threatened separation from the military because of overt homosexual behavior or behavior unsuitable to military life; (3) alcohol or drug abuse with overt relapse into drug or alcohol use following the diagnosis of HIV positivity (the substance is seen as an attempt to escape from the awareness of the stresses); (4) clinical trait or mental disorder, for example, anxiety or depression (affective disorders are frequently seen in this group of patients); (5) male youth are known to be at high risk for suicidal behavior (the young adult is most apt to experience the HIV diagnosis as a catastrophic threat to his unlived life).

A recent report of findings in HIV-positive air force individuals who made suicide attempts noted that of 650 HIV-seropositive U.S. Air Force individuals consecutively medically evaluated over a 12-month period, 7 had attempted suicide since diagnosis (1.08%), and one had succeeded (0.15%). Several findings differentiated attempters from a matched comparison group of 12 nonsuicidal seropositive individuals: (1) multiple psychosocial stressors, (2) social isolation, (3) substance abuse, (4) perception of external locus of control, (5) physical or serological evidence of disease progression, (6) and loss of effectiveness of the defense mechanism of denial. Presence of cerebro-spinal fluid abnormalities were not predictive in this series. Combinations of these findings were present in all of the suicide attempters. One attempt occurred immediately after learning of seropositive status; all others were several months later. It is suggested that the more of these factors present, the higher the risk of suicide in individuals who are infected with HIV (Rundel, 1988).

A recent study of HIV-infected males (Atkinson et al., 1988) revealed a high lifetime prevalence of specific major psychiatric disorders in ambulatory homosexual men with AIDS. The men had a lifetime rate of alcohol or nonopiate drug abuse of 22/56 (39%), and major depression rate of 17/56 (30.3%) that often preceded diagnosed medical illness or knowledge of HIV status.

TREATMENT ISSUES AND STRATEGIES

The four most turbulent periods for the HIV-positive patient are (1) at the time of the first testing and notification of the diagnosis; (2) when the family, work, and/or peer group learns of the diagnosis; (3) when there is concrete evidence of failing health and progression of the disease; and (4) when death appears imminent and unavoidable.

All patients (and family members if available) who have a positive HIV screening test are seen by a member of their mental health team. The soldier's commander or an equivalent substitute accompanies the soldier to his initial visits and on notification of the test result. This procedure insures that the identification of a person as HIV positive will not be experienced as an overwhelming event in the context of being abandoned and unprotected. This preventive measure allows for rapid, early development of a treatment alliance and builds the patient's confidence that his or her needs will be met.

At first there is disbelief and emotional numbing. The person often reports that he or she is in shock or numb. There is crying or a frozen, anxious affect. Depending on the underlying preexisting personality structure and the degree of preexisting mental health problems, the person will recover to some degree from the state of emotional shock and numbing with the help of empathic supportive psychotherapy, counseling, and information. By supporting defenses that promote rejoining to the existing social matrix, the person can maintain his or her sense of control and mastery. The person is encouraged to form a positive therapeutic relationship and develop a positive transference reaction. It is important to engage the patient at this point because there is an opportunity for crisis intervention. Carl Rogers noted that the necessary and sufficient conditions for psychotherapy are warmth, empathy, genuineness, and unconditional positive regard.

Once the patient has formed a trusting relationship with his or her infectious disease physician and a therapeutic alliance with the therapist, issues such as who to tell about the HIV infection, sexual behavior, the need for infection control and safer sex, drug use, family relationships, and dating come to the surface. If the patient trusts the therapist, there will be an exploration of behaviors with the idea of working with the therapist to preserve health and promoting altruistic goals. Losses are mourned. There is anger about the foregoing of many goals, for example, children of one's own, a military career, marriage, a long life, career goals. Many patients have the need of retaining their privacy at work and in their personal lives and fabricate a secret that they use as an explanation for their absences from work. Some strive to understand rejection and prejudicial actions against them. Some fear exposure of their homosexual preference. For some there are numerous incidents of poor judgment that come to the commander's attention or into legal action. Drug abuse relapse, AWOL, and DWI are frequent in those with past history of such behaviors prior to army service.

For some patients, severe characterological problems or strong antisocial traits make it difficult for them to cooperate with medical regimens or to give up risk-taking behavior and practice infection control. These soldiers will often get into legal difficulties on a command level. Once they become physically ill and incapacitated, they are usually more amenable to control of undesirable behaviors. Participation in AZT treatment and in the medical management of their infections and/or cancers is often the motivation for them to change their antisocial behaviors.

FAMILY ISSUES

Families affected by the HIV infection represent every ethnic group and walk of life. Problems will vary according to the socioeconomic status, ethnic background, and prior experience of prejudice. In addition, the mode of acquiring the HIV infection will be a significant factor. Those infected by blood transfusion or donor organs will not bear the guilt and remorse that is borne by those who contracted the virus by past risk-taking behaviors. The soldier may belong to a dysfunctional family, as this is usually found associated with substance abuse, a known cofactor in the acquisition of HIV infection.

Shame and fear of public rejection and fear of family disintegration are the main concerns of soldiers infected with HIV. School-age children face rejection by community and school. Adult children of HIV-infected parents fear rejection and humiliation. Some children become active in support groups and public education in an attempt to regain dignity and self-esteem. Others wish for privacy and anonymity.

Mothers who are infected and have advanced illness feel inadequate to care for their children because of fatigue and preoccupation with their health. Mothers who have breast fed their babies and subsequently learn of their HIV-positive status fear that they infected their child while trying to be nurturing and close. Separation anxiety and a pervasive mourning for the loss of their future are issues. The thought of having infected their child brings guilt and remorse. For those who have children who are not infected, the thought of having to give up their children is overwhelming. Many of these parents do not have extended families.

For some of the families there has been substance abuse as the risk factor, and the family situation with substance abusers is dysfunctional or disrupted. Tenuous marriages often end after the diagnosis of HIV. The anger about, and the fear of exposure to, HIV is enough to accentuate any latent ambivalence or discord and disrupt the marriage.

Case Vignette. This is a young military family. Husband and wife grew up together in a large metropolitan area and come from dysfunctional families, where child neglect and emotional abuse were the norm. The husband acquired HIV most probably from IV drug abuse as a teenager, a practice that was rampant in his neighborhood. The couple have been married 8 years. They have two young children under the age of 5. A year ago the couple were told they were positive for HIV. The mother was breast feeding her new baby, then 3 months old. She immediately stopped breast-feeding and both children were tested. Both have tested negative so far. The wife believes that she and her husband are going to die soon and has kept this a secret. When she shared her situation with neighbors and close friends, they turned away from her and her family and broke off contact. She is afraid of anyone in her new location finding out. She has not shared with her family, as they have already rejected her on several other occasions and were abusive to her as a child. The same situation is true of her husband's family. Both feel stressed and have no one to talk to. The older child has become aware that there is a serious health problem and expressed wishes to die with his parents rather than be left without them.

This case brings to the fore the tragic situation of the HIV-infected family. In this case it is likely that the children are not infected. There is significant pain and sorrow of these young parents. The lack of family support is usual in the HIV-infected population. There is usually a lack of protection and support, and this needs to be sought from community resources or distant relatives. Often the HIV-infected person is the supporter of others.

Case Vignette. This case is of a 40-year-old father of three who developed depression following diagnosis of HIV infection. The patient (Pt) has a wife and three daughters, who are HIV negative. Pt traces his HIV exposure to IV drug abuse, which he stopped before his marriage. Pt feels slowed down, has poor concentration and trouble driving, so he gave up his license. He has had several relapses into alcoholism since the HIV diagnosis, whereas he was hitherto in control. He has had an unsuccessful experience in the inpatient alcohol rehabilitation program but has moderate symptom relief with antidepressants and psychostimulants. It was with great caution that the psychostimulants were used, as there was a history of substance abuse including cocaine. Once it was decided to proceed with his medical retirement, several issues surfaced, such as the wife's insecurity concerning her husband's health and ability to care for the family. Pt's wife decided to return, with the children, to live with her parents. Suicidal thoughts, guilt, rejection, shame, and low self-esteem plagued Pt. His support system during this crisis was his treatment team and multidisciplinary unit.

This case illustrates the catastrophic impact of HIV infection on the family. Financial insecurity and concerns of losing the family member surface. There is guilt surrounding acquiring the HIV infection and fear of infecting the surviving spouse.

HOMOSEXUALITY

In addition to the legal predicament, the homosexual in the military carries a great risk of exposure and ridicule from "straight" soldiers. Homosexual behavior in the army is considered grounds for administrative separation and discharge from active duty. HIV seropositivity makes it virtually impossible for the soldier to conceal his sexual identity and preference. In some instances there is exposure of a homosexual lifestyle, and such soldiers are subjected to peer rejection, hostility, and alienation. Physical assaults against such soldiers have occurred. The HIV epidemic has increased the hostility toward homosexuals, and aggressive acts have been more frequent. Depression and stress of HIV diagnosis can lead to more risk taking and driven sexual behavior and relapse into drug abuse.

The myths that have been created about gay persons are problems themselves because they create inappropriate, negative, and stigmatizing attitudes toward homosexuality. Surveys indicate that approximately two-thirds of the American people feel that homosexuals are "harmful" to society and regard homosexuals with disgust, discomfort, or fear. Homophobia is often internalized and expressed as low self-esteem.

Societal rejection pushes homosexuals to form their own distinctive subculture. The HIV diagnosis brings to the surface issues regarding a homosexual lifestyle. There is fear of rejection by one's parents or by one's spouse and children. Often there is also a feeling of rejection by one's church and a discordance with one's religious beliefs. There is guilt, shame, humiliation and a profound sense of loss.

Case Vignette. M is a 23-year-old male recovering alcoholic and polysubstance abuser, with 3 years of outstanding service as an office administrator. M is the son of an actively alcoholic and rejecting father. M was diagnosed HIV positive 9 months previously and had a relapse of alcoholism after notification of test results. He reentered treatment in AA and later sought out patient therapy. He was treated with antidepressants and psychotherapy, and AA was continued on a regular basis. M could not accept the HIV diagnosis and felt that others would reject him. He wanted to tell his father about the HIV diagnosis but feared further rejection, as the HIV positivity would confirm, for his father, that his son was homosexual, and M was sure that his father would be critical and rejecting. M's mother and a circle of friends on the West Coast were the main support structure for the patient. At work M experienced disapproval by his commander and was passed over for better assignments and more interesting work. M began provoking the commander with his risk-taking behaviors. He relapsed into substance abuse, using poor judgment and failure to protect himself from the possibility of a positive drug screen. M's emotional need was to assert himself and rebel against the authority of his commander by forcing him to see his homosexuality. The situation improved when the dynamics of the situation were interpreted to M and he could take steps to relate to both his commander and father in more realistic ways, thus avoiding the punishment and rejection that he previously elicited.

This case demonstrates the many emotional issues that confront young persons with HIV infection. Relationships with family and authority figures and their place in society are conflicted and leave young persons feeling isolated and alienated and often suicidal. Treatment is essential to bring about a resolution to the overwhelming chaos.

PSYCHOTHERAPY

Psychotherapists draw from the wisdom and techniques of several schools of therapy. What is important is the evaluation and assessment of what the patient needs and the application of treatment in as skillful a manner as possible. Psychotherapy of the HIV-infected person and his or her family requires understanding of the HIV infection and knowledge in crisis intervention techniques as well as the usual techniques for more conventional treatment needs. The clinical hypothesis is the underlying guiding direction. The HIV-positive patient often needs such diverse interventions as crisis intervention and preventive interventions such as education, advice, psychological support, family therapy, and/or long-term individual psychotherapy. The therapist needs to be knowledgeable of the stresses and crises that are part of the HIV-positive condition and be prepared to offer ongoing treatment and contact. The stress and trauma of the HIV diagnosis is superimposed on the pressures of the developmental life stage and coexist with the state and trait psychiatric givens for each patient.

When treating the HIV-positive patient, it is best to use a fisherman's net approach so as to encompass the many facets of the condition. All psychotherapies, including brief psychotherapy, share the importance of nonspecific curative factors in their anticipated outcomes. These factors—abreaction, new information, and success experiences—guide all forms of medical treatment in which clinicians are striving to increase the probability that patients will experience relief of pain and suffering.

The psychodynamic life narrative is useful to treat a patient in a crisis situation. A powerful bond between physician and patient is formed and offers the possibility of a rapid relief from dysphoric symptoms. It is most effective in patients whose general adaptation has been stable and whose psychological homeostasis has been disrupted by a life event of real and symbolic significance (Viederman, 1983).

Psychotherapy issues often include a split in the transference between the therapist and the treating physician. Positive and negative transference feelings will shift. At times patients will experience paranoid feelings and anger toward the primary physician; as an authority figure, he or she is blamed for the patients predicament. Transference distortions are lessened with multimodal psychotherapy (collaboration with support groups, substance abuse treatments, social services, family members, art therapy, nutritionists, etc.).

Existential issues often focus on the need to accept a shortened life. The connection of death and sexual intimacy is perplexing and often the source of guilt. Issues and conflicts related to the sexual lifestyle need to be understood in the context of needs and wishes of the individual.

Managing the stress of the HIV diagnosis is crucial. There is extraordinary stress surrounding the diagnosis of HIV infection, the progression of one's illness, and the infection of a child or partner. Horowitz (1976) cites the following as typical phases of response to a stressful event: the individual usual responds with outcry (Oh God! Oh God! Oh God!), denial (It isn't true! You're joking! It's not true!), or affective numbing and repetitive thoughts about the event. As noted by Caplan (1964) and Lindemann (1944), these initial reactions to catastrophe are reflexive and probably serve some adaptive function. Outcry is accompanied by an automatic discharge like the flight–fight response described by Cannon (1932), and denial has a resemblance to dissociative mechanisms of ego defense. Caplan traces the sequences of responses from the dazed impact or flight–fight response to affective flooding, that in turn is followed by coping efforts.

Patients facing terminal illness who are able to defend well (major deniers) not only lower their anxiety and raise their hopes but also survive significantly longer. One should not confuse neurotic denial in nonemergency situations with "denial in service of the need to survive." Denial may also be used to master painful affects (Hackett & Cassem, 1970).

The phase of cognitive and affective integration is best examined by referring to the model of the ego described by Hartmann (1958) as the central, creative part of the personality that synthesizes, rationalizes, and makes do with whatever tools it has to bring to the individual the greatest possible peace and function during deviations (trauma) from the "average expectable environment." Integration is accomplished when the individual optimally balances mechanisms of defense with the capacity for the tolerance of negative affects and emerges with flexible yet realistic plans for dealing with trauma in the present and anticipating problems that may emerge in the future.

Integration depends at least partially on the stressed individual's ability to shoulder what Lindemann (1944) aptly terms grief work. Grief work is the process of experiencing the painful affects associated with mourning to gain emancipation from bondage to what is lost. The major obstacle to doing grief work is the individual's unwillingness to suffer the pain of mourning. The psychotherapist's task in such work is to encourage grief work and support the grieving individual.

Those patients who have difficulty experiencing their affects, (e.g., drug abusers) will need added help. Supportive psychotherapy, role-playing events, support groups, drug and alcohol treatments (AA, NA) and psychotropic medications are often added to psychotherapies.

COUNTERTRANSFERENCE ISSUES

Is there something about an epidemic that is like a magnet, that compels one to get caught up and that becomes larger than life? When there is great tragedy and loss, humans cling strongly to life and rebuild with great vigor after a disaster. We don't lose our faith but instead renew it. When confronted by a community disaster, a group or society may be imprinted by it; deny it; incorporate it or even relish its destructiveness; mourn the losses it brings; survive it; survive it with guilt; memorialize it. So also may the individual in the personal disasters of his or her life.

Psychiatrists are no strangers to patients who are stigmatized, undeserved, or chronically ill. Countertransference issues that have been identified by mental health workers are: (1) fear of the unknown, (2) fear of contagion, (3) fear of dying and of death, (4) denial of helplessness, (5) fear of homosexuality (homophobia), (6) overidentification, (7) anger, and (8) need for professional omnipotence (Dunkel & Hatfield, 1986).

The fact that an individual survived when another did not may lead to a feeling of elation and excitement. Yet this feeling cannot be justified in light of the deaths of others, and so guilt rapidly appears.

TRAUMA

Studies of psychic trauma led to the formulation of psychic trauma as being understood not in terms of the intensity of stimuli, but rather in relation to the psychic reality of the individual and how that person interprets and reacts to a traumatic experience. Thus, the traumatic memories, the nature of self, object, and world representations would be involved in the shaping of the impact of a potentially traumatic experience. In addition, affect tolerance has a major role in all traumas. Krystal (1984), in his genetic studies of affects, presents a scheme to understand the role of affects in traumatic situations. The "freezing" response seen in adult catastrophic patterns may be related to infantile affective responses. The developmental lines of emotions to be taken into consideration are "differentiation, verbalization, and desomatization."

STIGMA

Stigma is defined as something that detracts from the character or reputation of a person—a mark of disgrace or reproach. AIDS seems to be equated with sin, requiring retribution and punishment. Often patients will feel that they deserve to be infected as they did something wrong.

A few years ago, herpes was one of the major preoccupations in this country. But AIDS appears to be another story. For one thing, unlike herpes it is usually fatal. It also seems to afflict primarily homosexuals and intravenous drug abusers. The combination of these two facts has sparked in conservative religious thinkers round the country a very old answer—retributive justice.

Lex talionis, the law of retribution, is a theological perspective deeply etched in the hearts of many people. It takes a certain amount of hardening of the heart to remain loyal to this early Old Testament point of view. In Exodus, the plagues of Egypt were explained as just punishment for the sins of the pharaoh. Since that time, there seem always to have been enough well-meaning self-righteous individuals around to allow retributive justice to survive. The old formula has been applied to the victims of AIDS; they have done something wrong, and the hand of a righteous God is striking them down.

Ironically, in the Book of Job, an Old Testament work written centuries after Exodus, we find a sustained attack on retributive justice as the proper interpretation for the meaning of human suffering. In the opening verse we learn that Job is "blameless and upright."

In our time, Albert Camus, in his novel *The Plague,* appears also to have had a keen sense of the shortcomings of retributive justice as a mature and coherent response to the problem of suffering.

DISCUSSION

Our patients' lives have a tragic quality. The ending is foretold; life is telescoped into a brief time. We are presently powerless to change the fatal outcome, and thus feelings of pity and fear are provoked. We are in an unsuccessful race against time. Our own denial keeps us from being overwhelmed and forever saddened.

While natural disasters generate anger at God, at the world, at nature, a much greater anger appears in response to disasters that are seen as somehow the consequence of human error or vulnerability. These disasters seem to awaken all the primitive causal logic that someone must be to blame for death and destruction. Here blame is allocated either by formal inquiry into the disaster or in the minds of the bereaved and others affected.

Loss, the psychological event leading to the experience of being bereft, may be in response to something obvious and concrete, or it may be subjective and highly abstract, difficult to define, describe, or even acknowledge. The loss may be of the self, self-image, self-representation and feelings of self-worth, attractiveness, livability, special qualities and capacities, sexual interest, and positive self-attitudes such as pride, esteem, independence, or control. Important ideals may be lost as position in society or status. Developmental loss involving phases of security and predictability occurs, such as an adolescent soldier being deprived of the freedom of youth. Loss is simultaneously a real event and a perception by which the individual endows the event with personal or symbolic meaning. One may experience an event as a loss, such as loss of honor or face, when another individual would not describe it as such. In addition, each loss carries with it the threat of additional or future loss.

Having a serious life-threatening illness can bring losses and high stress or it can bring great change. Personal disasters involve the personal experience of loss. Forces of illness destroy or threaten to destroy the human body. The individual's own fantasies and explanations of destructiveness and his or her own guilt about destruction must inevitably be stirred. This confrontation with the destructiveness of man and nature may be fought against with defenses that are adaptive, so that it can be encompassed as only one facet of human behavior, but one that must be accepted as part of the self.

There may be grief for loss of innocence. Splitting and projection are seen when destructiveness is viewed only as part of others; or it can be internalized with depression, self-destructive lifestyle, even suicide; or to acting out of rage, violence, and destruction because impulses can no longer be controlled. These patterns are seen in the war veteran, but they are also seen in those who encounter personal disaster.

Personal disasters involve the personal experience of loss. They involve a loss of belief in the security of the personal and physical world and in one's own immortality. These losses must be mourned and grieved in the adaptation to personal disaster.

Personal disaster is not forgotten but stays with individuals as a reference point. They may change their lives following it, or they may attempt to repress it, but because of memories and anniversary phenomena, attempts to interpret the disaster remain an ongoing part of their experience.

Death is a part of the life cycle, an inevitable outcome of life that brings closure to a life story. Death can seem like castration when a man is cut down in the prime of his life, thereby rendered impotent to carry out his striving and hopes and to find fulfillment in love. Death is the reaper with a scythe who cuts off life. Death also provides a challenge and a test, particularly to men who must prove to themselves that they can face death and not run or flinch—the essence of bravery. Perhaps a person feels that he must conquer death by looking straight into its hollow eye sockets before he can feel man enough to live (Lidz, 1968).

SUMMARY

In summary, psychotherapeutic approaches draw from the wisdom of past experiences with catastrophic conditions and illness—from the literature on oncology treatment, the support of families with an ill child, and from our past experiences in dealing with stigmatized populations. The health care professional will experience less frustration and demoralization by setting humanistic and reachable therapeutic goals. Professional groups can widen their scope as to patient selection and include HIV patients as worthy of scientific interest and expertise.

Psychotherapists often deal with the narcissistic issues of loss of self-esteem and stigmatization. Existential issues are frequently encountered, such as Why me? facing death in youth, dying with the feeling of isolation and guilt, or rejection by the family. Countertransference feelings take many forms. There may be a sense of futility such as what can one do when death and a short life are inevitable. Professional groups can help reduce the sense of professional isolation of those that work with the HIV-positive patient by incorporating the HIV condition into curricula and scientific meetings and agendas.

REFERENCES

Abrams, D. I., Dilley, J. W., Maxey, L. M., et al. (1986). Routine care and psychosocial support of the patient with the acquired immune deficiency syndrome. *Medical Clinics of North America, 70*(3), pp. 707–720.

Atkinson, J. H., Jr., Grant, I., Kennedy, C. J., et al. (1988). Prevalence of psychiatric disorders among men infected with human immunodeficiency virus. *Archives of General Psychiatry, 45,* 859–864.

Becker, E. (1973). *The denial of death.* New York: The Free Press.

Cannon, W. B. (1932). *The wisdom of the body.* W. W. Norton & Co., New York.

Caplan, G. (1964). *Principles of preventive psychiatry,* Jason Aronson, Inc., New York.

Centers for Disease Control. (1981, June). Pneumocystis pneumonia, *Mortality and Morbidity Weekly Reports, 30,* 250–252.

Dilley, J. (1984). Treatment interventions and approaches on care of patients with acquired immune deficiency syndrome. In *Psychiatric Implications of AIDS,* American Psychiatric Press, Washington, DC.

Dunkel, J., & Hatfield, S. (1986, March). Countertransference issues in working with persons with AIDS, *Journal of Social Work,* pp. 114–117.

Frierson, R. L., Lippmann, S. B., & Johnson, J. (1987). AIDS: Psychological stress on the family. *Psychosomatics, 28,*(2), 65–68.

Hackett, T. P., & Cassem, N. H. (1970). Psychological reactions to a life-threatening illness. In H. Abram (Ed.) *Psychological aspects of stress* (pp. 29–43). C. C. Thomas, Springfield.

Hartmann, H. (1958). *Ego psychology and the problem of adaption.* International Universities Press.

Herbold, J. R. (1986). AIDS policy development within the Department of Defense *Military Medicine, 151*(12), 623–627.

Horowitz, M. J. (1976). *Stress response syndrome.* New York: Jason Aaronson.

Krystal, H. (1984). Psychological views on human emotional damages. In B. A. Van Der Kolk (Ed.), *Post-traumatic stress disorder: Psychological and biological sequalae* (pp. 10–12). Washington, DC: American Psychiatric Press.

Kübler-Ross, E. (1969). *On death and dying.* New York: Macmillan.

Lidz, T. (1968). *The person.* Basic Books, New York.

Lindemann, E. (1944). Symptomatology and management of acute grief, *American Journal of Psychiatry, 101,* 101–149.

Lomax, G. L., & Sandler, J. (1986). Psychotherapy and consultation with persons with AIDS, *Psychiatric Annals, 18*(4), 253–259.

Morin, S. F., Charles, K., & Maylon, A. (1984). The psychological impact of AIDS on gay men. *American Psychologist, 39,* 1288–1293.

Nichols, S. E. (1985). Psychosocial reactions of persons with AIDS, *Annals of Internal Medicine, 103,* 765–767.

Nichols, S. E. (1983). Psychiatric aspects of AIDS, *Psychosomatics, 24*(12), 1083–1089.

Rothberg, J. M., Bain, M. W., Boggiano, W., Cline, W. R., Grace, W. C., Holloway, H. C., & Rock, N. L. (1990). The stress of an HIV-positive diagnosis. *Military Medicine, 155*(3), 98–104.

Rundell, J. R. (1988). Frequent findings in HIV-positive suicide attempts. In *Proceedings of the American Association for Suicide Prevention.* Washington, D.C.

Shaw, S. & Rothberg, J. M. (1988). *A Suicide Prevention Program,* Proceedings, Amer Assoc Suicide Prevention, Washington, D.C.

Viederman, M. (1983). *The Psychiatric life narrative: A psychotherapeutic intervention useful in crisis intervention.* Psychiatry, Vol 1, No. 46 p 236.

Volberding, P. A. (1988). Caring for the person with AIDS, an integrated approach. *Infectious Disease Clinics of North America, 2*(2), 543–550.

Living with AIDS

Coping Processes and Strategies and Personal Resources among Persons with HIV-Spectrum Disease

DAVID D. CELENTANO and AMANDA BENEDICT SONNEGA

INTRODUCTION

Living and coping effectively with HIV-1 infection is an enormous challenge, not only because of the potential lethality of the infection but also because of the chronic nature of illness episodes, which often include frequent hospital stays, and the potential for social discrimination. For the asymptomatic seropositive person infected with HIV-1, the potential for a long latency period (the interval from seroconversion to first symptoms of AIDS) translates the threat of developing AIDS into a chronic stressor commonly leading to psychological distress. For those who are not infected with the virus but who perceive themselves as being at risk for infection or continue to place themselves at risk because of their high-risk behavior, the threat of AIDS is viewed as a profound stressor.

The psychosocial impact of HIV-1/AIDS has been widely discussed in recent years, as the health care community seeks to understand the changes

DAVID D. CELENTANO and AMANDA BENEDICT SONNEGA • Division of Behavioral Sciences and Health Education, Department of Health Policy and Management, The Johns Hopkins University, School of Hygiene and Public Health, Baltimore, Maryland 21205.

Living and Dying with AIDS, edited by Paul I. Ahmed, Plenum Press, New York, 1992.

that occur in patients' lives resulting from HIV spectrum disease. Although the importance of psychosocial research was recognized early on in the HIV-1/AIDS epidemic (Coates, Temoshok, & Mandel, 1984; Morin & Batchelor, 1984), a variety of important issues remain both in the medical and psychosocial arenas as we learn more about the natural history of HIV-1/AIDS. Why do some cases of AIDS progress to death faster than others? What is it about how people with AIDS interact with others that may be related to physical and mental functioning? What interrelationships are there between the immune system, stress, and psychological predispositions? Given the tremendous variety and sources of stress often affecting persons with, and those at high risk of acquiring, HIV-1, the growing reports of a broad spectrum of psychological functioning and distress give witness to the salience of these issues (Faulstich, 1987; Holland & Tross, 1985; Marzuck *et al.,* 1988; Ostrow, 1986; Perry & Tross, 1984).

There is a growing research and societal interest in how persons with AIDS or HIV-1 infection cope with their infection and/or illness and how they use support networks in order to attenuate distress and perhaps even prolong their survival. In this review, we draw from the existing literature on coping and psychosocial responses to HIV-1/AIDS to summarize current issues for future intervention and for a consideration of prevention strategies from a public health perspective.

In reviewing studies that may be relevant to the issue of coping with AIDS or HIV-1 infection, we found several distinct areas of literature. A variety of approaches have been proposed to investigate the relationships between coping, social resources, and HIV-1/AIDS, ranging from adjustment reactions to catastrophic stress (Morin & Batchelor, 1984), modeling the death and dying literature (Friedlander & Arthur, 1988; Nichols, 1985), and coping styles (Namir, Wolcott, Fawzy, & Alumbaugh, 1987). Published investigations range from individual case studies (e.g., Friedlander & Arthur, 1988) to prospective investigations of large cohorts (Ostrow *et al.,* 1989).

To organize the somewhat disparate literature, we begin with a review of studies describing emotional response to HIV-1 infection from a clinical perspective. They commonly consist of reports of the psychiatric morbidity associated with developing a potentially fatal disease but do not represent studies of coping *per se.* We then present a brief review of recent issues in coping research before proceeding to review empirical studies of coping with HIV-1/AIDS. Finally, we review studies that examine the effects of a variety of psychosocial variables that may relate to the issue of differential survivorship. Several investigators are using the multidisciplinary framework of psychoneuroimmunology in hopes of delineating mechanisms that might explain how emotions, coping, and personal resources account for variability in latency period and survival.

EMOTIONAL RESPONSES TO HIV-SPECTRUM ILLNESS

Early studies reported individuals' responses to HIV infection through observation, often in clinical settings. Early in the epidemic, researchers and health professionals began observing characteristics of gay men's response to AIDS. Typical psychological reactions to the threat of AIDS included denial, anger, depression, and self-hatred (Harowski, 1987). Morin, Charles, and Maylon (1984) have reported on hypochondriasis, somatization, and generalized panic attacks. Others have described patients' early responses to HIV-1/AIDS in terms of stages from denial and disbelief to acceptance and preparation for death (Forstein, 1984; Nichols, 1985).

In part, the recognition of the importance of psychosocial factors, and particular coping strategies, emerged from the recognition that suicidal thoughts and actions may be relatively frequent following informing individuals that they are infected with HIV-1 (Glass, 1988). A number of recent reports lend empirical support for this association. Marzuk *et al.* (1988) reported suicide rates 36 times in excess of the rate expected among men with AIDS in New York in 1985, while Kizer, Green, Perkins, Doebbert, and Hughes (1988) reported suicide rates 21 times that expected among young California men in 1986.

Perry, Jacobsberg, and Fishman (1990) investigated suicidal ideation before and following HIV-1 testing and found that overall, suicidal thoughts did not increase following testing. Rather, in the weeks following notification and counseling, rates of self-reported suicidal thoughts decreased significantly among the seronegative participants and did not increase among seropositive subjects. However, suicidal ideation persisted among 15% of both seropositive and seronegative patients. It must be noted, however, that this sample differs from many of the longitudinal investigations of the natural history of HIV-1 infection in that these volunteers had markedly higher rates of depression and substance abuse before testing, all of which are markers for suicidal risk (Perry *et al.,* 1990).

In the medical literature, there has been considerable interest in assessing patients' reactions to the diagnosis of AIDS from a death and dying perspective. Nichols (1985) delineated the emotional process from this stage perspective as encompassing the following steps. First, there is an initial crisis, marked by alternating phases of denial and periods of intense anxiety, in which the emotional reactions include shock, guilt, fear, anger, denial, sadness, bargaining and acceptance (Nichols, 1983). The second phase is a transitional state in which alternating periods of anger, self-pity, guilt, and anxiety overcome denial, a period in which self-esteem erodes and self-isolation may ensue, as well as severe displacement and loss of trust in the medical community. This is commonly followed by the acceptance state, sometimes referred to as "supportive denial" (Dilley, 1984), in which a new, stable identity develops as the patient learns his or her functional limitations and realizes that self-management of the everyday processes of life are still possible and necessary. A final stage, preparation for death, may be marked by an acceptance of mortality or by fear of total dependence on others (Siegel & Hoefer, 1981). The issue of suicide within this group cannot be avoided (Ostrow, Joseph, Monjan, & Kessler, 1986). While this approach fits well within the medical model of disease and intervention, it is predominately based upon anecdotal and observational reports with some concerns raised for the generalizability of conclusions drawn.

Weitz (1989) has proposed that dealing with uncertainty is one of the most salient problems for persons with HIV-1 infection. Using an ethnographic technique of semistructured interview, she obtained data on several sources of uncertainty for persons with AIDS. In general she found that, compared with other chronic diseases, AIDS imposes greater uncertainty for the following reasons: (1) AIDS patients are more likely to be aware that they are at high risk of AIDS well before diagnosis, (2) obtaining a diagnosis may be difficult because of the multiple illnesses that characterize the syndrome, (3) patients may have greater uncertainty regarding the predictability and severity of illness episodes, and (4) because information about AIDS continues to develop and change so rapidly, patients may have difficulty trusting medical advice.

PERSONAL RESOURCES IN HIV-SPECTRUM ILLNESS

The coping literature provides a useful starting place for a more systematic and empirical investigation of how HIV-1/AIDS affects patients' lives. Coping and social support are viewed in the psychosocial literature as being two complementary personal resources that are commonly viewed as mediating the effects of stress on psychological distress. Further, there is literature that demonstrates the positive influence of personal resources on the stress–psychological functioning–physical health continuum.

Generically, coping reflects an internal personal resource, reflecting traits and habitual ways of responding to environmental challenge, while social support refers to the external interpersonal networks that have the capacity to provide assistance (emotional and instrumental) in times of need. We begin this section with a short review of historical issues in coping research and present a rationale for considering use of social support as a coping strategy as a preface to exploring the literature on personal resources and HIV-spectrum illness.

Coping Processes and Strategies

The concept of coping has historical antecedents in ego psychology in which reactions to intrapsychic conflict were categorized under the rubric of defense mechanisms. Emphasizing traits within the individual, psychologists such as

Rappaport, Gill, and Shafer (1945), Cattell (1946), Allport (1966), and others attempted to describe predispositions to react to situations in consistent and enduring ways. Other theorists emphasized a focus on situational determinants of individual reactions (e.g., Mischel, 1968). Speilberger initiated the phrase "state–trait" to refer to an appreciation of the interaction between situational and dispositional determinants of individual reactions to stressful events (Speilberger, 1975).

Since most research on the effects of stress on physiological and psychological functioning has yielded consistent but modest correlations with health outcomes, many researchers have speculated that there were mitigating factors in the relationship between stressors and illness (Rabkin & Struening, 1979). It has been hypothesized that the individual's ability to cope with a stressor may be more predictive of health and well-being than objective events themselves (Antonovsky, 1979; Lazarus, 1981). Coping has therefore been proposed to be a mediating variable between stress and negative emotions generated by a stressor (Folkman & Lazarus, 1988).

Descriptions of coping strategies have been grouped into various conceptual domains. Most commonly (Moos, 1988) they are divided into problem-focused (functioning to alter the stressor itself), emotion-focused (regulating emotional reaction to the stressor), and appraisal-focused (altering the meaning of the stressor) domains. A common and historical assumption is that emotion-focused strategies such as denial and avoidance represent an immature or maladaptive coping style. Indeed, this style of coping with a health threat has generally been shown to be associated with poorer psychological functioning (e.g., Rippetoe & Rogers, 1987). However, in a review of avoidant versus nonavoidant coping strategies, Suls and Fletcher (1985) found that avoidant strategies could be effective in decreasing psychological distress during the beginning of a stressful experience. Furthermore, in dealing with uncontrollable situations, such as having cancer, Meyerowitz, Heinrich, and Schag (1983) have found that denial is a particularly effective coping strategy for some aspects of this experience both in the short and long term.

Early approaches to the study of coping focused on adjustment to a stressor and defined effective coping in terms of successful adjustment. Lazarus's model of coping has been criticized on grounds that the independent variable of coping and the dependent variable (the health outcome under investigation) are operationally and conceptually confounded (Dohrenwend, Dohrenwend, Dodson, & Shrout, 1984). That is, in his transactional model of stress, Lazarus proposed that the individual's perception that a stressor is threatening (primary appraisal) and that it exceeds his or her resources for dealing with it (secondary appraisal) leads to emotional distress. Coping is thus a response to perceived stress and is defined as "constantly changing cognitive and behavioral efforts to manage specific external and/or internal demands that are appraised as taxing or exceeding the resources of the individual" (Lazarus & Folkman, 1984, p. 141).

The implicit assumption is that most stressors (events or circumstances with an objective reality) in themselves are not stressful. In criticizing this perspective, Hobfoll (1989, p. 515) has pointed out that the transactional model is tautological, by stating: "Demand is that which is offset by coping capacity. . . . Yet coping capacity is that which offsets threat or demand." In response to criticisms of operational confounding, Lazarus and Folkman suggested that for a wide array of relatively minor stressors or daily hassles, the degree of subjectivity concerning the degree of stressfulness is large. Hobfoll notes that this issue remains largely unresolved.

Edwards (1989) has recently proposed a model of coping based on decision-making processes. He defines stress as "a negative discrepancy between an individual's perceived state and desired state, provided that this discrepancy is considered important by the individual" (p. 242). This discrepancy is considered important in determining motivations to cope with the stress. Coping is described as an outcome of stress and is defined as "efforts to reduce the negative impacts of stress on individual well-being" (p. 242). Edwards's model focuses on factors affecting the selection of coping strategies, such as the physical and social environment, personal characteristics, social information, and the individual's cognitive construction of reality. Information concerning these factors should be obtained when investigating how individuals cope with stress to clarify differences in strategy utilization across individuals and situations.

Both Edwards (1989) and Hobfoll (1989) have made the point that the selection of coping strategies may not always follow a rational model in which the individual will seek to maximize well-being. Citing research by Watson and Clark (1984) on negative affectivity, Edwards (1989) suggests that individuals may select coping strategies that "preserve a customary level of affect" (p. 252). Thus if an individual's affect is dispositionally anxious or depressed, coping may only serve to prevent more severe depression or anxiety in the stressful situation.

In a review of measures of coping processes, Cohen (1987) noted that inventories of coping can be generally grouped into trait or episodic measures of coping. Most studies, therefore, focus on either dispositional or situational coping. Some studies have shown that there is only modest agreement between coping styles and actual behavior in a stressful situation (e.g., Cohen & Lazarus, 1973). More recently, researchers have attempted to disentangle the relative effects of dispositional versus situational coping styles. For example, by increasing the number and complexity of coping styles measured, Carver, Scheier, and Weintraub (1989) have found significant agreement between dispositional coping style and coping acts in specified situations. Meyerowitz et al. (1983) have proposed that coping with a chronic illness such as cancer (and by analogy, HIV-1/AIDS), which presents varied stressful situations, should be measured using a situation-specific approach in which problems related to the illness are enumerated and actual coping responses to those problems are also assessed. This approach would allow investigation of the differential effectiveness of various coping strategies across situations.

Social Support

Social support has been conceptualized as the emotional or tangible aid or assistance that is provided from individuals in one's interpersonal network. This is especially salient in discussions of HIV-spectrum illness because of the disabling nature of the disease as it progresses, the interpersonal nature of acquiring HIV-1 infection, and the social isolation commonly seen among persons with AIDS, especially near death. Since social support is frequently referred to as a salient mediator in the study of psychosocial influences on the natural history of AIDS, its investigation is warranted in the study of the coping process.

Social support typically refers to the functions performed for an ill or distressed individual by persons in the social network, most commonly family members, friends, co-workers, and neighbors. House (1981) has categorized these functions to include instrumental aid (assisting with the normal daily functions of life), socioemotional aid (sympathy, affection, and affiliation) and informational aid (provision of advice, opinion, and fact). There is an extensive range of literature demonstrating that social support, and particularly the existence of confidants (intimate personal relationships), reduces (buffers) the impacts of adverse stress-producing events (Kessler & McLeod, 1985; Turner, 1983). Brown and Harris (1978) and Pearlin, Lieberman, Menaghan, and Mullan (1981) have suggested that social support bolsters self-esteem and perceived competence, thereby improving positive affect in the light of a stressful experience. Thoits (1986) suggests that this perspective ignores the chronic nature of many stressful exposures as well as the differential help provided by one's social network. She suggests that, in fact, rather than conceiving of social support and coping as independent mediators of stressful circumstances, social support should be viewed as a type of coping assistance. This approach focuses on the source of the stress and implies that the restoration of self-esteem is a secondary (rather than the primary) mechanism by which support operates. While there continues to be controversy in the field, there is little question as to the overall utility of an activated social support system in light of highly stressful exposures.

Empirical Reports on Coping and HIV-Spectrum Illness

No one theoretical perspective or measurement strategy has been widely used in the literature, and the empirical reports from the field have been spotty at best. Nyamathi and van Servellen (1989) comment that the literature fails to demonstrate a sound theoretical orientation, reflecting the nascent state of the field.

Although many strategies of coping have been identified, researchers have often found it useful to measure coping with specific threats associated with HIV-1/AIDS. Researchers in the Multicenter AIDS Cohort Study have used a self-administered questionnaire measuring coping responses used in dealing with the threat of AIDS. In order to make the domains of content for the coping strategies measured relevant for gay men, focus groups were held with gay men to find out how the HIV epidemic had affected their lives and how they were coping with AIDS (Joseph *et al.*, 1984). Items were based on the Folkman and Lazarus (1980) "Ways of Coping Scale" and were adapted to reflect the domains of concern revealed by focus group participants. Factor analysis of the scale resulted in four domains of content: health vigilance, denial/fatalism, collective/ gay orientation, and religious coping (Joseph *et al.*, 1984).

More recently, a few studies have reported on the effectiveness of various coping strategies in protecting against distress associated with HIV-1 infection. Namir *et al.* (1987) investigated the coping mechanisms used by homosexual men recently diagnosed with AIDS, and delineated the effectiveness of varying coping styles on psychological health status. Reflecting the conclusions of Christ and Weiner (1985) and Forstein (1984) that AIDS has a wide-ranging impact on social relationships, interpersonal functioning, physical and psychological abilities, and self-esteem, the authors sought to document ways of coping with a life-threatening illness. Three methods of coping derived from Billings and Moos (1981) were addressed: active-behavioral (attempting to master the situation), active-cognitive (a search for meaning in the event, reassessing the situation to cast it in more positive terms), and avoidance coping (efforts to avoid thinking about or behaving in direct response to the illness, including self-medication).

The subjects were 50 self-identified homosexual/bisexual (94% Caucasian) males, with a mean age of 36. The psychological correlates of the differing coping methods showed that men with AIDS who primarily used avoidance coping methods experienced greater psychological distress than those who were active in orientation. Avoidance was related to greater depression, anxiety, and lower self-esteem, with active-behavioral coping being significantly associated with better functioning on each of these measures. Active-cognitive coping demonstrated similar positive findings with psychological health, although generally not at statistically significant levels. Avoidance coping was also inversely related to social support networks, leading to a spiralling downward in social contacts over time. These data may be interpreted as supporting the assertion of Holahan and Moos (1987) that avoidance coping is a response to threatening situations when personal and social resources are scarce.

With respect to the physical health correlates of coping, less dramatic results ensued. While perceived health status demonstrated a consistent relationship with coping strategy (highest for active-behavioral, lowest for avoidance coping).

physicians' ratings of their patients' physical performance were uncorrelated with method of coping, and there were no associations with total number of medical symptoms or immunological functioning. Namir *et al.* (1987) conclude that avoidance coping was not the product of poor health; as such, intervention efforts to deter passive, helpless feelings and bolster self-esteem are warranted.

Psychological functioning is often entangled with the physical symptoms associated with disease progression as well as neurological manifestations of this disease. The Multicenter AIDS Cohort Study (Chmiel *et al.,* 1987; Kaslow *et al.,* 1987), a prospective investigation of the physical, immunological, and epidemiological nature of AIDS among nearly 5000 homosexual men in four U.S. metropolitan areas (Chicago, Baltimore/Washington, Pittsburgh, and Los Angeles), recently reported on the relationship between psychological functioning and HIV-related symptoms (Ostrow *et al.,* 1989). At enrollment into the study, HIV-1 antibody status was a less important predictor of depression (using the Centers for Epidemiology Studies Depression (CES-D) Scale) than were self-reported physical symptoms. Men who reported the absence of "confidants" (persons they could "talk to about serious problems") had more depression and other types of psychological distress (enervation, negative affect, and interpersonal sensitivity) than men with perceived support. The authors conclude that perceived physical symptoms may add to psychological distress, particularly among those with inadequate social support, a finding reported in other cohorts as well (Chuang, Devins, Hunsley, & Gill, 1989). While there is an explicit awareness that the nonspecificity of symptoms may overlap with the indicators of depression and anxiety, age and education effects noted were consistent with the psychosomatic literature.

Viney, Henry, Walker, and Crooks (1989) compared the emotional reactions of males who were HIV-1 positive with a matched comparison group of men with major life-threatening and disabling diseases (diabetes, epilepsy, multiple sclerosis, and coronary conditions) and a matched group of well men. The two ill groups demonstrated greater anxiety, depression, and helplessness on standard psychological tests than did the well group, and the group that was HIV-1 positive reported more indirectly expressed anger and competence than did the other ill group. Expressions of "enjoyment" in life differentiated psychological distress among men with AIDS: those with high reports of enjoyment had lower levels of depression. Overall, the emotional reactions of men with AIDS were similar to men coping with other illnesses. However, men who were HIV-1 positive were significantly more likely to express competence—to view themselves as able and effective—perhaps reflecting their successful coping efforts to date.

Empirical Reports on Social Support and HIV-Spectrum Illness

A key factor identified in much of the research to date underscores the importance of social support as a resource for bolstering the coping response in light of the stresses of HIV-1 infection (Namir, Wolcott, & Fawzy, 1989). Associated with the diagnosis of AIDS and notification of antibody to HIV-1 is the problem of social isolation, the response from the society at large, and the need for social support (Miller, 1986; Morin & Batchelor, 1984; Siegel, 1986). The mushrooming literature on social support suggests its importance in the investigation of coping with HIV-spectrum illnesses.

One of the first empirical reports on the importance of social support for AIDS was published by Donlou, Wolcott, Gottlieb, and Landsverk (1985). They investigated the role of social supports and resources among 21 homosexual and bisexual men with AIDS and AIDS-related complex (ARC). Contrary to the later published literature, they detected no advantage of social support for psychological distress or for self-esteem.

Emmons *et al.* (1988) analyzed the relationships between social network affiliation in the gay community and a variety of risky behaviors for acquisition of HIV-1 in a longitudinal investigation of the natural history of AIDS. In the Chicago arm of the Multicenter AIDS Cohort Study, there were no associations reported for social networks and any behavioral measure over time among men at risk for HIV-1 infection. However, ascribing to social norms for risk reduction was associated with decreases in the number of sexual partners over time.

A recent report on the importance of social support in the coping process among homosexual men provides substantive data on this relationship (Martin, 1988). In an investigation of a cohort of 745 New York City gay men, a direct relationship was found between bereavement and symptoms of traumatic stress response, fatigue, demoralization, sleep problems and sedative use, and use of psychological counseling services. Confounding factors such as perceived susceptibility to AIDS, HIV-1 antibody status, presence of symptoms of ARC, and sexual behavior history failed to alter this relationship. Martin (1988, p. 861) concludes that "the types of distress most reactive to AIDS-related losses involve intrusive and avoidant thoughts and emotions about AIDS itself . . . ; involve the depression, hopelessness, and helplessness associated with being demoralized; and involve the problems . . . that are so often reported by those suffering from affective disorders." Longitudinal data from this cohort (Martin, Dean, Garcia, & Hall, 1989) support these conclusions as well, demonstrating a cumulative impact of the stress response over time. The loss of lovers and friends to AIDS often depletes the network of emotionally supportive ties of the gay man, which may have been limited to only these to begin with.

Zich and Temoshok (1987) recruited gay or bisexual men with a recent diagnosis of AIDS or ARC from San Francisco who were administered a 2-hour psychological interview and completed a self-report questionnaire. A total of 50 persons with AIDS and 53 persons with ARC completed the study. For persons with AIDS (but not for persons with ARC), physical distress was associated with less perceived availability of social support. Both hopelessness and depression were associated with less perceived social support. Four types of assistance were rated (desirably) by these patients: emotionally sustaining behaviors ("someone to talk to"), problem-solving behaviors ("someone who offers suggestions"), indirect personal influence ("someone who conveys a willingness to help"), and environmental action ("someone who intervenes in the environment to reduce stress"). The most desirable type of help was the emotionally sustaining form, which was perceived as most readily available, and hence more frequently used, and was viewed as being of greater assistance than problem-solving types of help. Finally, perceived social support is directly related to both psychological distress and dysphoria, as well as to the number of reported symptoms and medical conditions.

The Impact of Psychological Distress on Physiological Functioning in HIV-Spectrum Illness

A burgeoning area of research that may have direct application for HIV infection is psychoneuroimmunology, the study of the interactions among psychological processes, the central nervous system, and the immune system. Because host vulnerability in HIV infection is most closely associated with immune functioning, psychosocial factors that affect immune functioning should be of great research interest (Temoshok, 1988).

Even as rates of disease occurrence and case fatality increase, there continues to be significant individual variability in viral latency among those infected. Indeed, most of the variance in length of survival from time of diagnosis cannot be accounted for (Turner, Miller, & Moses, 1988). In light of this, researchers have sought to identify cofactors that may affect the rate of progression of HIV-1 infection. In a review of studies of psychological influences on immune functioning, Kiecolt-Glaser and Glaser (1988) reviewed evidence to suggest that many psychosocial factors, including stress, bereavement, and loneliness, influence immune functioning, and they have proposed that these factors be considered as potential factors influencing immune functioning in HIV infection.

Solomon and Temoshok (1989) are currently following a cohort of people with AIDS to determine factors that account for such differences in survivorship. Preliminary results indicate that how long a person has been diagnosed with AIDS is the main determinant of immune functioning. They have found that lower scores on a scale of depressed/anxious mood were significantly correlated with higher absolute number of helper T cells and that higher absolute numbers of cytotoxic cells were significantly associated with less stress from sickness. When this measure of psychosocial functioning was controlled, higher numbers of helper T cells remained significantly associated with less stress from sources other than their current illness, less tension and anxiety, and other sources of stress. Absolute numbers of suppressor cells were associated with more fitness and exercise (again controlling for sickness), less fatigue, and withdrawing to nurture oneself (Temoshok, Solomon, Jenkins, & Sweet, 1989).

In a corollary study of people with ARC, the same researchers found that dysphoric mood was associated with better immune functioning. To understand this contradictory finding, Temoshok has suggested that as these patients were newly diagnosed as having a potentially fatal illness, their distress stimulated the immune response. This study points out one of the difficulties with using immune status and functioning as outcome variables: up-regulation of the immune system occurs as a result of antigenic challenge. Patients with early ARC could be experiencing opportunistic infections that stimulate an immune response. Because they are in the earlier stages of infection, their immune systems are still sufficiently intact to respond.

Kemeny *et al.* (1989) have reported preliminary data on bereaved gay men and immune function. The purpose of the study was to determine if depressive mood in bereaved men was associated with immune functioning. Results were mixed and differed for subjects who were HIV-1 positive and HIV-1 negative as well as for bereaved versus nonbereaved subjects. In subjects who were HIV-1 positive, depressive mood was not associated with immune status in bereaved men, but bereaved men had better immune functioning than nonbereaved men. In nonbereaved men, greater depressed mood was associated with poorer immune status and functioning. In subjects who were HIV-1 negative, there were no differences between the bereaved and nonbereaved, and depression was associated with altered T cells and natural killer cells in bereaved men.

POTENTIAL FOR INTERVENTION

Based on results cited above, individual appraisal and coping with the threat of AIDS may prove useful in mediating the potential effect of subsequent distress on immune functioning. Interventions focused on bolstering social supports or improving coping capacities could have positive effects on stress-related decrements in functioning in the patient with HIV, thereby decreasing threats to immune functioning. Although there are reports of interventions to help individuals at risk for infection reduce their risk behavior, few such interventions have been reported that aimed specifically at altering immune functioning in infected men. Coates, McCusick, Kuno, and Stites (1989) reported the results of a stress reduction intervention that was aimed both at improving immune functioning and reducing unsafe behavior in men infected with HIV-1. After 8 weekly sessions involving learning systematic relaxation, encouraging changes in health habits, and learning skills for managing stress, they found no significant changes in measures of immune functioning but did find positive benefits for risk reduction. They cite as possible explanations for null findings regarding immune functioning that, among other things, single measurements (before and after) of immune cells may not have been sufficiently sensitive, that the nature of the interventions may not have been intense enough to bring about significant clinical changes, and that the nature of the group setting itself may have been stressful for the participants.

Given the empirical findings concerning the effectiveness of various coping strategies and social supports in affecting well-being, a more realistic approach may be to develop interventions directed toward decreasing emotional distress and promoting well-being or enjoyment with the more distal goal of prolonging survival. Fawzy, Namir, and Wolcott (1989) developed and evaluated an intervention for persons with AIDS that involved encouraging problem solving and other active coping strategies, since these have been shown to be associated with better psychological functioning. The intervention consisted of 10 2-hour weekly sessions in which participants received training for problem solving and problem resolution. In addition, they stated that participants gave and received emotional support from one another. Participants showed a significant decrease in total mood disturbance following the intervention. A self-selected control group showed somewhat increased mood disturbance.

CONCLUSIONS

It is clear that there is variation in the impact of coping strategies and social support in the response to HIV-1 infection and in their mediating effects on psychological functioning. There may be some promise in pursuing research on the physiological effects of these mediating processes for HIV-spectrum disease, with psychoneuroimmunology being a critical, although methodologically complex, approach.

Most behavioral research on psychosocial factors in HIV-1 infection to date has been primarily observational. With a few exceptions (e.g., Fawzy *et al.*, 1989), even the longitudinal investigations of the effects of coping and/or social support on psychological functioning have not incorporated active interventions or attempted to affect coping styles or alter social support networks. Indeed, the literature on which interventions for these domains is based primarily seeks to effect short-term adjustment or recovery following only brief recuperative periods (Auerbach, 1989). The extent to which this is a useful paradigm for HIV-spectrum illness may be questioned, especially given the chronic and usually declining functioning among most patients as the disease progresses. However, at present this is the only avenue available, and innovative intervention strategies for bolstering coping efforts and creating (new) social support mechanisms for patients appear essential, especially in light of the relative lack of medical interventions with any demonstrated efficacy.

REFERENCES

Allport, G. W. (1966). Traits revisited. *American Psychologist, 21,* 1–10.

Antonovsy, A. (1979). *Health, Stress, and Coping.* San Francisco: Jossey-Bass.

Auerbach, S. M. (1989). Stress management and coping research in the health care setting: An overview and methodological commentary. *Journal of Consulting and Clinical Psychology, 57,* 388–395.

Billings, A. G., & Moos, R. (1981). The role of coping responses and social resources in attenuating the stress of life events. *Journal of Behavioral Medicine, 4,* 139–157.

Brown, G. W., & Harris, T. (1978). *The social origins of depression.* New York: Free Press.

Carver, C. S., Scheier, M. F., & Weintraub, J. (1989). Assessing coping strategies: a theoretically based approach. *Journal of Personality and Social Psychology, 56,* 267–283.

Cattell, R. B. (1946). *The description and measurement of personality.* New York: World.

Chmiel, J. S., Detels, R., Kaslow, R. A., Van Raden, M., Kingsley, L. A., Brookmeyer, R., & The Multicenter AIDS Cohort Study Group (1987). Factors associated with prevalent human immunodeficiency virus (HIV) infection in the Multicenter AIDS Cohort Study. *American Journal of Epidemiology, 126,* 568–577.

Christ, C. H., & Weiner, L. S. (1985). Psychological issues in AIDS. In V. T. DeVita, S. Hellman, & S. A. Rosenberg (Eds.), *AIDS: Etiology, diagnosis, treatment, and prevention* (pp. 275–297). Philadelphia: Lippincott.

Chuang, H. T., Devins, G. M., Hunsley, J., & Gill, M. J. (1989). Psychosocial distress and well-being among gay and bisexual men with human immunodeficiency virus infection. *American Journal of Psychiatry, 46,* 876–880.

Coates, T. J., McCusick, L., Kuno, R., & Stites, D. P. (1989). Stress reduction changed number of sexual partners but not immune function in men with HIV. *American Journal of Public Health, 79,* 885–887.

Coates, T. J., Temoshok, L., & Mandel, J. (1984). Psychosocial research is essential to understanding and treating AIDS. *American Psychologist, 39,* 1309–1314.

Cohen, F. (1987). Measurement of coping. In S. V. Kasl & C. L. Cooper (Eds.), *Stress and health: Issues in research and methodology* (pp. 283–305). New York: John Wiley and Sons.

Cohen, F., & Lazarus, R. S. (1973). Active coping processes, coping dispositions, and recovery from surgery. *Psychosomatic Medicine, 35,* 375–389.

Dilley, J. W. (1984). Treatment interventions and approaches to care of patients with acquired immunodeficiency syndrome. In S. E. Nichols & D. G. Ostrow (Eds.), *Psychiatric implications of acquired immune deficiency syndrome* (pp. 62–80). Washington, DC: American Psychiatric Press.

Dohrenwend, B. S., Dohrenwend, B. P., Dodson, M., & Shrout, P. E. (1984). Symptoms, hassles, social support, and life events: Problem of confounded measures. *Journal of Abnormal Psychology, 93,* 222–230.

Donlou, J. N., Wolcott, D. L., Gottlieb, M. S., Lansverk, J. (1985). Psychosocial aspects of AIDS and AIDS-related complex: A pilot study. *Journal of Psychosocial Oncology, 3,* 39–55.

Edwards, J. R. (1989). The determinants and consequences of coping with stress. In C. L. Cooper & R. Payne (Eds.), *Causes, coping, and consequences of stress at work,* New York: John Wiley & Sons.

Emmons, C. A., Joseph, J. G., Kessler, R. C., Wortman, C. B., Montgomery, S. B., & Ostrow, D. G. (1986). Psychosocial predictors of reported behavior change in homosexual men at risk for AIDS. *Health Education Quarterly, 4,* 331–345.

Faulstich, M. E. (1987). Psychiatric aspects of AIDS. *American Journal of Psychiatry, 142,* 82–86.

Fawzy, F. I., Namir, S., & Wolcott, D. L. (1989). Structured intervention for AIDS patients. *Psychiatric Medicine, 7*(2), 33–45.

Folkman, S., & Lazarus, R. (1988). Coping as a mediator of emotion. *Journal of Personality and Social Psychology, 54*(3), 466–475.

Folkman, S., & Folkman, R. (1980). An analysis of coping in a middleaged community sample. *Journal of Health & Social Behavior, 21,* 219–239.

Forstein, M. (1984). The psychosocial impact of the acquired immunodeficiency syndrome. *Seminars in Oncology, 3,* 77–82.

Friedlander, A. H., & Arthur, R. J. (1988). A diagnosis of AIDS: Understanding the psychosocial impact. *Oral Surgery, Oral Medicine, and Oral Pathology, 65,* 680–684.

Glass, R. M. (1988). AIDS and suicide. *Journal of the American Medical Association, 259,* 1369–1370.

Harowski, K. J. (1987). The worried well: Maximizing coping in the face of AIDS. *Journal of Homosexuality, 3,* 299–306.

Hobfoll, S. E. (1989). Conservation of resources: A new attempt at conceptualizing stress. *American Psychologist, 44,* 513–524.

Holahan, C. J., & Moos, R. H. (1987). Personal and contextual determinants of coping strategies. *Journal of Personality and Social Psychology, 57,* 946–955.

Holland, J. C., & Tross, S. (1985). The psychosocial and neuropsychiatric sequelae of AIDS and related disorders. *Annals of Internal Medicine, 103,* 760–764.

House, J. S. (1981). *Work stress and social support.* Reading, MA: Addison-Wesley.

Joseph, J. L., Emmons, C., Kessler, R. C., Wortman, C. B., O'Brien, K., Hocker, W. T., & Schaefer, C. (1984). Coping with the threat of AIDS. *American Psychologist, 39*(11), 1297–1302.

Kaslow, P. P., Phair, J. P., Polk, B. F., & Rinaldo, C. R., Jr. (1987). The Multicenter AIDS Cohort Study: Rationale, organization and selected characteristics of the participants. *American Journal of Epidemiology, 126,* 310–318.

Kemeny, M. E., Fahey, J. L., Schneider, S., Taylor, S., Weiner, H., & Visscher, B. (1989, March 20). Psychosocial cofactors in HIV infection: bereavement, depression, and immune response in HIV+ and HIV− homosexual men. *CDC AIDS Weekly,* p. 19.

Kessler, R. C., & McLeod, J. D. (1985). Social support and mental health in community samples. In S. Cohen & S. L. Syme (Eds.), *Social support and health* (pp. 219–240). New York: Academic Press.

Kiecolt-Glazer, J., & Glazer, R. (1988). Psychological influences on immunity: Implications for AIDS. *American Psychologist, 43,* 929–934.

Kizer, K. W., Green, M., Perkins, C. I., Doebbert, G., & Hughes, M. J. (1988). AIDS and suicide in California. *Journal of the American Medical Association, 260,* 1881.

Lazarus, R. S. (1981). The stress and coping paradigm. In C. Eisdorfer, D. Cohen, A. Keinman, & P. Maxim (Eds.), *Models for clinical psychopathology* (pp. 177–214). New York: Spectrum.

Lazarus, R. S., & Folkman, S. (1984). *Stress, appraisal, and coping.* New York: Springer.

Martin, J. L. (1988). Psychological consequences of AIDS-related bereavement among gay men. *Journal of Consulting and Clinical Psychology, 56,* 856–862.

Martin, J. L., Dean, L., Garcia, M., & Hall, W. (1989). The impact of AIDS on a gay community: Changes in sexual behavior, substance use, and mental health. *American Journal of Community Psychology, 17,* 269–293.

Marzuck, P. M., Tierney, H., Tardiff, K., Gross, E. M., Morgan, E. B., Hsu, M. A., & Mann, J. J. (1988). Increased risk of suicide in persons with AIDS. *Journal of the American Medical Association, 259,* 1333–1337.

Meyerowitz, B. E., Heinrich, R. L., & Schag, C. C. (1983). A competency-based approach to coping with cancer. In T. G. Burish & L. A. Bradley (Eds.), *Coping with chronic disease* (pp. 137–158). New York: Academic Press.

Miller, D. (1986). Psychology, AIDS, ARC, and PGL. In J. Green & D. Miller (Eds.), *The management of AIDS patients* (pp. 131–150). London: MacMillan Press.

Mischel, W. (1968). *Personality and assessment.* New York: Wiley.

Moos, R. H. (1988). Life stressors and coping resources influence health and well-being. *Psychological Assessment, 4,* 133–158.

Morin, S. F., & Batchelor, W. F. (1984). Responding to the psychological crisis of AIDS. *Public Health Reports, 99,* 4–9.

Morin, S., Charles, K., & Maylon, A. (1984). The psychological impact of AIDS on gay men. *American Psychologist, 39,* 1303–1308.

Namir, S., Wolcott, D. L., & Fawzy, I. F. (1989). Social support and HIV spectrum disease: Clinical and research perspectives. *Psychiatric Medicine, 7,* 97–106.

Namir, S., Wolcott, D. L., Fawzy, I. F., & Alumbaugh, M. J. (1987). Coping with AIDS: Psychological and health implications. *Journal of Applied Social Psychology, 17,* 309–328.

Nichols, S. E. (1983). Psychiatric aspects of AIDS. *Psychosomatics, 24,* 1083–1089.

Nichols, S. E. (1985). Psychosocial reactions of persons with the acquired immunodeficiency syndrome. *Annals of Internal Medicine, 103,* 865–767.

Nyamathi, A., & van Servellen, G. (1989). Maladaptive coping in the critically ill population with acquired immunodeficiency syndrome: Nursing assessment and treatment. *Heart & Lung, 18,* 113–120.

Ostrow, D. G. (1986). Psychiatric consequences of AIDS: An overview. *International Review of Neuroscience, 29,* 1–13.

Ostrow, D. G., Joseph, J., Monjan, A., & Kessler, R. (1986). Psychosocial aspects of AIDS risk. *Psychopharmacology Bulletin, 22,* 678–683.

Ostrow, D. G., Monjan, A., Joseph, J., VanRaden, M., Fox, R., Kingsley, L., Dudley, J., & Phair, J. (1989). HIV-related symptoms and psychological functioning in a cohort of homosexual men. *American Journal of Psychiatry, 146,* 737–742.

Pearlin, L. I., Lieberman, M. A., Menaghan, E. G., & Mullan, J. T. (1981). The stress process. *Journal of Health and Social Behavior, 22,* 337–356.

Perry, S., Jacobsberg, L., & Fishman, B. (1990). Suicidal ideation and HIV testing. *Journal of the American Medical Association, 263,* 679–682.

Perry, S., Jacobsberg, L., Fishman, B., Frances, A., Bobo, J., & Jacobsberg, B. K. (1990). Psychiatric diagnosis before serological testing for the human immunodeficiency virus. *American Journal of Psychiatry, 147,* 89–93.

Perry, S. W., & Tross, S. (1984). Psychiatric problems of AIDS inpatients at the New York Hospital: Preliminary report. *Public Health Reports, 99,* 200–205.

Rabkin, J. G., & Struening, E. L. (1979). Life events, stress, and illness. *Science, 194,* 1013–1020.

Rappaport, H., Gill, M., & Schafer, R. (1945). *Diagnostic psychological testing.* Chicago: Year Book.

Rippetoe, P. A., & Rogers, R. W. (1987). Effects of components of protection-motivation theory on adaptive and maladaptive coping with a health threat. *Journal of Personality and Social Psychology, 52,* 596–604.

Siegel, K. (1986). AIDS: The social dimension. *Psychiatric Annals, 16,* 168–172.

Siegel, R. L., & Hoefer, D. D. (1981). Bereavement counseling for gay individuals. *American Journal of Psychotherapy, 35,* 517–525.

Speilberger, C. D. (1975). State–trait process. In C. D. Speilberger & I. G. Sarason (Eds.), *Stress and anxiety* (pp. 183–205). New York: Wiley.

Solomon, G. F., & Temoshok, L. (1987). A psychoneuroimmunologic perspective on AIDS research: Questions, preliminary findings, and suggestions. *Journal of Applied Social Psychology, 17*(3), 286–308.

Suls, G., & Fletcher, B. (1985). The relative efficacy of avoidant and nonavoidant coping strategies: a meta-analysis. *Health Psychology, 4,* 249–288.

Temoshok, L. (1988). Psychoimmunology and AIDS. In T. P. Bridge (Ed.), *Psychological, neuropsychiatric, and substance abuse aspects of AIDS* (pp. 187–197). New York: Raven.

Temoshok, L., Solomon, G. F., Jenkins, S. R., & Sweet, D. M. (1989). Psychoimmunologic studies of men with AIDS and ARC. Paper presented at the annual meeting of the American Association for the Advancement of Science, San Francisco.

Thoits, P. A. (1986). Social support as coping assistance. *Journal of Consulting and Clinical Psychology, 54,* 416–423.

Turner, C. F., Miller, H. G., & Moses, L. E. (Eds.) (1989). *AIDS—sexual behavior and intravenous drug use.* Washington, DC: National Academy Press.

Turner, R. J. (1983). Direct, indirect, and moderating effects of social support on psychological distress and associated conditions. In H. B. Caplan (Ed.), *Psychosocial stress: Trends in theory and research* (pp. 105–155). New York: Academic Press.

Viney, L. L., Henry, R., Walker, B. M., & Crooks, L. (1989). The emotional reactions of HIV antibody positive men. *British Journal of Medical Psychology, 62,* 153–161.

Watson, D., & Clark, C. A. (1984). Negative affectivity: The disposition to experience negative emotional states. *Psychological Bulletin, 96,* 465–490.

Weitz, R. (1989). Uncertainty and the lives of persons with AIDS. *Journal of Health and Social Behavior, 30,* 270–281.

Zich, J., & Temoshok, L. (1987). Perceptions of social support in men with AIDS and ARC: Relationships with distress and hardiness. *Journal of Applied Social Psychology, 17,* 193–215.

7

Workplace Issues and Strategies Concerning HIV

IRENE JILLSON-BOOSTROM

In the past several years, the public and private sectors have initiated many approaches to prevention of HIV. Although few of these have been directed to the individual at his or her place of work, employers have taken measures which, under the rubric of prevention, have raised serious ethical and social concerns. This chapter presents a framework for consideration of prevention strategies in the workplace and suggests criteria for management and employees to use in selecting strategies appropriate to their circumstances. This chapter also provides information that could be used in addressing ethical issues that underlie both the prevention of HIV and services available to assist employees in coping with the epidemic.

Ethical conflicts with respect to prevention of disease and injury are not new to the workplace. In the past, the two most notable issues regarding public health at the workplace have been:

- Corporate responsibility for occupational illness and injury
- Prevention of substance abuse (e.g., screening policies designed to eliminate or reduce the extent of alcohol and drug abuse by public and private employees)

It has been said that workplaces are reflective of the individuals who are in positions of power. The history of individual corporations' responses to ethical issues such as those just mentioned is certainly indicative of the values held by corporate directors and managers. Usually, a company will respond similarly to a variety of issues within the framework of protective laws and the influence of employee organizations.

IRENE JILLSON-BOOSTROM • Policy Research, Inc., Clarksville, Maryland 21029.

Living and Dying with AIDS, edited by Paul I. Ahmed, Plenum Press, New York, 1992.

AIDS AT THE WORKPLACE: MYTHS AND REALITIES

To understand the underlying dimensions of ethical issues regarding AIDS at the workplace, one must bear in mind the myths and misunderstandings that are the basis for many assumptions about the virus. Many myths have arisen since the first diagnoses; we shall consider three that pertain to the workplace.

Myth 1: AIDS Is a Contagious Disease That Can Be Spread by Casual, Nonsexual Contact

In spite of documented evidence to the contrary, many individuals, including public and private managers, believe that AIDS can be contracted by casual, nonsexual contact. This is simply not the case; there have been no documented cases of infection resulting from such casual contact. In fact, studies of family members and loved ones caring for AIDS patients have shown no cases of infection due to this contact.

For example, in 1986, the U.S. Centers for Disease Control (CDC) issued guidelines intended to reduce fear about AIDS at the workplace and elsewhere. In those guidelines, the CDC recommended that employees who are HIV positive "should not be restricted from work unless they have another infection or illness for which such restriction would be warranted." The CDC went on to state explicitly that medical evidence supports their recommendation that "workers infected with (the AIDS virus) should not be restricted from using telephones, office equipment, toilets, showers, eating facilities and water fountains" (CDC, 1985, p. 681). Thus, it can be safely said that there is virtually no possibility of casual contagion.

However, it is important to reiterate that the two most common means of transmission are sexual intercourse and intravenous drug abuse. If one is having sexual relations with a co-worker or sharing IV needles with a coworker, one is just as at risk as others engaging in the same behavior. In addition, health care providers who work with AIDS patients, as well as laboratory workers who handle contaminated specimens and materials, are at risk. The CDC has issued specific recommendations regarding precautionary measures for use in health care settings.

Myth 2: Those Who Are HIV-Positive Are as Sick as Those Who Have Progressed to Having Symptoms of the Disease

This myth has resulted in job discrimination (both explicit and subtle) against HIV positive persons who *may never actually contract the disease or exhibit its symptoms* and who are perfectly capable of functioning on the job.

In fact, estimates of the rate of progression from HIV positivity to the disease vary widely. This results from the lack of a sufficient data base to develop valid estimates and the divergent epidemiological assumptions that are involved in such estimates. Current estimates in the United States range from a 35% to a 50% rate of progression from HIV infection to development of symptoms of AIDS in seven to eight years (Gordon, 1990).

To what degree are HIV-positive persons ill? No published studies have shown HIV-positive persons who have not actually developed AIDS symptoms to be more ill than those in comparable sociodemographic groups, nor any less effective on the job. A few studies have shown that HIV-positive persons may exhibit some stress resulting from concern about progression to the illness and from the need to change some of their accustomed behaviors that place them and others at risk (i.e., unprotected sex or IV drug abuse). However, no studies have shown that such persons exhibit significantly higher rates of stress-related illness than other workers facing other stressors such as divorce, death in the family, and occupational stress. Therefore, there is no valid reason to assume that HIV positive persons are any less capable of functioning on the job than their co-workers.

Myth 3: Once Someone Has the Disease, He or She Cannot Really Function at Work

Persons who have progressed to the disease stage (i.e., those who have been diagnosed with AIDS) have exhibited many different symptoms with varying degrees of severity at varying times, and they have differing life expectancies after diagnosis depending in part on the exposure group category; i.e., in San Francisco, where the largest proportion of diagnosed persons are homosexual/bisexual men, life expectancy in 1989 was 24 months. In New York, where the largest proportion of diagnosed persons are IV drug users or fall into other related categories, the median survival time is 10.3 months (Gordon, 1990; Smith, 1991). This makes it very difficult to generalize regarding the ability of those with symptoms to function at their normal level. However, many have continued to work effectively, some for several years, in their previously held jobs. Some who have continued to work require frequent and/or lengthy sick leave, but while on the job they function quite well. Based on available evidence, the World Health Organization (WHO) has determined that presence of HIV itself does not result in impaired occupational performance. The Presidential Commission on the HIV epidemic concurred with this finding (Watkins, 1988). Further, with the advent of treatments such as AZT, it has been possible to extend the "work life" of some individuals. In the future, more effective medicines may extend life and improve the quality of life and the functional capacity of persons with AIDS.

Many persons with AIDS or ARC have continued to function at their current jobs, or in jobs for which minimal or no retraining is necessary. In fact, allowing employees to continue to lead productive lives brings benefits such as the sense of well-being they get from continuing to work despite illness, the relatively high income they generate from employment (an average of $30,000 a year prior to the onset of HIV-related illness based on a 1989 study in California), and the taxes they pay. The cessation of work on the other hand, initiates one series of entitlements and hastens the day when others will begin (Yelin *et al.*, 1991).

This discussion of popularly held myths regarding AIDS in the workplace would seem to support the position that there is little or nothing to fear from having HIV-positive persons or those with AIDS as co-workers. If this is true, then why does so much fear exist? According to one professor of business ethics, "the fear of AIDS springs from very deep, sometimes irrational feelings about sexuality, chastity, and death, which we would rather not have invade the workplace" (Rowe, Russell-Einhorn & Baker, 1986, p. 28). Perhaps we would rather not have these feelings intrude upon our well-managed lives at all. For example, physicians have difficulty confronting death under many circumstances, and even those societies perceived as sexually liberated have seen prejudice, discrimination, and occasional violent action against the population group most at risk in this worldwide epidemic—that is, male homosexuals. [In the United States, male homosexuals or bisexuals who were not also IV drug abusers accounted for 63% of diagnosed cases as of the end of March, 1991 (Centers for Disease Control, 1991).]

WORKPLACE RESPONSES TO THE HIV EPIDEMIC: ETHICAL ISSUES

Of the many ethical issues that have arisen regarding AIDS in the workplace, the following predominate:

- Protection of individual rights, including for example, right to privacy, civil rights related to job discrimination, and confidentiality of medical and personnel records
- Perceived conflicts between individual rights and responsibilities and societal rights such as protection of public health
- Acceptance of or discrimination against marginal populations and individuals
- Shared burden of economic and other social costs of AIDS

How and in what contexts are these issues raised, and what reactions have there been thus far? The following are the contexts of most interest to employers, unions, and employees:

1. Testing job applicants and current employees for HIV seropositivity
2. Retaining and relocating employees who are known to be HIV positive or to have developed symptoms of AIDS
3. Company and union responsibility for HIV prevention and education programs and for support for HIV-positive employees and those with AIDS or ARC

The issues raised in each of these contexts are briefly summarized below.

Issues Regarding Testing for HIV Seropositivity

There is only one commonly available test for presence of HIV, the ELISA test. When this test is positive, a Western Blot test is used to confirm the result. The difficulty is that the validity of the ELISA test is increasingly being questioned by medical experts. A 1987 study found false-negative results with the ELISA test up to a year after initial contagion (Ranki, 1987). That means that an individual could actually have the virus in his or her system but show a negative result in the test. Further, use of such a test as a public health measure at the workplace is dubious, in view of the fact that casual contact is not a factor in spreading the disease.

Notwithstanding the questionable utility and veracity of the ELISA test (Valdiserri, 1989), in the United States, military recruits and employees of the Department of State and Agency for International Development are required to take the ELISA test. The stated rationale for each of these agencies is national security and, in the case of those posted in foreign countries, ensuring that adequate medical care is available in the event of onset of illness.

Required testing of certain groups of employees has been proposed in a number of public and private sector places of employment. Job categories for which mandatory tests have been proposed include, for example, surgeons, teachers, and emergency service personnel (e.g., ambulance drivers). The stated rationale for testing in each case varies, but generally concerns protection of public health, in spite of the lack of supporting data to justify such a rationale. In the case of teachers, for example, there is no evidence that either teachers or school children are at risk when in contact with a person who is HIV positive or who has AIDS or ARC. In the case of surgeons, the American Medical Association (AMA) has recently stated that "there have been no documented cases of transmission from physician to patient. However, the recent cases of possible dentist-to-patient transmission have caused some uncertainty about the risk of transmission under certain circumstances. Consequently, until the uncertainty about transmission is resolved, the AMA believes that HIV-infected physicians should either abstain from performing invasive procedures which pose an identifiable risk of transmission or disclose their sero-positive status prior to performing a procedure and proceed only if there is informed consent."

"The AMA further believes that physicians who are HIV positive and who must restrict their normal professional activities have a right to continue their career in medicine in a capacity that poses no identifiable risk to their patients" (American Medical Association, 1991).

The American Dental Association (ADA) has adopted the following policy in response to the possible transmission of HIV from an infected dentist to three patients: "An advisory opinion to the American Dental Association's Code of Professional Conduct urges dentists who become ill or impaired to limit the activities of practice to those areas that do not endanger either patients or dental staff."

"There has been only one documented case of transmission from an HIV-infected healthcare provider to patients during the past ten years. The ADA continues to believe that the recommended infection control procedures are effective in preventing transmission of infection."

"However, the recent case of possible HIV transmission from dentist to patient has raised some uncertainty. Until the uncertainty about transmission is resolved, the ADA believes that HIV-infected dentists should refrain from performing invasive procedures or should disclose their seropositive status" (American Dental Association, 1991). Neither the AMA nor the ADA has recommended testing for HIV positivity.

If the public health rationale for testing of job applicants or current employees is weak or invalid, then why are some employers either testing or trying to implement testing procedures?

One reason that may be relevant in the United States but not in other industrialized countries is the reluctance to hire or retain at-risk employees who have a chance of becoming ill and requiring expensive health care paid for in part by the company (self-insurance) or through private health insurance policies to which the company contributes.

Another rationale concerns protection of the employee who is HIV positive or who has developed symptoms of AIDS. That is, ensuring that his or her health is not "further" endangered, for example, by exposure to infection. In fact, little is known about cofactors that may play a role in progression from HIV positivity to the disease, or progression of the disease itself, and we know of no published studies of occupationally related cofactors.

Adverse reaction on the part of other employees or customers is another rationale used by companies as the basis for not hiring or not retaining HIV-positive persons or those with AIDS. In the United States, "a straightforward application of principles from other forms of discrimination law suggests that customer or co-worker preferences should not be given great weight" (Leonard, 1987, pp. 116–117). Comparisons have been made between AIDS discrimination cases and those in previous years concerning customer and co-worker preferences for female flight attendants and Caucasian health care workers.

Unfortunately, given the lack of a justifiable rationale for testing of employees or job applicants, one is left to conclude that prejudice against AIDS risk group members (as mentioned previously, in the United States this would be primarily gay or bisexual men and IV drug abusers) may be the most common implicit reason. This has been shown, for example, in both the types of questions that have been added to job application forms and interviews, and in new types of analyses of data regarding applicants. These include, for example,

- Probing questions of male job applicants over 30 years of age who indicate that they have never been married (living arrangements, social contacts, etc.)
- Probing questions of male job applicants who have any medical history of sexually transmitted disease, or who have been employed in certain types of jobs, including, for example, the fine arts and interior decoration (which also reveals prejudicial assumptions regarding work roles of male homosexuals)

Of course, fear of the unknown is another, perhaps more justifiable reason for testing job applicants and employees. AIDS has shaken the medical science and public health community, showing it to be vulnerable in the face of a new, horrific disease that has worldwide impact and for which there is no known cure. Information seems to change continually, both that which is based on biomedical science research and that revealed by the few behavioral science studies or opinion surveys that have been conducted.* For example, data regarding latency periods have changed over time, as have assumptions held by epidemiologists regarding the extent of the practice of at-risk sexual behavior such as anal intercourse among heterosexuals. Media reporting of information regarding AIDS, including the "changes" in knowledge on the part of AIDS "experts" has necessarily influenced public opinion, including the opinion of corporate managers and their employees, who derive most of their information from the popular press. In addition to the basic question of whether or not to test employees, there is the related issue of handling the results, including, for example:

- Where and how should results be recorded (in personnel files? corporate medical files? not recorded at all?)
- To whom should results be provided (health authorities? only the individual tested?)

---

* An example of new information that alters one's understanding of AIDS is the following. Two weeks after the early-October 1987 publication of the book *And the Band Played On,* in which the author revealed CDC data showing that the introduction of the virus in the U.S. was, almost definitively, the result of homosexual contact by a Canadian airline employee in 1979, the results of a startling *ex post facto* discovery of an AIDS case in 1969 was published. The individual was a teenager who lived in St. Louis, Missouri, and had never been outside of the Midwest (Shilts, 1987).

- How can confidentiality of results be ensured, if at all?

In the United States, a number of civil suits regarding HIV testing have been successfully filed by employees against employers, on the following bases:

- Infliction of emotional distress caused by requirements for testing
- Invasion of privacy (related to testing requirements and recording and reporting of results)
- Violation of confidentiality of medical and personnel records (related to recording and reporting of results)

Retaining and Relocating Employees Who Are Known to Be HIV Positive or Who Have AIDS

Antidiscrimination policies in both the United States and in Sweden should be sufficient to protect employees who are HIV positive or who have AIDS or ARC. However, there have been many cases of job dismissal in the United States, and there have been some cases of job discrimination in Sweden. The primary rationale used for job dismissal in the United States is essentially the same as that used for testing of job applicants or current employees, that is, protection of other workers. When these dismissals have been challenged by either the individual worker or the union involved, they have for the most part been overturned, on the basis of evidence discussed previously. Employees are simply not placed at risk by having a co-worker who is HIV positive or who has AIDS.

Another rationale regards ability to adequately perform one's work role. In the United States, when a person with AIDS is applying for disability benefits under Social Security, a Functional Ability Test is used to determine general ability to perform job functions. This is the only way to determine validly if AIDS or HIV positivity is affecting an individual's ability to function on the job.

Of some interest to employers has been published information regarding chemical changes in the brain of HIV-positive individuals. Such research is preliminary and has not been verified and, furthermore, has not been correlated with information regarding the *actual functional ability* of study subjects. Because this type of research has been linked with the diagnosis of dementia in AIDS patients, it is important to note here that dementia is not a problem for HIV-positive persons. In those AIDS cases in which dementia occurs, it is usually in the last few months or even weeks of life (although there is considerable variability). In these instances, the person is probably not capable of working in any case.

Even when an employee with AIDS shows signs of deterioration in ability to function, or is too frequently absent from work, it may be possible for him or her to be relocated to another position with the company, if he or she wishes to remain at work. This is easier, of course, if retraining is not required.

U.S. laws prohibiting job discrimination on the basis of disability and sexual preference have been interpreted as applying to AIDS, both for HIV seropositivity testing and for persons with AIDS. In addition, several states have enacted antidiscrimination laws specifically relating to AIDS (Leonard, 1987).

Recognizing the rights of employees who have the disease, some American corporations (such as Levi Strauss, the jeans manufacturer, Bank of America, and local telephone companies) have developed detailed policies concerning AIDS that include procedures for determining functional ability of those who have AIDS and job reassignment and retraining, if necessary. Preparation of new co-workers to accept the AIDS worker is usually a part of this process.

Company Responsibility for Prevention and Education Programs

As with other public health issues that concern the workplace, such as occupational health, it is increasingly important for corporations and unions to assume responsibility for prevention and education programs that are workplace based. This is true because of:

- Concern among employees about contact with HIV-positive persons and those with AIDS
- The need to protect the HIV-positive person and those with AIDS from harassment by other employees, and to provide them with preventive information and counseling should they seek such information
- The necessity of the workplace being a nonthreatening source of HIV prevention information for those who fear contacting governmental clinics at which anonymity cannot be guaranteed

In the United States, some employers have developed their own informational materials, for example, pamphlets and videos. Others have used materials developed by the U.S. Public Health Service, state AIDS agencies, or community-based groups such as HERO, a Baltimore-based HIV prevention organization.

In the United States and elsewhere, gay organizations have been in the forefront of developing prevention and educational materials and in efforts for evaluating their effectiveness. For this reason, even though corporate contact with these organizations may seem unusual, it has been viewed as essential by some companies. This is true because the materials often can be used for their work force in general (that is, they apply to the general population), and they have been shown to be effective in positively changing risk behaviors. Additionally, HIV epidemiological statistics have increased the awareness of bisexuality among American men and of the practice of anal intercourse among heterosexuals. The workplace may be a nonthreatening source of informational material for individuals who engage in such risk-taking behavior and who might not seek such information elsewhere.

If companies are developing AIDS prevention materials *de novo,* it is of the utmost importance that they be accurate and not contribute to employees' irrational fears. Thus, such materials should be reviewed in advance by recognized authorities in the field (including representatives of HIV-positive persons and those who have developed AIDS) and others as appropriate to ensure that the information is accurate and will be "received" by the company's employees. Because opinions vary regarding testing, risk behaviors, and other issues, obtaining the opinions of diverse groups is advised. One important question regarding prevention materials is the degree to which companies are willing to distribute information regarding safe sex practices, including the use of condoms. Because HIV is primarily a sexually transmitted disease, dissemination of preventive information that relates to safe sex practices is viewed by many HIV prevention experts as the most important means of prevention. However, sensitivities with regard to sex education need to be carefully considered by companies or unions planning HIV prevention strategies.

In disseminating prevention information, companies have issued it to all employees, made it available upon request, or arranged for group discussions at which the materials are distributed. Having group discussions has proven useful because many of the myths regarding AIDS are raised as questions by employees, and the setting allows for dispelling of the myths and discussion of employees' fears regarding them.

Some companies offer, through their medical or personnel departments, support for those who are known to be HIV positive or to have AIDS or ARC. This may include providing psychological counseling, guidance regarding safe sex practices; advice regarding nutrition, alcohol, and drug use, and other suspected cofactors; referral for testing if requested, and guidance concerning relations with other employees. It is important that this support not be imposed on the employee, but rather be available as requested. Corporations themselves may offer testing to employees who decide to participate, but also may refer employees to alternative testing sites, at which testing is completely anonymous.

The President's Commission on Human Immunodeficiency Virus reported that the National Leadership Coalition on AIDS, formed in 1987, has over 100 members from businesses, corporations, labor, voluntary groups, and religious bodies. The Presidential Commission believes that this private organization is an important force in the development of appropriate and humane policies regarding HIV, including prevention (Watkins, 1988). The U.S. Government Office of Personnel Management issued employment policies for federal workers in early 1988; these include guidelines for prevention programs (Watkins, 1988).

RECOMMENDED CRITERIA FOR DESIGNING OR SELECTING A WORKPLACE-BASED HIV PREVENTION PROGRAM

The following criteria may be useful for managers and employees in designing HIV prevention programs for use in their workplace, or in selecting one that has been developed for use elsewhere:

- The strategy should have clearly delineated goals and objectives that have been developed based insofar as possible on discussions among management and labor representatives.
- The strategy should address more than one risk factor to ensure that employees do not perceive the information as targeted to a group; this will help to alleviate stigmatization.
- The information included should be factual, based on the most recently available information from authoritative sources; where experts in the field disagree on "factual" information, this should be noted, and the arguments and their implications clearly presented.
- Medical and social support (e.g., the Employee Assistance Program representative, if one exists) should be involved in the development of the prevention program.
- Multiple prevention strategies that are culturally sensitive and that have been shown to be applicable to comparable populations can be used, but should be specifically adapted to the target population.
- Prior to implementation of the prevention program, the company should develop clearly delineated policies regarding HIV and employment, including those regarding job applicants and existing employees, and should arrange for referral for counseling, testing, and treatment for those who seek such services.
- The prevention strategy should be evaluated periodically by both management and employees, and should be revised as appropriate.

The Report of the Presidential Commission on the HIV epidemic included several recommendations regarding HIV at the workplace; the one that is most directly relevant to a discussion of coping issues is the following (Watkins, 1988): "Employees with any disease or disability, including HIV infection, should be treated with compassion and understanding and allowed to continue working as long as they are able to perform their job."

SUMMARY

The relatively constant nature of a society's ethical principles both facilitates and complicates one's ability to consider sensitive social issues such as those raised by the HIV epidemic and various approaches to prevention of HIV infection. On one hand, it is not likely that a sudden shift will occur in a society's ethical principles. Therefore, to a great extent, one can anticipate individual and collective reactions to challenges such as the HIV epidemic—challenges that test society's ability to equitably apply the values it holds, including those reflected in the basic tenets of its government (such as constitutional laws). On the other hand, one is not always assured that *apparent* egalitarianism and respect for humanity will be reflected in society's reaction to such a challenge, including the reactions of governments, the private sector, and individuals.

We are learning, through this disease, much about the dissonance between a society's explicitly stated ethical principles and the reality of individual and collective values that belie those principles when they are challenged. In the case of AIDS, both individuals and some governments have revealed deep-seated biases toward, and even loathing of, high-risk group members—in particular homosexual and bisexual men and drug abusers—irrational fear of death and disease, and disregard for individual rights. This has been reflected in national AIDS testing policies, in the delay in producing and distributing prevention information and in the types of information included in such materials, and in the dismissal of employees who are HIV positive or who have progressed to AIDS. While the Presidential Commission applauded the efforts of industry and labor in the HIV epidemic, it also acknowledged that severe obstacles to prevention and assurance of protection of human rights exist at the workplace, including confusion, fear, and lack of education programs tailored to specific situations. The Commission recommended specifically that "employers should work with employee representatives as well as area HIV education and health experts to tailor the HIV information programs to the needs of the work force" (Watkins, 1988, p. 183).

In the history of this epidemic, national governments for the most part have not been exemplary in their policies or in the process of developing policies. There is no cure for AIDS, and no vaccine to prevent it. While the world awaits miracles from the medical scientific community, companies—and unions—have an opportunity to serve as a positive force in prevention, while at the same time safeguarding the rights of employees who are HIV positive or who have AIDS.

REFERENCES

American Dental Association. (1991, January 16). Press release.
American Medical Association. (1991, January 17). *AMA statement on HIV infected physicians,* AMA Department of Public Information, Chicago.
Centers for Disease Control. (1991, April). *HIV/AIDS surveillance report,* pp. 1–18.
Centers for Disease Control. (1985, November 15). Recommendations for preventing transmission of infection with human T-lymphotropic virus type III/lymphadenopathy-associated virus in the workplace. *Morbidity and Mortality Weekly Report, 34,* 681.

Gordon, S. (1990). Sero-conversion staging and survival: Natural history of HIV infection. *Journal of American Podiatric Medical Association, 80*(1), 9–14.

Leonard, A. S. (1987). AIDS in the workplace. In H. Dalton & S. Burris (Eds.), *AIDS and the law: A guide for the public* (p. 113). New Haven: Yale University Press.

Ranki, A. (1987, September 12). Long latency precedes overt seroconversion in sexually transmitted human-immuno deficiency virus infection. *Lancet, 2*(8559), 589.

Rowe, M. P., Russell-Einhorn, M. & Baker, M. A. (1986, July–August). The fear of AIDS. *Harvard Business Review,* 28.

Shilts, R. (1987). *And the band played on: Politics, people and the AIDS epidemic.* New York: St. Martin's Press.

Smith, P. *et al.* (1991). The AIDS epidemic in New York state. *American Journal of Public Health, 81*(Suppl.), 54–60.

Valdiserri, R. O. (1989). *Preventing AIDS: The design of effective programs* (pp. 211–217). New Jersey: Rutgers, The State University Press.

Watkins, J. D. (1988, June). *Report of the presidential commission on the human immunodeficiency virus epidemic.* Washington, DC: U.S. Government Printing Office, 0-214-701:QL3.

Yelin, Edward H. *et al.* (1991, January). The impact of HIV-related illness on employment. *American Journal of Public Health, 81*(1), 79–84.

8

Coping with AIDS and Substance Abuse

BARBARA G. FALTZ

AIDS AND SUBSTANCE ABUSE

The rapid spread of AIDS presents enormous challenges for health care providers. There can be many difficulties for patients whose substance abuse places them at risk for contracting the disease, makes them particularly vulnerable to its rapid progression, and leaves them with poorer ability to cope with the complexities of its psychosocial and medical sequelae. There are numerous connections between HIV disease and substance abuse. These will be reviewed, and suggestions will be made for interventions addressing complex counseling issues that result from the simultaneous problems of HIV disease and alcohol or drug abuse.

The Risks

The first link between alcohol, drugs, and AIDS is the direct transmission of HIV through the sharing of hypodermic needles, syringes, and other injection drug paraphernalia. According to the Centers for Disease Control (1991), injection drug use is the primary risk factor for 22% of the people with AIDS. In addition, 7% of the homosexual and bisexual men with AIDS report a history of intravenous drug use. The second link of substance abuse with AIDS is the transmission of the virus by infected substance abusers to their sexual partners (Centers for Disease Control, 1989). Third, infected women who are the sexual partners of, or who are themselves, injection drug users can transmit the virus during the perinatal period (Centers for Disease Control, 1989a).

BARBARA G. FALTZ • CPC Belmont Hills Hospital, Belmont, California 94002.

Living and Dying with AIDS, edited by Paul I. Ahmed, Plenum Press, New York, 1992.

The effect of alcohol and drugs on the immune system has been widely researched. Although not directly linked to AIDS, alcohol, marijuana, cocaine, and amphetamines may be immunosuppressant (Klein, Newton, & Friedman, 1987; McGreggor, 1988). Additionally, there is increased sexual risk and needle-using behavior while under the influence of alcohol or drugs (Coates, Stall, Catania,& Kegeles, 1988; Stall, Wiley, McKusick, Coates, & Ostrow, 1986). Substance abusers who have made promises to themselves or others concerning behaviors that may increase risk of exposure to HIV are often not able to follow them due to intoxication or other drug-related states. Alcohol and drug abuse also interferes with the medical treatment of AIDS and can sabotage social service and mental health interventions. Financial problems, housing difficulties, and the exacerbation of emotional crisis situations are common consequences of substance abuse. They are particularly devastating accompanying a diagnosis of AIDS or ARC.

The Nature of Substance Abuse

The reality of being able to insure a steady supply of the desired drug or alcohol, the need to avoid confrontation about continued use and it's consequences, and the fear associated with possible illegal acts are daily features of the life of a substance abuser. If, for example, an addict has a $100 per day heroin habit, he or she would also need to obtain $36,500 per year just to obtain the needed drug. In addition, if he or she would steal merchandise to pay for this habit, the value of the goods stolen would have to be much greater than this amount, since those who receive and resell stolen property do not pay its true market value. The constant need to have funds available to get heroin coupled with the physiological cycle of intoxication alternating with the onset of withdrawal symptoms approximately every 4 hours makes the life of an active opiate addict incredibly stressful.

Additionally, substance abusers are already operating well outside the bounds of sound medical advice; they may be unwilling to trust or believe warnings concerning AIDS, especially if they do not perceive an immediate personal threat from HIV. There is also the additional component of denial of risk involved in continued substance abuse and its consequences. This denial makes AIDS-related health education interventions more difficult.

The Position of the Substance Abuser in Society

Because of their status as "outlaws" within society, most substance-abusing patients are not well served by the community groups that provide help to others. They are cut off from basic health care and social services. Even where such groups or agencies exist to serve them, substance abusers are less likely to be aware of them and less likely to trust them. They are unlikely to have medical insurance and are thus served primarily by public hospitals and clinics, which are often heavily burdened with AIDS patients. They are usually unemployed and have fewer financial resources to draw on.

Due to the position of substance abusers in society, medical and psychological complications of HIV disease are often not addressed adequately. Often they seek treatment only during acute episodes of an HIV-related opportunistic infection. Substance abusers are at a distinct disadvantage both in learning how to avoid AIDS and in coping with it when it occurs.

Underlying Health Issues

The substance abuser's underlying health is likely to be a strong contributor to the development of HIV disease. Poor nutritional status, use of immune-suppressing drugs, repeated bouts of infection and illness, and high stress levels pose a direct threat to the body's immune system. When a substance abuser encounters HIV, he or she does so with an already compromised immune system. Thus the course of the disease is often more rapid and more devastating.

Because of the increased vulnerability to HIV infection, it is essential to rule out the presence of substance abuse disorders in people with any HIV-related diagnoses when planning medical and mental health interventions. A thorough drug and alcohol use history, as part of a comprehensive psychosocial evaluation, taken in a direct and nonjudgmental manner is extremely helpful and appropriate for all patients with HIV-related risk.

SUBSTANCE ABUSE ASSESSMENT

Social users of drugs and alcohol can control the amount and frequency of use and can limit their use to enhance social interactions. They do not develop problems as a result of use, do not take risks when using that may endanger themselves or others, do not drink or use to get intoxicated. If there is a problem of any kind from use of alcohol or drugs and use continues, a substance abuse disorder may be present. If the use has not caused a problem but is coupled with a physically hazardous situation and it has been occurring for at least one month or repeatedly over a period of time, it is considered abuse (American Psychiatric Association, 1987). Appendix A is a tool for evaluating a substance abuse disorder. The suggested questions after each indicator of abuse can be used to determine if it applies to the patient being interviewed.

If there appears to be problematic use of alcohol or other drugs, the patient should be referred for further evaluation or for treatment to a substance abuse program. The immediate goal of the substance abuse assessment is to link the current crisis or presenting problem to the continuing drug or alcohol use. This is the "missing link" in the mind of the patient, who often wonders why all those unfortunate circumstances happen for no apparent reason. "I have so many financial problems" or "Why do I always wind up in trouble at work?" and similar statements demonstrate the occurrence of drug and alcohol use on the one hand and crisis after crisis on the other.

An evaluation can help patients see the reality of their substance abuse in a thorough and objective manner. At the least, a substance abuse assessment is also an occasion for patient education concerning drug and alcohol use. Whether or not patients seek help for their substance abuse problem, they need information about HIV prevention related to their current and prior behavioral HIV risk.

AN EFFECTIVE AIDS EDUCATION PROGRAM FOR SUBSTANCE ABUSERS

An effective AIDS education program for patients at risk for HIV as a result of their substance abuse must deal with all aspects of risk behavior. These include risks involving needle use, sexual transmission and impaired judgment secondary to drug or alcohol use, use of immunosuppressant drugs, and perinatal transmission. Education should include personal risk assessment and methods of preventing transmission based upon past or present risk behavior.

Education that fosters behavioral change and is nonjudgmental is most effective. It should include a problem-solving component to help patients determine how they will initiate needed behavioral change (Gibson, 1988). Additionally, fostering of the feeling of self-efficacy, that one can do something to prevent HIV disease, and the feeling of response efficacy, that there are concrete things that will work to prevent HIV, will facilitate the needed behavioral change. A checklist can be made and used as a teaching tool for patients at risk for HIV infection secondary to their alcohol or drug use (Faltz & Rinaldi, 1987). All patients with a history of alcohol or drug abuse could benefit from a repeated consistent education program.

EMOTIONAL COMPONENTS OF HIV FOR SUBSTANCE ABUSERS AND THEIR FAMILIES

Although HIV risk education and entrance into treatment for substance abuse disorders are goals for health care intervention, often an appropriate referral is not made. The combined problem of HIV disease and substance abuse raises critical clinical, ethical, and personal dilemmas for patients, loved ones, and health care providers. These can often lead to barriers to effective substance abuse treatment for those affected by it. This can be due to both patient resistance to seeking help and to difficulties on the part of treatment providers. When substance abuse treatment referral is deferred, the continued use that usually results can serve as a barrier to the successful implementation of medical and psychosocial interventions addressing HIV-related problems.

Substance abuse in a person with HIV infection or a diagnosis of AIDS or ARC can have profound consequences. The patient and loved ones are often traumatized by the diagnosis, and loved ones may be reluctant to confront the patient's substance abuse. Health care and mental health treatment providers may overlook substance abuse in persons diagnosed as having AIDS or ARC. They may perceive the HIV disease to be their most immediate concern and the substance abuse as an ancillary issue. Many of the difficulties with the dual problem of HIV disease and substance abuse are related to the inability of patients to cope with their new diagnosis as a result of continuing substance abuse.

Denial

The issue of denial is crucial when discussing patient resistance to substance abuse treatment and successful coping with HIV disease. Denial is the chief defense against seeing the extent of substance abuse or other illness and its consequences. Substance abusers also deny their risk for HIV infection and often deny illness with symptoms of AIDS. Often substance abusers wait until there is a medical or emotional crisis before seeking treatment. Therefore they do not take advantage of prophylactic treatment for opportunistic infections, research treatment protocols, or peer support groups.

"Denial" in substance abuse treatment is a term that can refer to many behaviors. Rationalization of use, minimizing of harmful results, deflection of attention from one's own problem to society's or someone else's, and blame on childhood experiences are examples of defensive behaviors that prevent the acceptance of the diagnosis of substance abuse. Although denial is expressed in various ways, it can be viewed as either the denial of the loss of control over use, the consequences of uncontrolled use, or both.

Denial of a substance abuse disorder will bolster the denial of risk for infection with HIV. Additionally, substance abuse evaluation and referral is most effective when a patient is becoming more accepting of the HIV-related diagnosis. Interventions that are caring, matter-of-fact, gently probing, and done with humor and directness are most effective in confronting denial. Confrontation that is punitive or that attempts to illicit guilt feelings is destructive to the therapeutic relationship.

Any presenting problem can be viewed as the event that can bring a person into substance abuse treatment and recovery. This is "hitting bottom," the time when it can no longer be denied that drinking or drug use is out of control. With early skillful intervention, this "bottom" can be "raised" so that a person need not wait until there are more serious consequences of abuse before awareness of the problem emerges.

Motivation

Motivation to enter treatment for substance abuse is essential. Some patients, even after a thorough evaluation, deny their abuse and are not motivated to seek treatment. In this case, it is important to outline the consequences of their choice and to keep the door open to treatment at a later date. One example of doing this would be to ask the patient to describe how bad it would have to be before he or she sought help. If they stated that they could stop use on their own, one could ask "What would you do if this plan doesn't work for any reason?" If motivation is lacking for treatment at the time, even after these interventions, it is important to remember that the process of the practitioner's interaction with the patient will be remembered by him or her. It will be recalled at a later date when something else is going wrong in his or her relationship with alcohol or drugs. Then there may be a call requesting a referral for treatment.

Coping with Manipulative Behavior

Manipulative behavior can be a frustrating feature of active substance abuse. The first aspect of manipulative behavior is an annoying or other inappropriate action. The second is the request for a favor, either stated or implied, that the patient is making. Flattery, intrusiveness, intimidation, inflammatory remarks, and bargaining are common ways a chemically dependent person can alienate or attempt to manipulate therapists and health care workers. Additionally, a patient may appear overly helpless or compliant or, conversely, may repeatedly question a professional's actions.

Each of these actions has as its goal the second aspect of manipulation— the request for a favor from the practitioner. Typical of the goals that a patient hopes to achieve are acceptance of their drug or alcohol use, increasing the amount or strength of the medication prescribed, access to services or funds, or justification for continued use. Justification can come when the patient "feels rejected" by a professional who may have been setting reasonable limits to manipulative behavior.

Practitioners dealing with the initial manipulative behavior need to ask themselves "What does this person want?" This helps defuse the behavior. When what the patient hopes to accomplish is established, it is up to the practitioner to decide what he or she wishes to do about the explicit or implicit request. The action taken by the provider should be based upon clinical judgment of the merits of the request rather than on the initial manipulative behavior.

Noncompliance and Continued Substance Abuse

The most troubling difficulties with substance-abusing patients are the lack of consistent compliance with recommended treatment and the continued use of drugs and alcohol. Use of contracts or agreements for complex problems such as pain management difficulties or noncompliance for substance abusers with HIV disease can be beneficial. For example, drug treatment programs clearly state their expectations and regulations to patients in writing either as a contract or in patient handbook. Patients are asked to stipulate that they have read these so that there is no misunderstanding of policy affecting them. Often, contracting is used for patients who relapse or who are noncompliant with substance abuse treatment program policy. Improvement is expected within a stated time and expectations are clearly presented. Consequences for continued noncompliance are also clearly defined. Contracts can be also applied to situations in mental health and medical settings. For example, use of a medication agreement can be useful with a manipulative or drug-abusing patient (Faltz, 1989).

Health care and mental health workers need to know what the consequences are for patients' unacceptable behavior toward themselves and their agencies. These need to be followed fairly and consistently. If patients are jeopardizing therapy by coming drunk or late to, or acting belligerent at, therapy sessions, or are unable to avail themselves of housing, medical, and social service interventions, this may also adversely affect the therapeutic relationship with an individual practitioner or agency. It is appropriate to discontinue a therapy session if a patient is intoxicated or to decline to see a patient who is late. Every effort should be made to confront the specific objectionable behavior, relate it to continued substance abuse, and, most importantly, offer substance abuse treatment to the patient.

Following through on stated policy or guidelines for an agency in an even-handed manner maintains the integrity of a program or agency. It gives clear messages to patients and a sense of fairness. It also frees practitioners to be caring toward substance-abusing patients because limits of what is allowable are clear for him or her.

Pain Management and Psychoactive Medication

Successful pain management for patients with AIDS and ARC is crucial. When there is a dual diagnosis of AIDS/ARC and a substance abuse disorder, average effective doses of opiates or other psychoactive medication may be inadequate. Additionally, medication for anxiety, depression, sleep disturbances, and to combat side effects of HIV-related medication is often prescribed. Problems arise for patients when medication is used more frequently and in higher doses than recommended and when it is used for indications for which it was not prescribed.

If there is medication misuse, a medication agreement—formalizing an understanding between health care providers and the patient for the therapeutic use of medication—can be extremely helpful. Symptoms of possible abuse of prescription drugs (Faltz, 1989) include those in which the patient:

1. Is feeling tired or having a clouded mental state.
2. Is feeling "hyperactive" or nervous.
3. Is anticipating the next dose ahead of time.
4. Is frequently asking for a higher dose or stronger medication.
5. Supplements medication with alcohol or drugs.
6. Approaches more than one doctor asking for medication.

If there is an inappropriate use of medication there can be an agreement by the patient to follow the prescription as signified, to discuss any medication problems with the health care provider, not to obtain medication from other sources, and not to self-medicate with alcohol or other drugs.

Co-Dependency

Co-dependency, or the reaction of a family member or a significant other to a person's continuing alcohol or drug use, can be exacerbated when there is HIV disease present. The persons affected by the abuse over a period of time have already become frustrated by their friend or loved one's behavior, broken promises, and lies. In an effort to cope with the abuse, they have often tried to arrange the environment to minimize use or have lectured and tried to control use in other ways. If there is true addiction, these efforts have not worked.

Family members of the AIDS patients who continue to abuse drugs and alcohol need particular outreach by mental health professionals. They need encouragement to care for themselves, to take needed food and rest, and to focus on their own feelings and needs. Gentle probing around co-dependency issues that is supportive of the family member can be helpful. Referral to self-help groups such as Al-Anon, Nar-Anon, and therapy should be made, if appropriate.

PROBLEMS OF HEALTH CARE PROVIDERS

On occasion, a health care provider can inadvertently be drawn into the process of addiction by his or her own behavior. A professional may also minimize or not talk about the problem, may avoid confrontation of the obvious abuse, or make excuses for continuing use. Often the provider tries to protect the patient from alcohol or drugs or the results of their use. They often encourage the use of will power to control the disease or a change of location or job or living situation. Finally, the provider may be punitive and gossip about the patient, or express anger or blame toward the patient. These behaviors, although understandable, jeopardize the therapeutic relationship.

Often there is a tacit agreement between a patient and health care provider not to mention the underlying cause of the hepatitis, AIDS, bleeding ulcer, or repeated admission for abscesses. Sometimes the need for treatment is addressed with cursory comments such as "You know you should cut down on your drinking" or "Using drugs can kill you." One question that comes up repeatedly when a hospitalized AIDS patient is also a substance abuser is "Why bother about the substance abuse?" People working with AIDS patients may feel that substance abuse is a "coping strategy," that treatment is strenuous and confrontive and will increase the stress on these individuals, and that the use of drugs is a personal choice, not a disease, anyway. These views are often the result of a misunderstanding of the nature of substance abuse or of the modalities used in treating it.

Substance abuse is often seen as a problem secondary to difficulties in the environment. When these difficulties are resolved, it is hoped that the substance abuse will go away. Similarly, substance abuse can be viewed as a problem resulting from an underlying mental health problem such as depression, low self-esteem, or excessive anxiety. The solution proposed is often insightful therapy or "talking it out" with a friend. Unfortunately, both the social and mental health approaches often do not work on a primary substance abuse disorder. The model of substance abuse as a disease that is chronic and progressive is used most commonly in substance abuse treatment. Such treatment focuses on patient education, counseling directed at arresting abuse and planning for relapse prevention. It is not punitive, certainly less stressful than the chaotic life associated with active abuse, and can be extremely powerful and releasing to an individual caught up in the grip of the disease.

Often, substance abuse is seen as a "moral" issue, in a fashion similar to judgments about HIV infection. This sometimes occurs among health care providers, who take to "lecturing" patients about their use or who can become punitive. They may be very supportive at first but later change after experiencing manipulative behavior or noncompliance by the patient.

At times, it appears that there are many pitfalls for the professional in approaching a patient who is actively using drugs and alcohol. It is possible to be both caring and effective. Interventions that encourage constructive expression of feelings, which express concern for the individual while holding him or her responsible for actions, are beneficial to the therapeutic relationship. Health care providers need to be consistent in their approach to substance-abusing patients.

This will help insure that patients are responsible for their behaviors and are informed about specific actions that are disruptive or not appropriate. This approach can help prevent common patient- and professionally generated barriers to successful substance abuse and HIV treatment.

TREATMENT APPROACHES FOR THE SUBSTANCE ABUSER WITH HIV DISEASE

Key concerns in approaching substance abusers with HIV disease are the evaluation of their knowledge about HIV disease, resources in the community, and health maintenance issues. Additionally, assistance is usually needed in finding ways to cope with emotions generated by the HIV-related diagnoses. Appendix B is a plan for early intervention with substance-abusing patients with AIDS. It outlines these key concerns and desired outcomes or goals of intervention. It also suggests initial helpful interventions.

SUMMARY

The relationship between alcohol, drugs, and AIDS and some of the barriers to effective dual treatment of substance abuse and AIDS-related diagnoses have been detailed. Practical strategies to improve the response of treatment providers in caring for this difficult population of patients have been offered. While there are many problems associated with the dual diagnoses of AIDS and substance abuse, professionals can intervene effectively by first recognizing how their own values and anxieties impact upon substance abuse treatment approaches. They can accept substance abuse as a problem that can be treated. Finally, they can evaluate substance abuse in HIV-infected patients and develop effective treatment approaches addressing it.

APPENDIX A: SUBSTANCE ABUSE EVALUATION TOOL

Name _____ Date _____

I. Drug and Alcohol Use History (Amount, frequency, route, length of time used).
   Alcohol:
   Stimulants:
   Opiates:

Barbiturates:
Abuse of antianxiety, pain, or sleep medication:
Hallucinogens:
Other:

II. Abuse Indicators
    1. Consequences of use (Presenting problems)
        a. Have you had any difficulty with your spouse, partner, or other relationships as a result of your use?
        b. Have any friends discussed your drinking or drug use with you?
        c. Have you had any housing or financial difficulties?
        d. Any work problems? Are you able to work?
        e. Health problems related to drug/alcohol use?
        f. Emotional difficulties when using?
        g. Other problems?
    2. Loss of control (Inability to control amount or frequency of use)
        a. Have you tried to stop using in the past?
        b. Have you tried to control the amount or frequency of use?
    3. Preoccupation (Increasing focus on drug/alcohol use and situations)
        a. Do you look forward to weekends (or whenever) to get "high"?
        b. Do you spend much time with people who don't use or drink?
        c. Do you try to make sure that you will have the opportunity to drink/use at social situations?
    4. Self-medication for emotional states
        a. Do you use when you are feeling sad, anxious, angry, or frustrated?
        b. Do you use to try to relax?
        c. Do you feel that you need a drink or to use drugs when things are not "going well?"
    5. Use while alone
        a. Do you keep your own "private stash" of alcohol or drugs?
        b. Do you use by yourself?
    6. Rapid intake
        a. Do you find that you want to use your drugs as soon as possible after getting them?
        b. Do you gulp drinks when you first start drinking to "get a buzz"?
        c. Is it hard to wait to use or drink?
    7. Protection of supply
        a. Do you try to make sure that there is enough alcohol to last the day?
        b. Do you hide drugs or alcohol from others?

8. Tolerance (Increasing use of drug or alcohol with the same level of intoxication)
    a. Can you use more drugs or alcohol than others?
    b. Has your use increased in the last six months?
9. Withdrawal symptoms
    a. Shakes? Tremors?
    b. Cramps, diarrhea?
    c. Feeling paranoid, fearful?
    d. Difficulty sleeping?
    e. Rapid pulse?
10. Blackouts
    a. Do you have periods that you can't remember what happened while drinking?

APPENDIX B: COUNSELING PLAN FOR SUBSTANCE-ABUSING PATIENTS WITH AIDS

I. Key concerns

1. AIDS awareness/education, focusing on quality of life issues, treatment options
2. Health maintenance and avoiding further disease progression
3. Resource/referral awareness
4. Dealing with emotions generated by the diagnosis, uncertainty, and the need for changes in behavior to extend and improve the quality of life, and reduce transmission of the disease

II. Desired outcomes

1. Patient will minimize risk behavior and avoid relapse
2. Patient will utilize emotional support provided by the counselor to encourage behavioral changes
3. Patient will be able to utilize appropriate community social services, medical, chemical dependency and alcoholism treatment, mental health, vocation, and legal resources
4. Patient will be motivated to continue to benefit from treatment for dependency

III. Initial intervention strategy

1. Check the level of understanding of basic AIDS information and implement an education plan based on patient needs

2. Confront denial or lack of commitment to minimize risk behavior
3. Offer hope for stabilization of health
4. Check the need and depth of motivation for referral to chemical dependency or alcohol treatment programs
5. Encourage continuing commitment to the recovery process in treatment for chemical dependency
6. Check the apparent need and then refer for medical follow-up, emotional or sexual counseling, or to support groups and other self-help programs
7. Help the patient verbalize feelings of anger, grief, and loss generated by the diagnosis, the need for change in sexual and drug use behavior, or the possible delay in childbearing
8. Reinforce the fact that taking action now may improve health and slow deterioration
9. Discuss "contagion" issues with patient and family members to allay fears of spread by casual contact
10. Encourage and support patient verbalization of such feelings as
    a. Fear of dying from AIDS
    b. Fear of having exposed others to AIDS or doing so through continued risk behavior
    c. Feelings of guilt over risk behavior in the past
    d. Feelings of loss over necessary behavior changes and possible postponement of childbearing
    e. Fear of what others will think or do or of being isolated and/or rejected
11. Compile and distribute a list of community resources to serve people with HIV concerns or AIDS/ARC diagnosis
12. Encourage the use of tools learned in recovering from chemical dependency in coping with this life crisis
13. Continue to confront the drug abuse as you would with other patients not diagnosed with AIDS
14. Emphasize positive things the patient can do to maximize health
15. Extend hope that with continued attention to health matters the patient can live longer, possibly extending life until more effective treatments become available
16. Emphasize what control the patient does have over the quality of life for as long as he/she lives
17. Encourage patient planning for care of family members and for financial/legal matters

18. Consult with physicians about any possible chemical dependency program modifications to help the patient stay in continued treatment
19. Set realistic expectations for yourself as a counselor and for the patient
20. Consult with physicians and other caregivers on medication issues in order to maximize benefits without abuse of prescription drugs

REFERENCES

American Psychiatric Association. (1987). *Diagnostic and statistical manual of mental disorders* (3rd ed., rev.). Washington, DC: American Psychiatric Association.

Centers for Infectious Diseases, Centers for Disease Control. (1989b). Update: Acquired immunodeficiency syndrome associated with intravenous drug use—United States, 1988. *Morbidity and Mortality Weekly Report, 38*(10), 165–170.

Centers for Infectious Diseases, Centers for Disease Control. (1991, February). *HIV/AIDS Surveillance,* p. 9.

Coates, T. J., Stall, R. D., Catania, J. A., & Kegeles, S. M. (1988). Behavioral factors in the spread of HIV infection. *AIDS, 2*(suppl 1), 239–246.

Faltz, B. G. (1989). Strategies for working with substance abusing patients. In J. W. Dilley, C. Pies, & M. Hilquist (Eds.), *Face to face: A guide to AIDS counseling* (pp. 127–136). San Francisco: UCSF AIDS Health Project.

Faltz, B. G., & Rinaldi, J. (1987). *AIDS and substance abuse: A manual for health care professionals.* San Francisco: UCSF AIDS Health Project.

Gibson, D. R., Sorensen, J. L., Lovelle-drache, J., Catania, J., Kegeles, S., & Young, M. (1988, June). *Psychosocial predictors of AIDS high-risk behavior among intravenous drug users and their sexual partners.* Poster presented at the IV International AIDS conference, Stockholm, Sweden.

Klein, T. W., Newton, C., & Friedman, H. (1987). Inhibition of natural killer cell function by marijuana components. *Journal of Toxicology and Environmental Health, 20*(4), 321–332.

McGreggor R. R. (1988). Alcohol and immune defense. *Journal of the American Medical Association, 256,* 1474–1479.

Stall, R., Wiley, J., McKusick, L., Coates, T. J., & Ostrow, D. G. (1986). Alcohol and drug use during sexual activity and compliance with safe sex guidelines for AIDS: The AIDS and Behavioral Research Project. *Health Education Quarterly, 13,* 359–371.

Dying with AIDS

Dying with AIDS

ALEXANDRA TEGUIS

VARIOUS STYLES OF COPING WITH DEATH

Consider the following scenarios (names have been altered except where people have expressly requested that their actual names be used):

1. Sally, a youthful-looking grandmother of 36, whose 18-year-old daughter contracted AIDS through a drug-using husband who "snorted," rather than injected, heroin and cocaine, describes her relationship to her 9-month-old granddaughter Meegan who has tested HIV positive. She relates that she barely interacts with her daughter (who currently resides with her and the baby) and that she has distanced herself, half-consciously, from her beloved Meegan. The infant has tested seropositive three times and it may not be known for another year whether the child will ultimately test "negative."

2. At Starcross Monastery in northern California, the Starcross Community members prepare to bury Aaron with his toys in the handmade coffin Brother Tolly has fashioned from native wood. The year-old infant died of respiratory complications from his AIDS. Emergency firefighters had refused to answer the distress dispatch, having decided in advance that they were unprepared for such emergencies. At the last moment before interment, the child's teenage mother, who had rendered the care of her child to Starcross, recanted, and requested that Aaron be buried in her town. Tolly and the others buried his toys anyway, and marked the grave with a cross (McCarroll, 1988).

ALEXANDRA TEGUIS • Manchester Community College, Manchester, Connecticut 06040.

Living and Dying with AIDS, edited by Paul I. Ahmed, Plenum Press, New York, 1992.

3. As Joey M. expresses his grief over having AIDS, lamenting his poverty he sobs uncontrollably, continually repeating, "$30,000 in my veins and up my nose, gone, gone, gone. Now I have nothing!"

4. A young mother of a 7-year-old hemophiliac son describes her reaction on being told of his AIDS diagnosis:

> A numbness had come over me. When you are told that someone you love is going to die, it's as if time skips a beat. And once the clock resumes ticking, nothing is the same. Your voice belongs to a stranger. Your eyes linger on some inconsequential detail; a smudge on the doctor's glasses; a speck of color amid others on the floor. When the person who is dying is your child, you know that things will never be the same again. That the pain will stay inside you forever. (Oyler & Oyler, 1988, p. 213)

5. PWA Chuck Morris recounts his experience of resolving unfinished business at a residential weeklong workshop experience.

> Elisabeth Kübler-Ross is very fond of talking about the Hitler in us. And we all have a Hitler in us. We also all have a Mahatma Gandhi in us. But we can't keep in touch with that Gandhi because so often people press buttons that bring out the Hitler. And those are all things that go back . . . garbage that we carry with us for ten, twenty, forty, sixty years. The purpose of [externalizing] is to get back to that initial experience and get rid of it, so we can stop reacting to people in that old way. We get rid of that unfinished business so we can get back in contact with the Mother Theresa in us. Because that's our natural state. (Serinus, 1986, p. 43)

6. Nancy Phelps is an R.N. on a dedicated AIDS unit with 28 patients in a large metropolitan hospital. We ride the elevator together as she leaves her shift more exhausted emotionally than physically. She is leaving on a long-overdue week's vacation (nurses in this work typically delay and accumulate more time off because of the intense and intimate nature of the caregiver–patient relationship, similar to a wartime triage ambiance). She has a great deal of anxiety even before her tropical vacation begins, anticipating a number of deaths before, or upon, her return. She has already encountered 50 deaths from AIDS in this last year alone. She describes her AIDS nursing as the most intense in her entire nursing career, except for her experience of triage in Vietnam 22 years ago.

7. The following describes how Cleve Jones, founder of the national AIDS Quilt Project, called "Remember Their Names," journeyed from despair to hope and healing.

> In April 1986, Cleve [Jones] told a nationwide television audience that he was antibody positive to the AIDS virus on a "60 Minutes" program about San Francisco's response to the AIDS epidemic. He wanted, he says, to help demystify the disease. Four weeks later, two men, calling him "faggot," stabbed Cleve in the back as he neared his home in Sacramento. During his three months of recuperation, Cleve had time to think about organizing the Quilt, an idea that had long been floating around his head. Some friends thought the idea was morbid; others simply couldn't see how it would work. (Ruskin, 1988, p. 19)

Jones continues:

> "The Quilt has helped me turn my back on cynicism. . . . I used to be constantly aware of hurt, pain and evil people are capable of. The Quilt has helped me believe that in all of us there really is something that is very good. It's O.K. to get angry, it's O.K. to get impatient, it's O.K. to have fights, but it is important not to give up on people." (Ruskin, 1988, p. 19)

Is it possible to go from immobilizing shock to depths of despair and subsequent reinvestment of energy into healing, and even hope? Cleve Jones, finding himself paralyzed by the deaths of most of his friends in 1984, describes this sense so eloquently.

> "To me, Castro Street is populated by ghosts. When I walk to 18th Street from Church Street to Eureka Street, a distance of eight blocks, just looking at all these houses and knowing the stories behind so many of the windows, makes me feel so old. To know that's where Shane died, that's where Alan died, that was Bobby's last house, that's where Gregory died, that's where Jimmy was diagnosed, that's the house Alex got kicked out of . . ."
>
> By the time of Marvin's death in late 1986, the grief was overwhelming. "I began to believe that there was no hope," he says "and that everyone I cared about was going to die from this disease. I lost my sense of humor, and I lost my ability to fight back." (Ruskin, 1988, p. 18)

Cleve, although healthier than many diagnosed HIV positive, was able to convert that despair through proaction. His old spirit returned with the launching of The NAMES Project.

> "I had become numb," he recalls. "When somebody you know dies every day, what do you do? You try to stop feeling and stop remembering. But I don't want to stop remembering Marvin Feldman and all the other friends of mine that have gone. They shaped my life and I love them and I don't want to forget them. I had to find a way for me to hold on to those memories and everything I cherish about those people." (Ruskin, 1988, p. 19)

8. It is estimated there will be close to 20,000 HIV-infected children in the United States by 1991. Multiplicity of losses in AIDS leads us to speak of *dying families* as well. We often only regard the perspective of the family losing a child through death via AIDS; we seldom look at this from the dying child's perspective.

> In the not-quite-four years of his life, Jimmy has lost his home, his mother, his father, two sisters, two brothers, maternal and paternal grandparents, aunts, uncles and cousins, staff members to whom he was attached, and, progressively, his health. Some of his family was lost to death, some just don't come to visit anymore. Jimmy knows the names of all his family, living and dead. He remembers them, and likes to talk about them. The people who work with Jimmy aren't always comfortable with that, especially when he talks about his mother. Often, the subject gets changed, and staff are cautioned not to discuss her death. (Dubik-Unruh, 1989, p. 10)

9. Paula is a 14-year-old high school freshman. She has come to the family caregiver support group because she is anxious and insecure about revealing to

her friends that her father has AIDS. She walks the tenderloin district of her small city in search of her father, who is continuing to shoot crack, cocaine, and heroin. Frequently, she enlists her uncle and grandfather in her attempts to locate him by cruising the tenderloin slowly in their car, passing the prostitutes and the johns in search of father. At a time when Paula should be enjoying the moratorium of adolescence, being carefree and trying out new roles, she is on a daily rescue mission, hoping she can stop her dad from what she feels could be his last fix.

What all these scenarios have in common is that each person, in every instance, is undergoing some aspect of the grief process.

Additionally, all the scenarios point to the enormous number of people the pandemic affects. It involves an extended kinship system the likes of which perhaps have never been experienced with any other terminal illness (with the possible exception of plagues and epidemics at the turn of this century in America). In a lateral sense, it extends outward to those who have taken in babies or adults with AIDS (hospitals, support groups, hospices, and reconstructed families, as well as families of origin). It also affects vertical systems, where a mother mourns her own impending death while she mourns the death of her child, and a grandparent mourns the loss of both of them.

The stories also speak of the multitude of other losses, each necessitating its own grief process: physical ones, emotional ones, material ones, and intellectual and spiritual ones—overlapping, overwhelming, and pyramidal.

It might be well to summarize elements in the grief process as outlined by Kübler-Ross, keeping in mind that it is only intended as *one* paradigm, a guide, similar in most features to others. Although it has been criticized by some as implying a lockstep approach to the dying trajectory, universally applicable to all who encounter death, it was never conceived in that manner (Kalish, 1981a,b). Indeed, in my 10 years of staffing countless grief workshops with Dr. Kübler-Ross, I have never witnessed her presenting the material to be implemented via a cookbook approach. Her broad-based thanatological philosophy is much too humanistic, and her individualized approach belies such intent. She has railed against such pat distortions of a system meant merely to serve as a guide for further understanding. All too frequently she hears of well-intentioned professionals asking if a patient has reached "bargaining" yet!

The multiplicity of other losses at varying points accompanying an AIDS diagnosis would make it unlikely, in any case, that a forward sequential progression would occur in an orderly manner. Explication aside, most people who simplistically and academically interpret the grief stages have never had the opportunity to directly experience the validity of the model for the thousands of people who have found it to be veridical for them.

Additionally, though Kübler-Ross has published 14 volumes since *On Death and Dying,* in which she originally postulated her thesis of the grief model, countless individuals have described its healing aspects and their ability to identify with the similar feelings and experiences it sets forth.

The model is herewith presented in order to acquaint the reader with a broader context of interpretation.

THE GRIEF PROCESS

The stages of grief are universal to any loss, whether physical, mental or symbolic:

1. Denial and isolation
   "No, not me!"
2. Anger, scapegoating or rage
   "Why *ME*?"
3. Bargaining, survivor guilt, atonement
   "Yes me, but!"
4. Depression, withdrawal
   "Yes me"
5. Acceptance
   "Yes me" (Kübler-Ross, 1969, 1975)

Here are some key points to keep in mind regarding the grief process:

1. It may apply to whole countries, entire cultures, or subcultures (such as AIDS caregivers), as well as to individuals.
2. This sequence is by no means cast in stone. People can go back and forth or remain at any one point for weeks, months, or years. There is no right or universally appropriate time for healing grief. People also can partially be in several phases at any one point in time.
3. Given any family constellation, each person may be at a different point and may progress at different rates, or remain at one particular phase.
4. Although particular behaviors may seem odd, the process itself is normal and necessary for healing to occur.
5. Healing/acceptance (even partial) involves reorganization and redirection of energy and subsequent reinvestment in living each day fully!

CULTURAL RESPONSES TO THE GRIEF PROCESS

Kübler-Ross has recently recounted how her model of the grief process has applied to our own society over the past several decades (Kübler-Ross, 1983b). In a retrospective analysis, she describes how, in the decades of the fifties and early sixties, we as Americans were experiencing extreme denial of our fallibility, our mortality, and our spiritual, or "higher," nature, the arrogance of which led us to develop high-technology medicine, life extension, new life-form patenting, and even life-suspending technologies. This was the era of burgeoning interest in transplantation and harvesting of body organs; of the capability of indefinitely maintaining people on life-support systems (with its attendant legislation mandating new and technologically based definitions of death); and cryogenics (freezing corpses until cures have been found, at which point persons could be "revitalized" and healed, in an ultimate postponement of the death event!) (Kübler-Ross, 1983b). She adds that we really believed in our grandiosity, that with "high tech" and sufficient money, we could "conquer" even death. This ego- and ethnocentric attitude also led us to deplete our natural resources and posed a serious threat to the very survival of earth and its inhabitants. Later, as we now know, (perhaps we might consider it as a form of acceptance by converting anger and despair into assertion) groups like Physicians for Social Responsibility led the rest of us to awaken and assume a proactive stance in preserving the environment. Dr. Kübler-Ross also viewed the simultaneous events of the war in Vietnam and the killings at Kent State as playing huge roles in raising consciousness regarding our vulnerability. We as a society were no longer able to maintain the myth of the personal fable (typically ascribed to youth, who in *their* grandiosity and denial believe that by virtue of strength, health, and energy, they are impervious to harm, even death).

Kübler-Ross contends that both the riots and the hedonism of the 1960s were expressions of the phase of anger. Many attempted to reject society's path by turning back the clock and living alternatively or communally on the fringes of America.

The stage of depression in the 1970s closely followed, in which people often made a conscious decision not to have children ("to go to school wearing gas masks") (Kübler-Ross, 1983). The events at Kent State represented the nadir of despair as well as the catalyst for action and hope. The university law school and medical school closed, as well as all the seminaries in Chicago. Then came the moratorium and the teach-in (Kübler-Ross, 1983).

Dr. Kübler-Ross articulates:

> It was the first time in my life in the United States that I had seen a Southern Baptist minister sit next to a rabbi; the medical director sat next to the black cleaning woman; we were literally brothers and sisters for the first time. One after the other we started to talk, to evaluate where we were. Was there anything we could do? And after a day and a night of endless moratorium, with everybody coming up to speak: poor, rich, Black, and white, an old woman from 63rd Street, an old Black woman whom I'm sure never even went to high school, got up and said something very profound: she said, "I think we have talked enough. Maybe it's time now to stop cursing the darkness and go home and light a candle. It is possible that if all of us, just this room full of

people, would go home and do one good thing, anything positive instead of negative, then it is not too late to change the tide." (Kübler-Ross, 1983, p. 2)

And this, Dr. Kübler-Ross maintains, was the turning point of converting despair into hope, resignation into action, and of living more fully and consciously.

SOCIETAL STRATEGIES FOR COPING WITH CATASTROPHIC IMPLICATIONS OF AIDS

Assuming the validity of Kübler-Ross's concept that, indeed, entire societies experience the grief process, let us look at a few grief stages in the context of the AIDS pandemic and describe how an entire culture, or large numbers within our culture, might react to the grief surrounding AIDS.

Denial

How might we express denial as a nation? Most of us feel that we have no direct connection to the two highest risk groups—homosexual/bisexual men and IV drug users—and thus are "safe" from the ravages of AIDS.

One might even propose a new grief substage as applicable in traumatic events. It occurs as an aspect of shock in which, in addition to being numbed by reality, we feel overwhelmed and inundated by the reality and become terrified, thus closing ourselves off to contacts and new input. One researcher calls this often media-induced reaction AFRAIDS, a kind of "social disease" that encourages the person to fear AIDS, its potential consequences, and the risks that are presented to others (Miller, 1987).

The general population, including health professionals, also may express denial by behaving in, or expressing attitudes to, situations involving AIDS in a completely different manner from that which they convey in abstract attitude questionnaires. Poling and colleagues (1989), citing numerous recent studies (1986 through 1989) elaborates:

> Persons with AIDS portrayed in standardized, written vignettes were viewed with much greater negativity, harshness, and avoidance than [were] persons portrayed identically but said to have leukemia. . . . Alarmingly, AIDS patients relative to leukemia patients were also rated as less deserving of sympathy, less deserving of health care, more deserving to die, and of less loss to the world if they did die. . . . Respondents . . . were markedly less willing to interact even in conversation with an AIDS patient than [they were with] an identically described patient with a disease other than AIDS. (Poling, Redmon, and Burnette, 1989, p. 64)

Denial is expressed by separating ourselves from those groups we feel in some way are at much higher risk, and yet, if one were to visit the AIDS Quilt, one would realize the tapestry of AIDS is created from "common threads."

> The AIDS Quilt specifically speaks to the diversity of lives affected by the disease. Although the remembrances sewn into each quilt panel can only hint at the person's life, and although the entire quilt records only about 10 percent of the nation's AIDS deaths, the disease's undiscriminating nature is easily seen in the range of the people memorialized. They include a Colorado stockbroker, a mother of four teenagers in Atlanta, an Olympic athlete, a prize-winning Chicago journalist, a biker from Nevada, and a Stanford University professor. Some quilt panels name celebrities like Rock Hudson and Liberace. Others name people who were living on welfare, struggling to keep off the streets. There are policemen, schoolteachers, farmers, doctors, playwrights, ministers, chefs, lawyers, artists and politicians. There is a quilt panel for the hairdresser who styled Joan Mondale's hair during the 1984 Democratic Convention, and there is one for the respiratory therapist who tended Ronald Reagan after the 1981 assassination attempt. There are sons and daughters, mothers and fathers, lovers, brothers, friends and grandparents. (Ruskin, 1988, p. 12)

Anger

In our effort as a society to vent our anger at the disease or at the elusive and mutable virus itself, that attacks *healthy* cells, we see AIDS as the "enemy" in a war that seems incapable of being won. Susan Sontag feels that *any* disease if feared and hated enough (as well as mystery-laden) is viewed as being morally as well as medically contagious and is used metaphorically. Despite the probable dismay of Susan Sontag, who abhors adversarial jargon to describe events like AIDS and TB, the *analogy* of and, indeed, the *metaphor* of war once again enters our descriptive vocabulary (Sontag, 1978, 1989). There are even studies currently that describe posttraumatic stress disorders in a high proportion of maternal AIDS caregivers, a concept that, in fact, came into being as a direct result of the Vietnam War (Trice, 1988).

Consistently in the description of the pandemic we hear of "battling" the epidemic using "combatant" drugs, entering the AIDS "battlefield" and fighting the "enemy." Indeed, a "biological holocaust" task force formed in 1974 by Lyndon LaRouche spoke of developing a "war plan" modeled on the National Disaster Medical System (NDMS) designed by the Emergency Mobilization Preparedness Board (EMPB) created by President Reagan in 1981 to deal with unusual "surge" medical demands such as those resulting from nuclear war or natural disasters. This health care system, which was based on a plan developed by the Defense Department in 1980 called the Civilian–Military Contingency Hospital System (CMCHS), now consists of a network of 83,000 hospital beds, both civilian and military, in the United States as well as overseas (Hamerman, *et al.,* 1986).

This reaction, considered by some as hyperbolic, would be mere fantasy were it not for the fact that we have already established precedence for isolating those with contagious diseases. People with leprosy (due in large part to "leprophobia") were placed in the barbwire-enclosed U.S. government-operated leprosarium in Carville, Louisiana, in 1921 (Gussow, 1989).

The danger in addressing *any* threat to our sense of inner security as a "war" is that we tend to blur distinctions between our rage at the disease or the epidemic and our displaced anger at those who suffer from it, ultimately regarding *them* as "the enemy."

Bargaining

One possible example of our country's "bargaining" might be the implementation of mandatory premarital screening for HIV using the ELISA test. Thirty-five states now have such mandatory testing. Not only is it cost-ineffective, but it targets a relatively low-risk traditional sample. One study indicates that it would tag 1,200 new cases—0.1% of those now infected—but would incorrectly identify 380 people—actually free from infection—as infected, even when further tested by the Western Blot. Also, it would falsely reassure close to 120 people with false negatives (Brandt, 1988).

Another, more powerful and constructive mode of bargaining has been for society as a whole, particularly high-risk groups and those groups peripheral to them, to institute drastic and fairly immediate changes in risky behavior; indeed, many, finding a distinction between intimacy and sexuality, are expanding their domain of interpersonal relationships and discovering "new" (in actuality, "old") ways of relating (Becker & Joseph, 1988; Murphy, 1988; Ulene, 1987).

It may be evidence of our denial, however, that much of our population, particularly the young and affluent, even those injecting drugs recreationally or periodically, do not consider themselves at risk and, therefore, see no need to alter behavior (Fineberg, 1988).

Acceptance

Acceptance seldom means approving of what exists but, rather, mobilizing energy, often after hopelessness and despair, to make the most of the "in between."

Witness what occurred in the San Francisco community when the Quilt Project began.

> While seven volunteers shared the Project's single borrowed sewing machine in a room that was initially without lights, Cleve taped a sheet of butcher paper outside the front door with the announcement: "This is the new home of The NAMES Project and this is our wish list . . ." They needed everything from sequins, beads, fabric and glue to extension cords, computers, telephones, lights and furniture. At the end of the list, Cleve added "back rubs, hugs and money."
>
> The Castro was quick in responding to The NAMES Project's call. Within two weeks, The Project had received ten sewing machines, including three industrial models, and the storefront building owners donated the space rent-free. (Ruskin, 1988, pp. 9–10)

If, indeed, Kübler-Ross's concept prevails regarding groups, subgroups, and societies experiencing stages of grief, we may each ask ourselves at what point we, as members of various group identities, presently find ourselves.

IS THERE A BEST WAY FOR INDIVIDUALS TO COPE WITH DEATH?

Denial

PWAs may experience either first-order denial, for example, denying the diagnosis even exists, calling it "cancer" instead, or secondary denial, that is, agreeing with the diagnosis but negating the progressive or catastrophic nature of it (Lazarus, 1981). It may be that numerous factors contribute to this minimizing or negation: the long (possibly 10- to 15-year) incubation period for the illness; the 6-week to 1-year window within which the antibodies reveal themselves on the ELISA test; the symptom-free status of those HIV-infected (for every diagnosed PWA, 2–5 people have ARC, and 20–50 are HIV positive (Melchreit, Hadler, & Weinstein, 1988). In addition, the worried well, those people at risk but "well," or asymptomatic, live in limbo, in the "grey zone," and vacillate between high anxiety and denial (Baumgartner, 1985; Lopez & Getzel, 1984). The nature of repeated relapses and remissions and discoveries of new abatement approaches, such as AZT, DDI, and aerosolized Pentamidine mist, also maintain denial and a yo-yo effect of alternating denial and acceptance.

Denial is certainly adaptive. It maintains hope and possibly insures probability of surviving the emergency stress response; indeed, "well-defended" people show lower levels of the corticosteroid secretion that accompanies the fight-or-flight response (Lazarus, 1981).

Anger and rage are probably the most underestimated aspects of the grief process because most of us consider them "negative" or "abnormal" emotions. With AIDS, people often blame themselves for one reason or another, for the disease. The need to address this issue, particularly, but by no means exclusively, by gay or bisexual men or women or drug users, may help explain why workshops that focus on self-love and self-esteem by means of working through anger are so needed and responded to. Louise Hay's "Healing AIDS" workshops may draw 700 PWAs, and Sally Fisher's seminars attract hundreds. She terms AIDS as *A*nger *I*ncorrectly *D*irected at the *S*elf, while others use self-help approaches to describe the acronym as *A*ccelerated *I*nner *D*evelopment of the *S*elf (e.g., Fisher, 1987; Hay, 1988; Melton & Garcia, 1988).

One PWA described the source of his anger this way:

> I feel anger about myself and how I feel about healthy people. I see so many people doing things that could hurt themselves and they act like they don't care. Now that I

know I only have a short time left, this really makes me mad. I'm mad at myself because I should have better prepared myself for this. There is so much I want and need to get done and now there is no time left. There are days I wish it would hurry up and be over with and other days when I wish the doctor would say it was a mistake and I'm not dying. There are other things I try to focus on, but the anger keeps coming back. (D. Smith, 1986, p. 6)

Anger

Because many of us have pushed down or not worked through our *own* anger around AIDS, we must be cautious about projecting this onto PWAs.

It is the height of professional arrogance for us to assume that we can determine the passage of one grief phase to the next. Just as we express individual differences in progression of the rate of healing for our physical wounds, we likewise vary greatly in our transitions, both affective and behavioral. Although we can "nudge," or offer to assist in, the possibility of viewing affairs from an alternative vantage point, we must always respect the right of the person to remain where he or she is for however long he or she needs to be there.

> I guess I've been spending a lot of time trying to decide what I did to deserve this. But I don't ever seem to come up with any answers. But I guess when it comes to something like this, there aren't any answers. I still have trouble separating the disease from me. I mean I'm still the same person as before, but I don't *feel* the same. (D. Smith, 1986, p. 7)

Bargaining

Bargaining has many facets. Sometimes it involves subjecting oneself to painful and undisclosed treatment protocols; sometimes it involves promises to God (or self) that one will change one's lifestyle; at other times it involves survivor guilt: surviving when others developed AIDS, and beyond this, agonizing or wanting to atone for *what one may have chosen or needed to do in order to "survive,"* like isolating or separating oneself, or leaving one's child to the care of others.

> I guess telling my roommate about my AIDS was one of the worst parts. I thought he needed to know even though we didn't have anything sexual. He just needed to know so he could decide things for himself. Unfortunately, it meant he packed up and moved out the next day. Next I thought I better tell my parents. They sort of knew about my lifestyle, as much as they wanted to know anyway, but how do you tell your parents that your lifestyle is costing you your life? My father couldn't or wouldn't understand anything about my lifestyle or choice. I could see he was hurting but he couldn't speak about it then *or* now. My mother took it the hardest. She never really approved or disapproved of my lifestyle as long as I didn't expose my younger brother and sister to it. We cried a lot that first night. *I* was the one that decided to move out a long time ago and I don't really expect they'll let me come home now. I guess in the long run

it'll be easier for them not to see me during whatever will happen at the end. (D. Smith, 1986, p. 6)

Many PWAs, in an attempt to overprotect their parents as well as themselves, delay sharing the diagnosis of AIDS until the later stages. This is especially true when there is great fear of judgement of lifestyle and the disease or after long separation from family. No one is really protected; in fact, they feel a greater sense of hopelessness and helplessness. I have heard countless parents mourn the fact that if they had only known earlier they might have been able to be of greater help (Peabody, 1986).

Depression

A major source of depression, both reactive as well as anticipatory, is loss of control of functioning (75% of people with advanced AIDS have CNS disturbances and often some degree of dementia; Baumgartner, 1985), of treatment, of mobility, of energy, of autonomy. It is critical for us as caregivers to encourage as much autonomy as possible. If, because of our solicitousness, and wanting to rescue, we disempower PWAs and further enhance their sense of impotency, they may become further depressed and hopeless (Lopez & Getzel, 1984). Allow them to feel their sadness ("AIDS Patients Who Take Control," 1990; Lopez & Getzel, 1984; Nichols, 1985).

The following illustrates that an individual can progress from transient reactive depression to a point of acceptance once he or she has acknowledged feelings of despair and desperation.

There were and there are still days I think about suicide. I know it would be the coward's way out but that doesn't mean much right now. So far the biggest thing stopping me is the insurance money. I know if I kill myself, my parents won't get the money to bury me and hopefully have some left for themselves. I think I owe them that much for everything I've put them through. (D. Smith, 1986, p. 7)

Acceptance

Acceptance may take numerous paths. One way may be to actively seek out experiences in which one can cathartically work out one's unfinished business of relationships. Once one discharges the energy bound up in holding back feelings, one is able to use that energy to live more fully.

Chuck Morris poses the important questions that result:

How do we live now? How do we live a fulfilling life? How do we get rid of unfinished business? And most importantly, how do we learn to love people unconditionally? (Serinus, 1986, p. 41)

Tom Chaudoin corroborates this:

But the most important part is the spiritual aspects: *hope* and *love*. I think that love, "unconditional love" as Elisabeth Kübler-Ross would say, is a very, very powerful healing tool. I said to a friend recently, "All of a sudden I feel a lot of love for other people, but I don't really know how to express that or give that to them." And my friend said, "By letting other people love you, you're giving love!" That happens a lot more in my life than it used to. And I feel very hopeful and optimistic. (Serinus, 1986, p. 51)

Not everyone, however, reaches acceptance with such consciousness or energy. Many reach that point quietly as they disengage and go inward, choosing to be with only one or two closest people, and speaking very little. It reminds me of the last person in a baseball stadium shutting off banks of floodlights one by one, until the din is gone and only that sense of peace remains.

The important point is that we take our cue totally from the experiencing person and respect that most of us die in character with how we have lived our lives. Many who have reached acceptance and prioritized their lives may feel that they wish to arrange their property disposition and their funerals in detail. Others, having let go completely, transcend all material concerns (Moffatt, 1987; Levine, 1982, 1984).

Other PWAs reach acceptance slowly through support groups, where just *being* in the presence of others without judgment or necessity of explanations engenders a degree of acceptance.

Andree Walton, a woman who acquired AIDS through transfusion, describes how the group served her:

I was interested in doing work in substance abuse, chemical dependency, and child abuse or working with adult children of alcoholics. Now I just want to get my affairs in order: the fate of my book collection, provisions for my son, and my funeral arrangements so that the people I care about won't be burdened by them. (Laventure, 1988, p. 9)

The efficacy of such groups rests on the premise that sharing one's traumas, grief, and "war stories" lifts some of the stigma and shame and assists in the resolution of loss. The pioneering work of Lindeman with survivors of the Coconut Grove nightclub fire demonstrated the survival purpose of sharing unusual traumatic events (Lindeman, 1965).

Walton continues:

Three times a week I sit in a small room surrounded by men who have this disease. They have allowed me the honor of joining them, of expressing my deepest pain without fear of judgment or rejection. In turn, they have come to express themselves as openly as I do. There is a deep and abiding spiritual intimacy, a growing and sacred bond that is created.

Before I found and was found by this fellowship, there was a small group of friends who sustained me. Now there is a larger group that has taught me that this disease and its experience transcends all barriers. (p. 9)

We are at the very front of this war. We struggle and cry out in pain and frustration to each other, to our families, friends and the world. We comfort and care for each

other. We watch, helpless and with horror, whenever one of our number slowly fades.
If our collective and separate prayers are answered, there is a gentle and peaceful death.

We grieve our collective tears and remember those times of laughter and joy with
one another. These memories sustain us as our numbers diminish. (Laventure, 1988,
p. 9)

Irene Smith, a massage therapist from San Francisco, has been one of the
pioneers to bring touch and extraordinary emotional healing to so many, as a
result of her hospital volunteer massage programs, Service Through Touch. In
the Kübler-Ross book on AIDS, Irene articulates the humbling and honoring
effect of accompanying someone through the journey into acceptance.

He totally opened up my heart. I have never had the unconditional love inside of
me opened to such a level!

The K.S. lesions started growing internally and Peter started on twenty-four-hour-
a-day oxygen six months before he died. Peter said his doctor told him his lungs were
about 75 percent lesions six months before he died. Peter moved into a Shanti [Hospice]
residence and began to deteriorate quite rapidly, but he never lost his love and lust for
life. He was quite an extraordinary man, who absolutely refused to stay inside. You
have to understand that Peter was extremely ravished by K.S. [Kaposi's sarcoma]. [He
had] one of the most severe cases that I have seen. One of his eyes had [been] radiated;
granted, the lesions on the eye had disappeared, but the eye had closed due to the
radiation. Occasionally, it was open so that there was just a little bit of slit through
which he could see, but most of the time it was completely covered over.

He asked if we would drive by his home where he had lived for thirteen years
before he moved into the Shanti residence. He had been a stained-glass worker and all
of his belongings were in that house. We helped him out of the van and up on the
front porch so he could visit with his cats—one of them, Moon-gold, he had had for
eight years. One of us had to walk right behind Peter with the portable oxygen on our
shoulders. We all got seated on the front porch and started calling the cats. When he
called, "Kitty, kitty," the cats were a little bit scared. It was very difficult for him to
get near them, and at one point I had tears in my eyes and thought, "Oh, God, please
let the cats come and say 'good-bye.' " Peter sat on the porch and he finally coaxed
Moon-gold onto his lap and talked to her. He told her how much he loved her and
how much he missed her. Then he cried and told Moon-gold good-bye.

We were there for about fifteen minutes when Peter said, "Okay, I'm ready to go
to the park." The three of us got into the van and went out to Golden Gate Park,
where he wanted to go to his very, very favorite spot, which was a hill with a waterfall
and a little lake with ducks. Now you've got to understand that it was the middle of a
very hot sunny afternoon, and the park was filled with senior citizens and all kinds of
little ladies taking their afternoon walks. We got out the wheelchair, the oxygen, and
put Peter in the wheelchair and started wheeling him through the park. He stopped
and looked at the flowers, the trees, the ducks, and he stopped and talked to every little
lady walking through the park. He would say, "Hello, my name is Peter, isn't it a
beautiful day!" It *was* a beautiful day! (Kübler-Ross, 1987, p. 253)

When Irene had met Peter back in 1983, his grief work, in great part, involved
working through anger with "Mother Earth," as he described her. He had cursed
her because of what he viewed she had done to him and others. In his healing
process, he had come to terms.

As we were wheeling past the hill that day in the park, he said, "Oh, stop, I want to lie in the grass." So we stopped the wheelchair and I took a blanket and my jacket and put them on the grass, and Peter crawled on his stomach onto the grass.

I sat down and, at first, he put his head in my lap. Then he asked me to move and he put his face into the grass and lay there for quite some time, and the afternoon chill came. Since Peter had pneumocystis, I began to worry about the chill, so I mentioned it to him and he said, "No, leave me alone, don't worry, I'm not getting chilled, I just want to lie here." Peter lay there and talked to Mother Earth, made peace with her, and told her that he understood that it was not her fault, that he loved her, and that it was okay. When he had finished, we got him up and put him in the wheelchair, then we wheeled him back to the van. We got into the van, and he said, "Okay, I want to see the ocean." We drove to the ocean by way of the ice-cream store and the apple-pie store.

At the ocean, Andy got out for a couple of minutes while Peter and I sat in the van. He turned the country and western music up a little louder. He didn't say a word, just sat and listened to the ocean. We would look at each other and smile, and he would say, "Oh, God, Irene, isn't it a beautiful day. I feel fantastic! I feel fantastic, isn't it a beautiful day! (Kübler-Ross, 1987, p. 254)

Acceptance of death never means one likes it but that one can arrive at a greater sense of peace with its inevitability.

John Shine is a trusted colleague and staff member at London, England's Lighthouse AIDS Center, which provides residential hospice and home care for about 30% of Great Britain's PWAs. He provides a stunning example of what "coming to terms" with AIDS can provide at its fullest resolution of a peaceful death. He shares:

I first met Graham about two and a half years ago in one of our groups. He was a very beautiful man who had been diagnosed with Kaposi's Sarcoma, and the first question he was asked by his doctor was "who is your next of kin?" Needless to say, Graham was mortified at such a question. He could have ended up, like many others, as just a statistic programmed to die. But Graham was a searcher, and came along with another friend who had AIDS, who had recommended that he join one of our groups. It was ironic that Graham, who was such a beautiful man, and put a lot of store in his looks, should end up with such a disfiguring disease which caused more lesions on his face than there was normal skin. It was also ironic that he would rather be dead than ugly.

Graham died last week, and shortly before this he told us that these last two years have been the best years of his life. I remember in 1985 introducing Graham to one of our groups, and asking him the question? what was good about having AIDS? Out of his mouth fell one of the pearls of wisdom of which we would hear many. He said: "I realize that this diagnosis of AIDS presents me with a choice: the choice to either be a hopeless victim and die of AIDS, or to make my life right now what it always ought to have been." Many of us at London Lighthouse have been privileged to share with Graham his tears and fears, along with an enormous sense of fun and laughter. Just two days before he died, he arranged his funeral in every detail. He then finally decided to let go, and I took responsibility for his medical care in the last 24 hours of his life. He was able to die in the comfort of his own home, surrounded by the very people he always wanted to be there when he died.

> We set the room up with candles and incense, and played music that he liked very much—in particular "Room with a View"—and what a view we had in that room! We had made up beds on the floor all around Graham's bed, for his friends to sit or lie. By this time he was unconscious, but very peaceful, and we were explaining everything to him as we went along. His friends enjoyed taking part in his nursing care, and his mother never left his side. She lay next to him on the bed all through the night. I remember being particularly moved by her comment that Graham had never had so much love as in these last two years. He is the second son that she has lost, as well as her husband, and I told her how courageous I thought she was to be holding the son that she had once borne, while he died. She was a wonderful model of the healing process, and as she cried with Graham she just grew stronger and stronger. She herself was a woman who found it very hard to cry until she came on one of our workshops. It seemed ironic that she was now telling us that we must cry! There were lots of tears, laughter and sharing with Graham.
>
> I remember remarking to Graham's mother about how beautiful he was looking, how he was gradually becoming more baby-like in his appearance. He died so peacefully that it was hardly noticeable. We just stayed with him; there was nothing more to do. The candles burned on, the music played and people cried. Graham's wishes were to be carried out to the full. (Shine, 1989, p. 7)

There is no "best" way to cope with death. There is only the way that each person develops as a manner of "coming to terms" within their capacity at any given moment. We must at all costs accept that place where the person functions and be humble enough and flexible enough and as unconditional as possible. We must remember this is their journey through life, death, and the transition, and we need to drop our agenda(s) if we are to heal emotionally along with them. As Irene Smith points out, "AIDS is about looking at ourselves" and "AIDS is sometimes about looking all our fears in the face" (I. Smith, 1988).

Reverend A. S. Pieters, a PWA in remission, articulates an underlying message of wholeness: "When I gave myself permission to believe that I would die someday, *then* I was able to live. It is only in accepting death that we truly find life" ("An AIDS Survivor," 1989).

To Rev. Richard Dunphy, of the Society of Jesus, a sense of completion may be attained by persons with AIDS confronting a healthy sense of guilt from devaluing their body, by reducing some people to objects, or by having closeted their spiritual life. He suggests that the diagnosis focuses the need to live in the present, and one day at a time (Dunphy, 1987).

Dunphy ends his article with an account of a man who reflected spiritual wholeness just days before his death:

> I will probably be in the hospital for another week. I am confident I will recover from this illness. I am blessed with many good friends. Their love and support sustain me. I have had from four to ten visitors each day as well as phone calls, and I know I am in their prayers. Fr. Carlos came today and served communion. God has many hands. . . . I never thought of AIDS as a blessing, but how I've chosen to respond, how my faith is growing and deepening, most certainly is, I believe my faith is the most important thing. My doctor can cure my infection, but my faith in the love of Christ can heal

me. Even if my AIDS is not healed in this life, I know that my transformed spiritual body will be whole and healthy forever. (Dunphy, 1987, p. 63)

COPING WITH THE PAIN OF LOSS

Elsewhere in this volume I have outlined just a few of the numerous multiple losses that accompany AIDS. I shall merely list them here to remind us of the overwhelming odds against masterful or optimal coping: loss of self-esteem; secrecy and privacy; occupational and financial status; pride; optimistic outcome, as with other serious illnesses; youth and vigor; progress in healing old destructive patterns, such as addictions; physical comforting and contact; isolation, exclusion, and rejection; sense of reality (with dementia); of one's entire peer group (multiple and traumatic deaths, with no opportunity in between for homeostatic recovery); feelings of control; support of the family of origin; of secondary gain related to benefits of illness, as contrasted with a disease like cancer (e.g., compassion); of future hopes, dreams, goals; of a sense of perspective regarding what might constitute adequate coping (Lopez & Getzel, 1984).

OPENING COMMUNICATION

The best way to open communication is to let the PWA set the pace and guide the way. We must be sensitive both to nonverbal symbolic language (similar to parables and metaphor) as well as to verbal cues. We must also be prepared for the possibility that *we* may not be the person's first choice with whom to open the door to sharing (Furth, 1988). Be vigilant for any cues, whether they come in the form of dreams, imagery, hallucinations, or from art or "deathbed visions," as they may provide springboards for further openings. One elderly man, having been married for 49 years, was not sure his wife was able to release him to die or that she could adjust to his death. Since he had discomfort with and difficulty broaching the subject, and since he kept fluctuating in and out of dementia, one evening, after a long period of silence he asked, "Emily, are you afraid of a candle?" She said, "No, I'm *not*. Why?" He replied, "That's good." He died peacefully at home in his sleep one week later, Emily by his side. In their religion, when a person died, the family or spouse traditionally lit a 7-day votive candle in memory of the deceased. Emily later derived much solace in acknowledging a higher communication and awareness in that last rare moment of her husband's lucidity.

CARING FOR CAREGIVERS

Caregivers often represent the extended, reconstituted, or even substitute family for the PWA. Health caregivers often attain a level of greater intimacy and attachment than with their other patients. We can thus see the positive role that separate "caring support groups" can play for both staff and patients.

Miller describes one recent study's findings that AIDS staff had markedly higher rates of depression, anxiety, and stress, related less to the number of years in their AIDS work than to the *intensity* of their involvement (Miller, 1987). According to a study by Wegscheider-Cruse, 83% of all nurses are firstborn children of alcoholics. They are often selfless servants, having come from family systems where they devotedly took care of other family members, and those beyond family as well (Schaef, 1987).

This fact impacts on *our* grief as caregivers, as we encounter a pandemic that appears to have no paucity of sufferers and multiplicity of losses. It behooves us, then, to examine our own work on losses, to prevent burnout that results from "caretaking" as opposed to "caregiving" (e.g., Kelly & Sykes, 1989; Macklin, 1988; Martin, 1988; Trice, 1988). The following are some characteristics of caregivers who endure in working with people with AIDS or other life-threatening illnesses:

1. They live in the moment. This constitutes mostly living in the present, not the future, not the past, as well as devoting full attention to the task at hand, whether it be play or sports or shopping or meditation.
2. They know their limits—saying *no* is an essential part of this, as well as delegating responsibilities to others and "letting go" of control (One test of the success of this task is to ask if something will matter in 2 years and to eliminate it if the answer is "no").
3. They have developed both effective coping strategies for stress and internal objective stress "monitors," which signal them when (more hopefully before) the system is experiencing stimulus overload.
4. They see the larger perspective of their work as an outcome of some philosophical or spiritual framework.
5. They have done their grief work, which may involve an assessment of their motivation for choosing their particular field.
6. They maintain a sense of humor and balance; they respect and acknowledge the gallows humor of patients as a valid form of coping.
7. They balance their lives out so that their identities do not solely revolve around their role as caregivers.

Once caregivers have processed their own grief, they are in a much better position to truly assist the bereaved families of PWAs they have lost, such as is indicated in the following guidelines set forth by Kaplan:

1. Do allow them to express as much grief as they are feeling and are willing to share.
2. Do allow them to talk about their loved one as much and as often as they want.
3. Do talk about the special memories and endearing qualities of the one who has died.

4. Do reassure them that they did everything they could, that the medical care their loved one received was the best, or with whatever else you know to be *true and positive* about the care given to the one who died.
5. Don't say, "It was God's will," "I know how you feel," "Time will heal."
6. Don't say, "Be strong; others need you."
7. Don't simply say, "How are things going?"
8. Don't avoid mentioning the deceased person's name out of fear of reminding the bereaved of their pain. (Kapleau, 1989, pp. 317–318)

Krandall Kraus also gives some hints about caregiving for caregivers:

1. Reserve *one hour* everyday just for yourself; something that involves only you, and makes you feel healthy and good about yourself.
2. Say "no." Don't give excuses.
3. Say "I'll have to get back to you." Don't make "yes" commitments on the spur of the moment.
4. Ask for help and "delegate responsibility." (Laventure, 1988, p. 13)

CHILDREN AND DEATH

A mother of a child with AIDS remarks, "Ben had lived only a short 94 months. He had never driven a car. Never gone to a prom. Never held his own child. And now we're saying he *never would*" (Oyler & Oyler, 1988, p. 208).

This awareness, coupled with children's awareness of their own impending death, forces us to focus on this most painful of circumstances. It is critical that we are most open and completely *honest* not only with the child with AIDS, but also with his or her siblings (Dagle, 1990; C. B. Kelly, personal communication, Oct. 10, 1986; Kübler-Ross, 1983a).

Dagle, in describing long-term potential effects on siblings, points out the importance of considering magical thinking. She cites potential later problems as a consequence of dishonesty or exclusion, as follows:

1. problems with shame, self-worth and intimacy
2. feeling haunted
3. disconnected from emotions and feeling emotionally bankrupt
4. feeling of being unloved
5. harboring the perfect sister-love relationship fantasy, e.g., that there was never any fighting
6. strong dependency needs
7. pervasive sense of sadness and loneliness
8. anniversary depression
9. inability to trust others; testing them
10. need to be in control and perfectionistic. (Dagle, 1990, p. 3)

Children's Common Reactions to Death

Doyle (1980) most succinctly describes children's typical responses:

1. Children usually take longer than adults in going through the phases of grief. A child may grieve for many years, largely because they are not regarded as capable of registering the event in terms of mature logical processes.

2. A child over six months of age is deeply affected by the death of anyone close to him/her, especially parents, brothers, and sisters.
3. Children under six years cannot conceive of the finality of death. They expect the loved one to return.
4. Children often express their feelings about a death in indirect, delayed, and disguised ways. Often a bereaved young child seems neither to know nor to care about his loss, but such appearances are deceiving.
5. Between six and nine years of age the *permanency* of death is generally accepted, but the *inevitability* of death for the child and his loved ones is likely to be too difficult for him to face.
6. In many cases, children cannot move out of the first phase of reaction to a death. They continue to protest, the anger at separation, and refuse to face the finality of the loss. The phase of despair and disorientation may come only after several years, with hope and reorganization coming even later. (Doyle, 1980, pp. 28–29)

Doyle further succinctly suggests parental strategies:

1. Do not tell children what they will later need to relearn. [This involves two processes: "undoing" the myth and reteaching accurate facts, adding to the complexities that the child must contend with at an emotionally laden time.]
2. Allow the child to give vent to her emotions. Allow her to share yours. . . . *Assume* that guilt exists and talk about it. Children feel more guilty than adults since, in their experience, bad things happen to them when they are naughty. In addition to a sense of guilt which they may associate with given acts, in many cases by parents with AIDS, they may also feel a sense of shame in the form of low self-worth, simply by being AIDS-connected.
3. Suffering and death should not be linked with sin and punishment [particularly since the child, steeped in magical thinking, may already think he caused AIDS].
4. Do not teach the child as if you have the final answers that he must accept. Do not be afraid to say, "I don't know."
5. Help the child to unburden her feelings through remembrance and release. (Doyle, 1980, pp. 30–33)

In a special crisis section of their book *How Do We Tell the Children,* D. Schaefer, a funeral director, and C. Lyons, an outstanding educator, present an extraordinary depiction of children's reactions:

Be prepared for resistance from others. People may say of your children:

- They don't know what's going on.
- Wait until later to tell them.
- Make up a story.
- Don't say anything.
- Send them away until the funeral is over.
- Why do you want to put them through this?

Consider saying to these people:

- I really could use your help; I believe that what I am doing is the right thing for my children and me.
- You can help me by reinforcing what I am telling them, or by saying nothing. Don't undermine my effort. (Schaefer & Lyons, 1986, p. 118)

Anger

Anger is perhaps the most underestimated aspect of the grief process, even in children. Schaefer outlines the importance of knowing this:

> Anger is common at the time of death; it can be very damaging to the family. Understanding it and anticipating it helps parents deal with both their own and their children's anger.

Children may be angry at their parents for:

- not telling them that the person who died was so sick
- spending so much time with the sick person
- just because they need someone to be angry with

Children may be angry at themselves for:

- wishing the person would die
- not visiting or helping the dying person
- not saying goodbye, or "I love you"

Children may be angry at others for:

- not taking care of the person who died (the doctors for not treating him adequately)

Children may be angry at the person who died for:

- not taking care of himself or putting himself in danger
- leaving, dying, abandoning them
- causing such family upset
- using up the family money
- not telling anyone he was sick
- causing the family pain and stigma
- not fighting harder against death

Children may be angry at their brothers and sisters for:

- no apparent reason
- grieving differently (some children cry, others don't)
- not wanting to talk about the death
- seeming more privileged (others can go to the funeral, but they can't). (Schaefer & Lyons, 1986, p. 130)

Guilt

Many people feel guilt about a death. This might stem from anger—

- How can I be angry at the person who died?
- How can I be alive when he's dead?

From the feeling that you didn't do enough—

- I should have told the rest of the family that he was sick.
- I should have visited him before he died.

And from all the "shouldn't haves"—

- I shouldn't have left the hospital. (Schaefer & Lyons, 1986, p. 131)

Guilt and a feeling of responsibility go hand-in-hand. Children can feel responsible for a person's death for a number of reasons:

- They may have been told something that they misunderstood and took to heart ("you're driving me crazy"; "you'll be the death of me yet"; "you're killing your father").
- Because they often see God as a rewarder or punisher, they may feel God has punished their bad behavior by causing the person's death; also they may feel if they had prayed harder the person wouldn't have died.
- They connect events that don't belong together ("If I had sent a 'get well' card maybe he wouldn't have died").
- They indulge in magical thinking ("If I wish hard enough, he'll come back"; "I got mad and wished that he would die").

This is why it is so important that children understand why the person died. Remember, your child may think he is responsible for the death, and tell him this is not so. (Schaefer & Lyons, 1986, p. 131)

ACCEPTANCE AND LETTING GO

Both acceptance and letting go are ultimately a greater challenge for the *rest* of us who will be facing this task over and over, should we choose to respond.

A quote by Mother Theresa above Cleve Jones's desk at the Quilt Project expressed the challenge of AIDS to each of us:

There is a light in this world, a healing spirit more powerful than any darkness we may encounter. We sometimes lose sight of this force when there is suffering, too much pain. Then suddenly, the spirit will emerge through the lives of ordinary people who hear a call and answer in extraordinary ways. (quoted in Ruskin, 1988, p. 19)

Perhaps the ultimate acceptance as healing is expressed by those of us touched directly or indirectly by AIDS' affliction who, once awakened, can never return to our former state of sleep. If each of us were to light just one candle, we would not only eliminate the need to curse the darkness, but by our very commitment, we would illuminate the way for others to begin their journeys, both inner and outer ones.

AIDS AS BLESSING, AIDS AS CURSE

Is there any aspect of the spectrum of AIDS that we might learn from? Is it conceivable that AIDS is in *any* sense a gift? I personally have been humbled and honored by virtue of being allowed to accompany dying and living people on their various journeys inward, both psychologically and spiritually. I stand in awe of the courage and resiliency of the human spirit. In addressing AIDS as "the ultimate challenge," not only of our lifetime, but possibly for our planet, Kübler-Ross describes it as both "a curse and a blessing" (Kübler-Ross, 1987). She considers AIDS as affording us our greatest opportunity to drop our separateness and to practice unconditional love and regard.

Indeed, AIDS, by *its* very nature, is unconditional—as a global pandemic it affects every color, creed, race, religion, age, nationality, and sexual identity.

Every few decades we find ourselves at war with a different nation, only to find ourselves, a decade later, befriending those very peoples, and making reparation to their scarred environs. Could it be that AIDS affords us the opportunity to abort this cycle and see our *common* purpose and our *common* dreams?

If so, then our moral imperative seems clear: to regard without judgment; to trust without bounds; to tear down walls held fast by the mortar of fear; and to love one another unconditionally, reclaiming the inner child.

REFERENCES

AIDS patients who take control benefit psychologically and physically. (1990, January). *Your Personal Best,* p. 3.

An AIDS survivor who turned hopelessness into hope. (1989, April). *Your Personal Best,* pp. 14–15.

Baumgartner, G. H. (1985). *AIDS, Psychosocial factors in the acquired immune deficiency syndrome.* Springfield, IL: Charles Thomas.

Becker, M., & Joseph, J. (1988). AIDS and behavioral change to reduce risk: A review. *American Journal of Public Health, 78*(4), 394–410.

Brandt, A. (1988). AIDS in historical perspective: Four lessons from the history of sexually transmitted diseases. *American Journal of Public Health, 78,*(4), 367–371.

Cunningham, C. (Ed.). (1989, May/June). The gay men's health crisis newsletter for volunteers and supporters, pp. 00–00.

Dagle, L. (1990). Lecture on sibling death, Manchester Community College, Manchester, CT, March 19.

Doyle, P. (1980). *Grief counseling and sudden death: A manual and guide.* Springfield, IL: Charles Thomas.

Dubik-Unruh, S. (1985). Children of chaos: planning for the emotional survival of dying children of dying families. *Journal of Palliative Care, 5*(2), 10–15.

Fineberg, H. V. (1988, October). The social dimensions of AIDS. *Scientific American, 259,* 128–134.

Fisher, S. (1987). *AIDS and anger* [Audiotape]. Los Angeles: Northern Lights Alternatives.

Furth, G. (1988). *The secret world of drawings.* Boston: Sigo Press.

Gavzer, B. (1988, September 18). Why do some people survive AIDS? *Parade Magazine,* pp. 2–5.

Gussow, G. (1989). *Leprosy, racism & public health.* Boulder, CO: Westview Press.

Hamerman, W. J., Grauerholz, J., Tennenbaum, J., Freeman, D., Lillge, W., Rosinsky, N., Shapiro, E., Burdman, M., Pauls, R., Cleary, C., Spahn, J., & Kellogg, B. (Eds.). (1986). *An emergency war plan to fight AIDS and other pandemics prepared by the EIR Biological Holocaust Task Force.* Washington, DC, (P.O. Box 17390, Washington, DC, 20041): Executive Intelligence Review.

Hay, L. (1988). *Heal your body.* Santa Monica, CA: Hay House.

Kalish, R. (1981a). *Death, grief, and caring relationships.* Monterey, CA: Brooks/Cole.

Kalish, R. (1981b). Dying with cancer. In P. Ahmed (Ed.), *Living and dying with cancer.* New York: Elsevier.

Kapleau, P. (1989). *The wheel of life and death.* New York: Doubleday.

Kelly, J., & Sykes, P. (1989, May). Helping the helpers: A support group for family members of persons with AIDS. *Social Work,* pp. 239–242.

Kübler-Ross, E. (1969). *On death and dying.* New York: Macmillan.

Kübler-Ross, E. (1975). *Death: The final stage of growth.* Englewood Cliffs, NJ: Prentice-Hall.

Kübler-Ross, E. (1983a). *On children and death.* New York: Macmillan, *xix,* 279.

Kübler-Ross, E. (1983b). *Death, dying and transition,* from a transcription of a workshop lecture tape, San Juan Bautista, CA, March 26th. Headwaters, VA: Elisabeth Kübler-Ross Center.

Kübler-Ross, E. (1987). *AIDS: The ultimate challenge.* New York: Macmillan.

Laventure, A. (Ed.). (1988, Autumn). *PWA Voice,* Vol. 1, no. 3, pp. 1–16.

Lazarus, R. S. (1981). Costs and benefits of denial. In P. Ahmed (Ed.), *Living and dying with cancer* (pp. 178–201). New York: Elsevier-North Holland.

Lindemann, E. (1965). Symptomatology and management of acute grief. In R. Fulton (Ed.), *Death and identity.* New York: Wiley. (Reprinted from *American Journal of Psychiatry, 101,* 141–148, 1944.)

Lopez, D. J., & Getzel, G. S. (1984). Helping gay AIDS patients in crisis. Social casework. *The Journal of Contemporary Social Work, 65(7),* 387–394.

Macklin, E. (1988). AIDS: Implications for families. *Family Relations, 37,* 141–149.

Martin, J. L. (1988). Psychological consequences of AIDS-related bereavement among gay men. *Journal of Consulting and Clinical Psychology 56,(6),* 856–862.

McCarroll, T. (1988). *Morning glory babies.* New York: St. Martin's Press.

Melchreit, R., Hadler, J., & Weinstein, B. (Eds.). (1988, April) *Connecticut responds to AIDS, A report of the Department of Health Services AIDS Prevention Programs,* Connecticut Preventable Diseases Division, D.H.S. Publication, Hartford, CT.

Melton, G., & Garcia, W. (1988). *Beyond AIDS. A journey into healing.* Beverly Hills, CA: Brotherhood Press.

Miller, D. (1987). *Living with AIDS and HIV* (with a guest chapter from Chris Carne). Basingstoke, England: Macmillan.

Moffatt, B. C. (Ed.). (1987). *AIDS: A self care manual.* Los Angeles: AIDS Project Los Angeles.

Murphy, F., & Curran, J. (1988). *AIDS and the human immunodeficiency virus in the United States, 1988 update.* Atlanta: Centers for Disease Control.

Nichols, S. (1985). Psychosocial reactions of persons with the acquired immunodeficiency syndrome. *Annals of Internal Medicine, 103(5),* 765–767.

Oyler, G., & Oyler, C. (1988). *Go toward the light.* New York: Harper & Row.

Peabody, B. (1986). *The screaming room.* San Diego: Oak Tree Publications.

Poling, A., Redmon, W., & Burnette, M. M. (1989). Stigmatization of AIDS patients by college students in lower division psychology classes. *Journal of College Student Development 31,* 64–70.

Ruskin, C. (1988). *The quilt: Stories from the names project.* New York: Simon & Schuster.

Schaef, A. (1987). *When society becomes an addict.* New York: Harper & Row.

Schaefer, D., & Lyons, C. (1986). *How do we tell the children?* New York: Newmarket Press.

Serinus, J. (Ed.). (1986). *Psychoimmunity and the healing process.* Los Angeles: Celestial Arts.

Shine, J. (1987, December). Room with a view. *Leading Lights,* pp. 1–16.

Smith, D. R. (1986). Who will bear the burden when serious illness strikes? Unpublished senior thesis, Eastern Connecticut State University.

Smith, I. (1988). *Christmas with Chuck* [Videotape]. San Francisco: Service Through Touch.

Sontag, S. (1978). *Illness as metaphor.* New York: Farrar, Straus & Giroux.

Sontag, S. (1989). *AIDS and its metaphors.* New York: Farrar.

Trice, A. (1988). Posttraumatic stress syndrome-like symptoms among AIDS caregivers. *Psychological Reports, 63,* 656–658.

Ulene, A. (1987). *Safe sex in a dangerous world.* New York: Random House.

Whitmore, G. (1988, January 31). Bearing witness. *New York Times Magazine,* pp. 14–54.

10

Living with AIDS
Surviving Grief

ROCHELLE GRIFFIN

INTRODUCTION

Working with people who are seriously ill or dying involves supporting them to live their lives fully and with quality. An important part of achieving this quality of life is learning to face pain, anger, and fear in the grieving process so that we are free to experience love, hope, and inner peace.

This grief/growth process is based on a philosophy that emphasizes wholeness of being, whereby the physical, mental, emotional, and spiritual are equally important aspects of health and wellness. The challenge is to bring these aspects into harmony, through which we can experience love, hope, and peace within ourselves and with others in any stage of life. The emphasis is upon quality of life, not quantity or length of life; I stress healing, not curing.

My work has grown from leading general support groups for people with AIDS to specific aspects of the mind–body connection: psychoimmunity and the healing process. At present, together with Geoff Hopping from London, I facilitate about eight 5-day residential workshops per year in the United Kingdom and Holland stressing the mind–body connection for people with HIV/AIDS, their loved ones and caregivers. I also have initiated a weekly "Mind–Body Dialogue" group, which is a place to continue individual and community growth work. Often I am asked by people who have become too ill to continue participating in the group to visit them at home or in the hospital for support in emotional discharge and spiritual consciousness. My work is expanding rapidly to include a number of professional health care organizations.

ROCHELLE GRIFFIN • Stichting Vuurulinder/Fire Butterfly Foundation for Conscious Living and Dying, 5328AS Rossum, The Netherlands.

Living and Dying with AIDS, edited by Paul I. Ahmed, Plenum Press, New York, 1992.

All too often, professionals are trained to focus only on one aspect of the mind–body connection: medical people address the physical and mental issues, psychologists address the emotional issues, and priests or ministers are consulted on spiritual issues. This is not a vision of the person as a whole being. Most of us in the health care profession have been trained to function at a practical level in "doing" something, like offering solutions to a problem, instead of simply "being" there and feeling comfortable with that. As a result we are uncomfortable with the silences, as our own feelings of fear, inadequacy, and helplessness arise. We have learned to take the lead instead of allowing the persons who are ill to take charge of their life and following their lead. We talk about "patients" instead of people, thereby distancing ourselves from our own feelings so that we feel less involved.

There is no prerequisite for working with seriously ill people as I do, but it is extremely important to feel comfortable with the physical, emotional, mental, and spiritual aspects of wellness. This does require a devotion to one's personal growth work, including regular emotional discharge and willingness to seek spiritual nourishment. One needs to be fully aware of what one's personal needs and motivations are and how to fulfill them before attempting to support others in this very intense final phase of life. This growth process will take a lifetime of training! I believe that one needs to practice what one teaches and be a model in that sense.

One of the greatest needs of people facing a catastrophic disease is to be listened to and to be heard. There are several aspects of listening: what is being said; what is *not* being said; the symbolic language; and the silence of the pauses. To be able to hear at all of these levels we must regularly cleanse ourselves of our own fears to be fully present for another person; we need to cleanse our heart with our own tears by allowing it to break in sadness from time to time, only then can it be open and loving; we need to learn to discharge anger in a safe manner and place so that it can be recognized as a positive energy sometimes necessary to bring about change; and we need to devote time and energy, on a daily basis, for our own spiritual nourishment. This ongoing process requires continual attention and care from all persons involved in this work.

GRIEF PROCESS

The well-known psychiatrist, Dr. Elisabeth Kübler-Ross, pioneered in working with terminally ill people and confronting the existing taboos about death and dying. She describes the grief process as having five stages: denial, anger, bargaining, depression, and acceptance.

I believe that all feelings, including fear, anger, sadness, shame, guilt, helplessness, uncertainty, as well as love and acceptance, can be a part of the grief process. One of our greatest challenges in life is to learn to recognize and express these feelings.

This is not an easy process, because most of us have learned to think of these feelings as negative. Who is not familiar with the message "Big boys/girls don't cry"? Crying is often thought to be a sign of weakness or breakdown, a feeling that should be hidden and shameful. Anger is also an emotion that we have been taught to avoid or fear. Yet as we become more dependent upon others through disease or handicaps and are filled with fear and uncertainty about where the disease may strike next, we will probably feel a great deal of anger. Often this anger will be projected onto others, often our loved ones. A short time ago I heard a man yelling at his sister because she had brought the wrong pair of pajamas to the hospital. He wasn't really angry about the pajamas, but it was the only way he knew how to release his anger at his growing dependence and at the elusive virus in his body. It is important to recognize this anger for what it is and not take these outbursts personally, and it is important to recognize and express these feelings ourselves so that we can start to accept them as part of our humanness.

All too often we think of grief only in connection with illness and death. However, grief can be recognized in all stages of life, anytime that major changes take place. Change means letting go of what is familiar, and it brings uncertainty about the future. We can experience grief in connection with moving; changing schools or jobs; getting married and divorced; having a baby or "losing" children when they grow up and leave home. Often, the feeling associated with these changes is not recognized as grief nor expressed as such. It is my experience that most people have experienced some form of physical, emotional, or sexual abuse by one parent or both sometime during their lives that often constitutes a sense of loss of love and safety. All of these experiences contribute to our personal losses, for which we must grieve so that we can let them go and get on with living.

During an illness we can experience grief each time we are confronted with a change in medication, a new infection, admission to the hospital, and whenever we feel a lack of control or increasing dependence. Only when we take sufficient time and space to work through these feelings can we reach a period of acceptance. Particularly with people with AIDS, where the disease itself is so unpredictable and changing, the emotions are very intense and often explosive. People struggle through this grief process repeatedly, from denial to acceptance of their situation, as their independence is lost due to new opportunistic infections. Acceptance is not the last phase in the grief process, but a new beginning. It is essential to learn to stand still at the points of despair, because only by doing so we can we recognize times of pleasure and peace as well. Young people in particular need a lot of support and understanding throughout this process.

People with AIDS are often confronted with multiple grief processes. The one who is ill is not only struggling with his or her own loss of personal independence and body functions but often grieving for an ill or dead lover as well as for friends and community. The caregivers are often grieving for the people they are caring for at present as well as those who have died and for their own friends who may be ill. In this we must understand the utter importance of learning to recognize and express our own grief.

AIDS VERSUS OTHER DISEASES

AIDS confronts us with a complicated conjunction of physical, psychological, and social factors. Most of us have been raised with two big social taboos: sex and death. We carry the fear of each within ourselves, and because AIDS is connected to both, the fear is that much greater. To date there is no cure for AIDS. The majority of those who are ill are young people in the prime of their lives. They have not had much experience with disease or with death and they are not prepared for this. Due to the danger of (re)infection with HIV and because it is sexually transmitted, there is a great feeling of guilt and shame. Following diagnosis it is very difficult to have contact with others for love, intimacy, or sex. The fear of rejection is great, and many men experience (temporary) impotence. For many gay men, AIDS has become a second coming-out; for others, it is a double coming-out, for their homosexuality as well as for AIDS.

Due to the nontraditional lifestyles of many people with AIDS, there is often a stressful or nearly nonexistent relationship with families. Sometimes the bond with friends is unstable or not the kind that can survive serious illness. These factors increase the difficulty of long-term intensive care that most people with AIDS eventually require. Generally, AIDS is not a disease from which people die suddenly or swiftly. It is a long, slow process of increasing debilitation, characterized by dramatic changes in health due to the many opportunistic infections that enter the body. People with AIDS are often repeatedly seriously ill, and they may be near death several times. Together with these many changes, a whole range of emotions is experienced. There is much fear, which quite possibly is the most infectious aspect of AIDS.

The diagnosis of AIDS is a crisis. How an individual learns to cope with a crisis situation is dependent upon his or her personality and experience, as well as his or her relationships with friends and family.

NEW TRADITIONS

In no way do I want to minimize this terrible disease and the enormous tragedy it has caused. However, many people with AIDS develop inner strength and a sense of spirituality, following their personal struggle with pain, anger, hopelessness, grief, and fear. This growth process gives rise to spiritual insight and wisdom that usually comes at the end of a long life. Many of us with a gay or lesbian lifestyle have distanced ourselves from the traditional means of spiritual support through the churches, which have often discriminated against us. We have chosen to emancipate ourselves from traditional thoughts and values. We have become more and more militant and have sought freedom in other challenges: new lifestyles, relationships, sexuality, and political consciousness. In the confrontation with AIDS, we have also sought a form of spirituality that fits our creative and progressive lifestyles. This seems to parallel the development of "New Age" thought throughout the world.

The manner of dealing with death and burial are also reflected in these nontraditional lifestyles. Many more people are choosing to die at home in familiar surroundings. Luckily, more professional and volunteer services are able to help realize this for people without a partner or family as the main source of support. Following death, the doctor is called to write the death certificate. A nurse, assisted by a partner, family member, or volunteer, washes and dresses the body. In Holland, embalming and making-up the body are rare. There is a growing tendency to keep the body at home in the casket, sometimes until the day of burial or cremation. Refrigeration elements are used inside a casket in warm weather to facilitate this.

Burial or cremation services may reflect nontraditional lifestyles: "The Rose" by Bette Midler, "That's What Friends Are For" by Dionne Warwick, and "So Fragile We Are" by Sting have become favorite funeral songs. These songs express our fragility, our need to overcome our fear of life and death, and the importance of mutual support out of which hope and strength may be discovered. Once, we were invited to join in a sacred dance around a casket that spilled over with flowers from our own gardens. Some choose a single color for everything, like red or white, for the casket, flowers, and cars. Sometimes, instead of formal speeches, each person is asked to toss a single rose into the open grave and say out loud what the dead person has meant to them. Some people with AIDS have felt that there should be a celebration of life at the time of their death and therefore arrange to have a catered reception for their friends and family. There are many individual, creative choices through which we can demonstrate our emancipation even beyond death.

EUTHANASIA

Most people with AIDS think about euthanasia or suicide at one point or another. Particularly with the newly diagnosed, euthanasia is a much-repeated topic of discussion in the groups. Each person's viewpoint about his or her quality of life and euthanasia is strictly personal and demands respect. Thoughts about euthanasia are nearly always based upon fear. Fear of physical or mental suffering, pain, dementia, blindness, and paralysis is common. Fear of becoming a burden and dependent upon others is great. However, the greatest fear of all is that of dying alone.

In Holland, although euthanasia is illegal, under some special circumstances, the physician may not be prosecuted for administering it. *Euthanasia* may be defined as willingly and actively terminating the life of a person at his or her explicit request. The use of pain medication, by increasing the dose and thus speeding death, is not considered euthanasia. Nor is stopping certain medical treatment, even if death occurs as a result. The "special circumstances" that a physician must adhere to are the following: the patient must have enough information to make an informed decision; the patient must agree to each step of medical treatment; the physician must previously consult with at least one colleague who interviews the patient; the physician must keep a medical journal, where the various consultations with the patient and second physician, as well as the process of the euthanasia, are recorded. Euthanasia may only be performed by a physician; the patient must be suffering physically and/or mentally without any hope of improvement through any medical treatment; the patient must state in writing that his or her request for euthanasia is a voluntary, well-informed, and durable decision. The euthanasia request may not be a sudden decision or one made under duress by anyone other than the patient. The death certificate must state the cause of death as "unnatural." If the above-mentioned requirements are met, the physician will probably not be prosecuted in court, although police and court investigations will be made.

I respect every person's choice in what he or she experiences as a quality of life worth living. In my experience, it is just in the last phase of life that much personal growth and healing take place. For this reason I do not promote euthanasia; however, I do not withdraw my support if a client does choose it. Again, the request for euthanasia is most often based upon fear. Therefore, I offer to people with AIDS an alternative to euthanasia; my support in any way they may need it in order that they not meet the challenge of AIDS alone and isolated. This service mainly involves working together, in a workshop, group, or individually, in recognizing and discharging fear and other overwhelming emotions in the grief process so that the ill person can take charge of his or her own life. The promise that someone will be there throughout this period is very often enough support that a person will want to get on with living.

My experience with physicians, at home and in the hospitals, is that their willingness to practice euthanasia is often based on their own fear of death and suffering, their feelings of helplessness at not being able to offer any cure for this individual, and their own sense of hopelessness about the terminal nature of AIDS. Euthanasia is something specific that they can offer, and often it is a very well-meant gesture. However, there is a tendency to offer euthanasia in the early stages of AIDS and sometimes even to people seropositive for HIV. I have had the opportunity to work closely with patients of most of the general practitioners, who have a large population of HIV-infected patients, as well as with the HIV specialists in all of the hospitals in Amsterdam. I have also been invited to address HIV and the grief process at several symposia for professionals. As a result, I believe that some of the doctors are gaining a better understanding of the stages and importance of the grief process. They are recognizing anger and depression, for instance, as part of normal grieving and as feelings that need to be experienced and expressed. Consequently, I find myself being consulted more often by these doctors. They invite me to talk about the grief process to their patients who are considering euthanasia. Sometimes I can facilitate some understanding of their own feelings so that the question of living or dying gains a different perspective. I am very honored by the fact that some of these doctors and nurses are also starting to seek help through me in the expression of their own feelings of grief.

CASE HISTORIES

I would like to illustrate the manner in which I work with people during their last stage of life (names and some circumstances have been changed to protect the identity of the surviving families and friends). Most of the people with AIDS that I describe have participated for at least a year in one of the support groups that I lead. As the participants become too ill to continue to come to sessions, the group celebrates their graduation by having a last group session at their home. At that time we give them a small gift as a reminder of the group. It may be a small crystal which, hung in a window, creates rainbows dancing on the wall, symbolizing hope, or a candle to remind them of the warmth and light shared together. My offer to continue regular visits is usually welcomed. My main function during these visits is to help the person recognize and express his or her feelings as well as facilitate spiritual development. Sometimes I am asked to help solve some practical problems or to negotiate conflicts with caregivers or family members. The most vital part of my function is to insure that the person dying retains control over his or her life and that his or her wishes are heard. Another function I fulfill is that of cheerleader, encouraging and reassuring them that they are doing just fine and looking beautiful in their dying process.

Michel

Michel lived alone, had few friends, and had little or no experience in sharing his thoughts or feelings with others. Apparently he contracted HIV during his single sexual experience in the sauna. Although hesitant at first, he participated in the support group for nearly 2 years. As he became too weak to attend the group, we held the last session at his home in celebration of his graduation. Michel asked me to visit him once a week from then on until his death. To ensure that we had quality time alone together, I visited him every Tuesday afternoon for several hours and arranged for the nurse to go shopping during that time. Gradually Michel became too weak to get out of bed and weighed less than 30 kilos. In the homecare administration book, I read that for several days Michel had not spoken to his caregivers and sometimes was confused and seemed to be filled with fear, even screaming out occasionally. Some of the caregivers thought that he was hallucinating.

On this particular afternoon, he had wet his bed, so the first thing that I did was change the bed, wash Michel, and make him more comfortable. Then I sat quietly next to his bed in silence, waiting to see what this visit would bring. Michel opened his eyes occasionally, but he didn't speak and was quite restless. After some time, I asked how he wanted to spend the time with me that afternoon. He said that he wanted a relaxation and visualization exercise. Yet, during this, his restlessness increased. Suddenly, he said loudly, "I'm angry!" and he hit his tiny balled fist on the blanket. I encouraged him to continue to say the words that came to him and use his fists to hit a pillow that I held in front of him. His anger was about his total dependence upon others, his body that wouldn't function, and his feelings of losing control of his life. After he had released his anger, he sobbed deeply for a long time. He asked me to get a mirror so that he could look at his own face, something he hadn't done in several weeks. I held the mirror to enable him to touch his face. He gazed at his reflection in surprise and said that he didn't recognize himself. He asked me why other people hadn't told him that he looked so awful, so thin, so like a concentration camp prisoner. I told him that I could see he had become terribly thin, but that I also could see he had become very open, and that in itself was beautiful. He was beautiful just the way he was at that moment. Gently I lifted his blanket, and he looked at his thin legs. He caressed them with wonder. I asked him what he felt and he said: "This body is worthless now, but I feel just fine! I'm really O.K." I assured him that he was just fine and doing exactly what he needed to be doing right then. He laughed with pleasure and spoke of the many people that he had loved in so many different ways. He talked about how he had been loved by others and that he still wanted to tell several important people in his life that he did love them.

Michel, in his anger and sadness, grieved over the loss of his body functions and investigated his body and feelings. Michel was relieved and accepted his situation as it was, at that moment, and he ended with a feeling of love and peace. As I got ready to leave that day, he called out to me with gleaming eyes: "I'm not going to die yet! See you next week!"

At my next visit, he was too weak to talk, yet he made me understand that he wanted me to lie next to him. I cuddled up to him, took him into my arms and softly caressed him. I spoke to him about love and how much he had meant to other people. From time to time he smiled and occasionally he squeezed my hand. He whispered that he had finished his job and had been able to see those last few people that he had spoken of the week before. He had been able to say "I love you" to everyone that he had wanted to. I told him that it was almost time for him to let go and make his transition. He said he was no longer afraid of death and if there was a life after death, the many people who had preceded him in death would be there waiting to greet him. It would be a celebration. If there was no life after death, the stillness would also be welcome. Two days later I received a phone call saying that Michel had just died in his sleep very peacefully.

This is an example of caring for a dying person. First, the ill person is made physically comfortable. It is not possible to talk about emotional or spiritual issues, if that person has been incontinent and is lying in a dirty bed! Next, the recognition and expression of feelings is stimulated, so that following the emotional discharge, a sense of peace and love remains. Together we look back at his or her life, at what he or she can be proud of, and also at what may still be unfinished before he or she can let go. It is important to continually assure the dying person that they are doing fine and proceeding exactly as can be expected at this moment, here and now.

All too often people near a dying patient say things like: "He's getting worse. It's going badly. He's suffering. It's taking so long." Comments like these are obviously a person's projections, and they demonstrate that person's own feelings of helplessness, lack of control, and discomfort with death. This attitude can contribute to unnecessary panic and unrest at the bedside of a dying person. Unfortunately, this can lead to unnecessary last-minute hospitalization and for requests for euthanasia by the family or others. In several situations I have witnessed the danger of this attitude, particularly when the physician is also uncomfortable with death and dying.

Peter

Peter had been shy and retiring before his AIDS diagnosis. His illness led to the loss of his job and health care benefits, about which he was filled with anger. He had participated in the group for nearly 2 years and had developed into a spokesman against discrimination and for human rights issues. Eventually, Peter became too ill to continue with the group. He was extremely thin, yet he wanted to continue to live alone as long as possible. Although I respected his attitude, I also encouraged him to start making a list of friends and others who he would like to spend time with and who could help with shopping, cooking, and the like, so that eventually we could set up a schedule of regular visitors who could help him. He was just about finished with this list when he got a surprise visit from a friend on a Sunday afternoon. The friend panicked and insisted that Peter be hospitalized immediately. The friend was shocked at Peter's condition and felt that he could not spend another night home alone. Peter phoned me and asked me to come and stay with him for a couple of days to prevent a hospitalization that he didn't want. He wanted help in rediscovering his own sense of peace. I agreed and moved in for a few days. Together we made a rotating schedule of friends and volunteers to help. Peter did not feel that he could rely on his family very much: his mother was ill, and he had not had any contact with his brother for several years. His family would visit on the weekends, however, to relieve the volunteers. Throughout this period we reflected upon his life and relationships, and we laughed and cried together. Peter held a deep belief that there was a life after death, and he had no fear of death itself. He was adamant that he would never consider euthanasia. Yet, I wondered what was keeping him from dying, as he was so frail. Never had I seen anyone hold on to life so strongly. When the schedule became functional, I left for home, agreeing to visit Peter twice a week and to keep daily contact by phone. The following week, a minor crisis occurred that could have been treated at home, but one of Peter's caregivers panicked and arranged to have him admitted to the hospital. Peter was too ill to protest. The hospital staff agreed that there was not really anything they could do for him and that he might as well go home in a few days. The homecare team together with the family, Peter, hospital staff, and I talked and arranged to have him moved back home. I stayed with Peter for a day until the schedule was again operational. The time for a short vacation that I much needed was rapidly approaching. I told Peter that I was planning to be away for one week. I had confidence that he would be just fine with the help that we had arranged. He agreed and wanted me to enjoy my free days. I said goodbye, fully expecting not to see him alive again.

When I returned from vacation, I was surprised to hear that Peter had requested euthanasia. A volunteer, together with Peter's family, had already spoken to the physician, who agreed to visit the next afternoon. The family expected euthanasia to be performed then and were already sorting through some of Peter's belongings that they wanted. When I arrived the next morning, Peter clung to me and asked me not to leave him. As I tried to sort out all that had taken place in my absence, I came to realize that while Peter had had several crises and had nearly stopped breathing, his family had become increasingly irritated with and critical of the volunteers. The volunteers were ready to quit, and knowing that Peter did not want to go to a nursing home, the subject of euthanasia had been brought up. The general feeling was that Peter's dying was taking too long, and everyone was fed up and angry. The tension was very palpable in Peter's apartment, so I decided that first and foremost we needed to create a sense of peace and tranquility there for Peter; later we could decide what to do about the practical care. I lit some candles, put his favorite music on the CD player, and Peter asked me to lead him in a relaxation exercise. The family retired to a corner of the room. Because I knew he had had trouble with his breathing and had been frightened of suffocating, I decided to focus on a "letting go of breathing" exercise. Peter relaxed and the apartment became peaceful and quiet. Peter talked to me about letting go and how earlier in the week he just hadn't felt ready to. He said that he was ready then and again asked me to stay with him. I agreed to stay that whole day and promised to stay longer if necessary. The physician arrived and specifically asked him if he wanted euthanasia, and Peter simply said "no." The doctor said something to the effect that Peter was so alert and calm now that his dying could take another week or two. I asked to speak to the physician alone before he left, wanting to be sure that he would respect Peter's wish to die in his own manner and not that of the family or caregivers, who seemed to be overwhelmed at that moment. Meanwhile, Peter's mother asked to see the doctor in the next room. Peter motioned for me to come to him, and he took my hand. He smiled at me, squeezed my hand, and turned his head toward the window. As I listened to the silence, I wondered how I was going to fulfill my promise to stay with him during the coming days. Suddenly I realized that he was no longer breathing.

I called out to the doctor and to Peter's mother, who hadn't been gone for five minutes. The family was irritated that I hadn't called them in sooner. The doctor supported me by saying that there had been no way of knowing exactly when death would occur and that he was also taken by surprise. As I left that day, I wondered what was really going on between those family members.

Before his death, Peter had asked me to speak at his funeral and had arranged for one close friend and myself to organize it as he wanted it to be. I agreed and tried to do so with the spirit of Peter in mind. As I was leaving the service, an old friend of Peter's, whom I didn't know personally, asked if I could drop him off at the train station. On the way, this man told me about a part of Peter's past that Peter had never shared with me. I understood his incredible timing of dying in the only five minutes during which he felt at peace that day!

I believe that this is an important illustration of how the people surrounding a dying patient, each in his or her own unrecognized grief process, can influence the course of events so much that euthanasia may be seriously considered. In this case, the family was suffering, not the man dying. If euthanasia had been performed, it would have been for them, not him. The response of the family clearly demonstrates how their own feelings of helplessness and anger can be projected on caregivers. I learned how very important it is to be absolutely clear about my own role within the circle of care surrounding a dying person. Peter's timing renewed my sense of peace with the universal order and underscores the necessity of truly listening to what is being said as well as to what is not being said! Peter was a great teacher for all of us.

Issac

Issac's lover had died of AIDS about 2 years before Issac himself was diagnosed. Issac became one of the first participants in the group and was a great inspiration to all of us. He had a wonderful way of quickly working through his anger, sadness, and fear, so that all of the many challenges he was presented with became exciting adventures. Issac's enthusiasm and love of life were terrifically infectious!

On Christmas Day, Issac quite suddenly lost nearly all of his sight in his right eye due to CMV (cytomegalovirus). He phoned me that morning and just asked me to listen as he screamed and swore and finally sobbed deeply. I offered to come to his home, but he said no, that would not be necessary. He phoned a taxi and went to the hospital, where he asked to be given a crash course in IV injection of chemotherapy to slow the spread of the CMV. Knowing Issac well, the hospital staff cooperated. His goal was to participate in the Red Cross vacation week for people with AIDS that was to start 3 days later. He succeeded in his goal, and when I saw him there later that week he was quite comfortable with giving himself the IV chemotherapy. When I asked about the star-shaped glitters glued to his black eye patch, he replied: "That's so when people ask me why I'm wearing the patch, I can reply with 'It's because I see stars!' and then we can laugh."

Besides CMV, Issac was challenged with severe neuropathy, which made him dependent upon a wheelchair, Kaposi sarcoma, epilepsy, and an undiagnosed intestinal infection that gave him diarrhea for more than a year. Each of these challenges he met with an equal amount of creativity. The one challenge that he felt he could not resolve was with his mother. He had a very deep, loving relationship with her, but she did not feel that she could cope with his death, and thus she did not visit him as often as he would have liked. She lived in another country, so frequent visits were out of the question anyway. She had been admitted to a mental hospital for a while following her last visit, and she was still a day patient there. Issac phoned and told her that he needed to see her soon. She agreed to come after being reassured that she would not be the only one caring for him. Issac had asked me to spend a couple of days with them to guarantee the continuity of his care. When she arrived, I spoke to her a little while alone. She was very worried about the fact that her friends had told her not to share her feelings with him. She thought that she had to "keep a stiff upper lip" the whole time she was there, and that was why she had not dared to come. She had nearly fainted at the airport on the way. I told her there was no reason why she shouldn't share her feelings and that I believed she could trust Issac to help her. She could also count on me if she wanted to. Later that night, after she had gone to bed, Issac asked me to help him discharge some of his fear through screaming. He was very clear about what he needed to do and about what was helpful for him, after which we both slept deeply. Of course, we had worked together many times before so this was familiar to him.

The next morning, Issac's mother came into his room where we were already having tea. She was very nervous and hadn't slept well. She sat shyly in a chair near his bed. Issac moved over and invited her to sit next to him. He put his arms around her and softly spoke to her about releasing her feelings. He said that he knew she was terrified of her emotions, and that he wanted to help her. I was ready to leave this very private scene, but Issac said to me: "Would you please get the towel? That worked best for me." Suddenly I understood that he wanted me to do a session with his Mom right then and there! As I asked myself if I wanted to do this and if it was safe enough, I also realized that this was a unique opportunity for all of us. I knew that Issac was very clear emotionally that morning following our late-night session, so I decided to go ahead, all the while wishing I could be a fly on the wall just to observe this scene! I asked her if she wanted to do this and she agreed. I got a towel, a tool that I sometimes use for people to hold on to while they look at their fear and other feelings. I explained the utter importance of recognizing and experiencing our feelings, especially as we are confronted with illness and death. As Issac held his mother against his chest, she took the towel and without any coaching from me, she started to scream. This lady screamed and screamed and cried as she held tightly onto the towel. Many feelings that she had kept bottled up for months and years started to come out. As she paused to catch her breath, she grinned and said: "This is great!" After a while, I realized that the home nurse would be arriving soon and we had better end this session for the moment. Issac suggested that his mother and I continue working together in her room downstairs. He would be involved with the nurse for awhile anyway. Issac's mother wanted very much to continue, so we moved downstairs and I was able to quickly grab my bag of tools to facilitate the expression of more feelings. This wonderful 69-year-old lady really worked on her business! She got in touch with her deepest feelings of abandonment and anger following the long-forgotten rape she'd experienced as a child as well as her husband's suicide 15 years before. She recognized similar feelings toward her son about his impending death. As she faced these feelings and allowed herself to express them she started to feel better than she had in a long time. Throughout the next few weeks I worked with both Issac and his mother several times in this manner.

From the beginning, Issac had wanted to die at home, and a team of professional and volunteer caregivers were operational, coordinated by one of Issac's best friends. The team seemed to be functioning well. One morning Issac phoned me and asked me to come over right away. He said that he wanted to go to the hospital and I was the only one who would understand why. When I arrived, Issac was adamant about wanting hospitalization, saying that the nonprofessional helpers were too unhandy in caring for him. I felt a great deal of tension at his home, but no one could tell me what had initiated this sudden change in behavior. Issac's mother told me that she thought Issac had had some conflict with the friend that was coordinating the home care. I phoned the home physician and the hospital and made the necessary arrangements. As it happened, I was on my way to the university hospital anyway, and by chance, I ran into Issac's specialist. We were both confused by Issac's behavior, and the specialist suggested I reassure Issac that he could be admitted the next day if he still wanted to be and that meanwhile I go back there to sort out the conflict. As it turned out, Issac's friend had tried to limit the very minimal amount of oral morphine Issac was using for pain relief, believing that he was "enjoying the high." The friend refused to listen to Issac's appeal for pain relief, and thus a conflict ensued. Issac told me that in the past the two of them had tried some drugs together and his friend had gotten more involved in drugs than he had wanted to and thus was wary of them. Issac believed that his only way to a peaceful death was in the hospital, where he didn't really want to go. I was able to convince the friend to go home for a couple of days to rest, as he had hardly slept during the whole week at Issac's house. I assured Issac that I would stay with him until we could get round-the-clock professional nursing care, as he indeed preferred that to hospitalization. A sense of peacefulness returned, and very quickly Issac became weaker. I stayed for a day, until the nurses were well acquainted with Issac's needs, and then I left for home. As Issac neared death, he and his mother spent more and more time together sharing feelings and experiences. The next day, Issac died in her arms as she sang a favorite childhood song to him. Both had experienced much healing and peace in their relationship in these precious 5 weeks that they spent together. Following the funeral, Issac's mother shared with me that she felt so strengthened by this whole experience, that when she returned to her home she hoped to help other parents of people with AIDS to manifest this kind of healing.

Issac's story illustrates the necessity of sharing feelings and shows the healing that can take place between family members. Issac taught us to listen to, respect, and protect the needs of dying people, because they know what is best for themselves. Issac's story demonstrates how our personal motivations and our own unfinished business (the friend's fear of drugs, in this case) can disturb the peacefulness of dying.

Charles

Charles could be described as a real loner. One of Charles's greatest difficulties was participating in the group and sharing at that level. Yet the exchange of information and support by people in a similar situation were vital to him. Charles was very articulate, and early in the onset of his disease he made it clear that he wanted to be in control of his death and made arrangements for euthanasia. He was confronted with an onslaught of various debilitating opportunistic infections, and each time he bounced back and chose life, much to my surprise after all the talk about euthanasia. Eventually Charles started to go blind from CMV. He was hospitalized and awaiting treatment when I visited him. Sometimes it was difficult to make contact with him, and I often just sat near him in silence. He always asked me to come again, so I presumed that he liked my company. On this particular day he seemed especially quiet, yet restless. He did not want to talk, but as I got up to leave he grabbed my hand. Very quietly he told me that the ward doctor had been coming in every day and saying to him: "Charles, you have to face the facts now. You're going to die within a few weeks at most, and you need to get your affairs in order." The ward nurse had also joined this campaign in trying to get Charles to talk. Everytime she brought in medication or the bedpan she reminded him that he was about to die. He told me that he was getting ready to ask for euthanasia during the following week, but that he needed his own time and space to get ready.

Charles told me about a dream he had been having. He spoke as though he were living the dream, so I asked him where he was at that moment. He replied that he was somewhere about 1000 kilometers west of Cape Verde. I didn't understand at first, but then I asked him if he meant that he was in the Atlantic Ocean? He affirmed this. I tried to imagine how that felt, floating alone in the middle of the great ocean. I guessed that he was feeling very depressed and alone—appropriate feelings for someone losing not only his sight but also his life. Charles confirmed this. I asked him if he could see anything nearby in the water. He said: "Yes, I see something! It's a tree trunk floating nearby." When I asked if he could make it to the tree trunk, he said: "Yes, I'm holding on to it now." I told him that he seemed to me to be doing fine and experiencing a depression that was a natural part of a normal grief process. I left that afternoon with a sense that this man was in a very deep and very appropriate depression. Because he had found the tree trunk, I felt confident that he had some support to hold on to. I also felt that because we had been able to communicate at this level, Charles would phone me if he wanted to talk anymore. I went out to find the doctor and nurse who were not allowing him the space he needed to be still and to be aware of his losses. Both of them were surprised at his clarity. They had thought he was in massive denial of his situation because he wasn't talking to them. I explained what he had said to me so they would not bother him anymore. The next day when I went to see him he had quite a few visitors, but he quietly drew me to his side and whispered: "I'm still in the ocean holding on to the tree trunk, but I see some gulls flying overhead." I understood his sighting of birds to mean that he was nearing land, and that was giving him a sense of hope. I also thought that he was nearing death, as birds often symbolize the soul freed of the constraints of the body. A couple of days later, the day before the euthanasia had been planned, I visited Charles one more time. I asked if he was sure that he wanted to go through with it the next day. "Yes," he said, "I'm still holding on to that tree trunk, but a beautiful shore is in sight and I'm nearly there!" We shared the memories of his many accomplishments and he felt proud of his life. He seemed happier and more relaxed than I had ever seen him. Eventually I took my leave, feeling that he was in a good place. The following day, he died as he had planned, surrounded by his family.

Charles's story illustrates a great misunderstanding of the grief process by some health care professionals. In this case, they had heard of the "stages of grief" but were unable to actually apply the theory to Charles's situation. Thus they used the label "denial" to impose their own needs on this patient's acceptance of his death, without listening to his needs. As far as this case of euthanasia is concerned, no one can know what Charles may have discovered on that shore if he had waited to reach it, or perhaps in death he did reach it. Yet, who are we to judge his decision? I feel confident that Charles died at peace with himself and with his family.

I would like to point out the use of symbolic language, as Charles and I conversed about his dream of floating in the ocean. Dream imagery can be a very powerful tool in understanding a person's feelings when he or she finds it difficult to recognize or communicate them. We need to train ourselves to hear and to communicate symbolically because it can be a means of bringing sub-conscious thoughts and feelings into consciousness.

Frank

Frank and his lover, John, joined the group at its onset. John had been diagnosed with AIDS a year earlier, and Frank had just heard that he was se-ropositive. Very unexpectedly, John died several months later. Only then could Frank finally admit to how ill he felt himself. Shortly after John's funeral, Frank was diagnosed with AIDS. Caring for John had really worn him out. A deep depression followed, as Frank considered the quality of his own life, his fear of dying alone, and his options, including euthanasia. I encouraged him to work through the fear as well as his anger and sadness, hoping that he would find a reason to want to live in the process. One day Frank called me and said shyly: "I've found someone to love me again, whom I care for very much!" He hadn't thought that would ever happen again. Frank made a clear decision to live out his life with the most quality possible. He was plagued by much pain and paralysis from neuropathy, and his eyesight continually worsened due to CMV. Frank's greatest fear was of becoming blind, and he discharged his feelings about this repeatedly. Throughout this period Frank had many sessions with me.

Frank also decided to look for a new doctor, a general practitioner who would be willing to support his desire to die at home, pain-free and fully conscious, as I had told him was possible. On his first visit to the new doctor, Frank talked about this desire. Much to his surprise, the doctor pulled a bottle of pills out of his drawer and slid it across the desk, saying: "This is your guarantee for a 'soft' death . . ." Frank was taken aback, but he took the bottle home. Frank phoned me crying, feeling very much misunderstood. I suggested that together we meet with this doctor so that Frank could make his desires known. Frank made the appointment for the following week. Meanwhile, the doctor stopped in to visit Frank at his home on Friday evening and asked for the bottle of pills. He said that he needed it for another patient. Both Frank and I were flabbergasted! Is this careful preparation for euthanasia? Is this in adherence to the strict euthanasia guidelines? I decided to wait for our appointment with the doctor the following week before asking him all of my questions. As the meeting began, I had difficulty controlling my anger, but I tried to listen to what this doctor had to say. Gradually, I understood that the doctor felt terrifically helpless in the face of so many young people dying, and it was obvious that he had real trouble in making contact with others. He didn't listen to what Frank was saying, nor did he make eye contact with either of us. The doctor repeatedly stated that he would deliver another bottle of pills the next day, but Frank insisted that he didn't want them in his house. Frank was contented knowing that the doctor would help with euthanasia if necessary; however, Frank didn't think that he would want it. My job was to make sure that the doctor finally heard Frank. In listening to their conversation, I understood that this doctor was sincere in trying to help his patients in the only way that he knew how. In understanding this I was able to feel more compassion than anger for this man. When the doctor left, Frank and I joked about how he would teach the doctor a lesson in living and dying when the time came!

Quite suddenly Frank became totally blind. He phoned me sobbing loudly and wanted to come to my house to work with me as soon as possible. I wondered if he was going to ask for my support for euthanasia. The next day when I picked him up to go to my house in the country, Frank had already decided that his blindness was going to be the next challenge to meet. He asked for my help in arranging for a crash course in the use of a white cane, a subscription to spoken books from the library for the blind, and an experienced blind person to teach him how to get around in his own home!

During the following month, Frank's general condition deteriorated rapidly, with several crises that included admission to the hospital. When it became clear that no more treatment was available, Frank's boyfriend took him home to die. A roster was set up among friends, family, and caregivers. When I arrived home from vacation later that week and visited Frank, he nearly jumped into my arms when he realized that I was really there. He said: "I'm glad you're here, now we don't have to talk about death anymore, we can talk about life!" He asked me to lie down with him, and as I held him in my arms, he started talking about how happy he was and how proud he was of his many accomplishments. At one point I asked him if, during any of the many crises that had occurred, he had ever been aware of a great white light that he may have felt attracted to? He affirmed that he had experienced this twice recently. One time in the hospital, there had been a lot of commotion and he had seen this light. He felt very drawn to it, and as he moved toward it he felt himself relax and feel peaceful. He realized that this was how it felt to die, and also that he didn't want to die yet. He had a sense that his job wasn't yet fulfilled. I asked him if he had had a sense of being surrounded by love and peace, and Frank affirmed this. He described the second occurrence of the light as more of a sudden flash, almost a discharge, whereby he became very relaxed and peaceful. He said, "I realized that I could choose not to come back, but I needed to for the people around me. No, mostly for myself." I asked Frank if he would be ready to go toward the white light if he experienced it again. He said, "Yes, I'm looking forward to it." He said that he felt very calm and peaceful. I left that afternoon promising that I would be back soon.

The next day, Frank was weaker and his breathing was more labored, but he was fully awake. The doctor was already there when I arrived, and I was surprised to learn that the doctor wanted to increase the pain medication. I didn't sense that Frank was having more pain. The doctor patted Frank's arm and told him: "Just remember that we have a deal, and anytime that you don't want to go on with this, I can help you." Frank turned to the doctor and said, "You're fired. I won't be needing you anymore." The doctor left, saying that he would be back the next day, ignoring what Frank had said. Frank asked me to join his two best friends on the bed. He said that he didn't want any more medication. We talked and laughed together, sharing memories. I asked Frank if he could repeat to his friends what he had told me about the white light. He agreed, but he thought that he had already told them about it. They assured him that he hadn't, but instead said they had seen something in Frank that they described as fear and restlessness. Frank said that was because he had had to fight so hard to come back from the light and that he was afraid if it happened again, he wouldn't have the strength to come back. He proceeded to describe in great detail his two experiences with the white light. All of us sat there filled with wonder and a sense of peacefulness. After awhile Frank said that he was tired and wanted to rest. We said goodbye and I left for home not long after that. The next morning, Frank's boyfriend phoned me saying that his breathing was much more irregular and labored. He felt that Frank was near death and that I should come. When I arrived, Frank's mother and his two friends were on or near his bed, and the "death scene" as Frank wanted it was complete. We shared memories together, sometimes laughing, sometimes crying, but a sense of peacefulness settled over the apartment. Meanwhile, the normal daily routine went on: the cleaning lady arrived and one of the volunteers stopped by for the grocery list. The doctor stopped in and assured us that "this could take many hours and maybe even days" and that he would be available 24 hours a day should we want him. We assured him that we felt Frank was doing just fine and that we were patiently allowing him to die. We sang some of Frank's favorite songs and played his music, realizing all the while that his breathing was becoming more irregular and shallow. Suddenly it was quiet. Frank's breathing had stopped. He had died peacefully, exactly as he had hoped he would.

Frank's story illustrates, again, the necessity of really listening to and taking care of the needs and desires of the person who is ill. Here we were confronted with a very sincere, well-meaning doctor who felt helpless to offer anything other than a quick end to suffering as he himself perceived it. Several weeks later I spoke to this doctor, and he admitted that he had never seen anyone die in such a beautiful and peaceful manner. I have encouraged him to participate in one of my workshops to look at his own issues. I was grateful that I hadn't shown my anger to this man. I believe that he may feel safe enough to come to a workshop.

I often ask dying people if they have been aware of a bright, white light, and many people answer affirmatively as they approach death. I believe this phenomenon is something we can all be more aware of if we dare to ask the questions. Dying people can teach us so much about life.

I am well aware that not everyone can or will come to the end of their life in a manner similar to those I have described. Not everyone can accept impending death as fully as some of these exceptional people have done. I want to emphasize the fact that we, the healthy caregivers, may not judge what is the right or wrong way for a person to live out his or her life. And each and every person needs to be free to die as best fits him or her. As caregivers to dying people, it is essential that we follow and support the person in his or her own process. Sometimes we are able to offer stimulation or assistance in the discharge of feelings, sometimes not.

PROFESSIONAL CAREGIVERS

I am aware that my personal and professional attitudes differ greatly from the traditional patterns adhered to by most professional caregivers. The scope of my work as a facilitator for people with AIDS touches each aspect of the wholeness concept: the physical, emotional, mental, and spiritual aspects of wellness. Giving up the "role" of professional caregiver is not easy—that role offers protection and clarity. It is difficult to just "be present"; we want to be "doing" something. It is hard to deal with silences; we are afraid of them and want to fill them up with talk. I try to support the person who is ill as one human being to another, from heart to heart. I feel privileged and honored to serve as I do.

It is very important to integrate my work, which is a philosophy of life, as much as possible with my private life, and I do not separate the two. Often I become close with people with AIDS that I have met through my work. Sometimes I take them home with me to my house in the country. For some, this is time to work out their feelings in my screaming room. For others, it is a place to rest and share mealtimes or an escape from the hospital, from a new diagnosis, or painful treatment. This is not always easy for my partner. At one point, my partner asked me why we kept getting so close to people that we knew had a limited life expectancy. My partner didn't always like to share all of that grieving and certainly not all of the funerals! However, we both have come to realize that our lives have become richer as a result of this experience. There are fewer barriers that need dealing with to get really close to many of these people. Our contact with them may be very short, yet more intimate and loving than with friends that we have had for years.

Working with people with AIDS has been an absolute challenge to all of my previously held beliefs. It is of vital importance that each and every one involved in this work start to recognize and express their feelings so that they can be integrated into our lives. I want to emphasize that this is my personal style and my way of life. It is important that each of us, whether healthy or ill, caregiver or care receiver, develop our own style in learning to grieve and grow, while we respect one another's needs in meeting the challenge of AIDS.

11

A Personal Perspective on Living and Dying with AIDS

Anthony J. Puentes

INTRODUCTION

AIDS. When you hear the word it probably sounds frightening. Any discussion of the disease brings about a variety of responses. Fears about death and disease are among the most common reactions. Eventually, one reflects on what is shown in the media, what is taught in school, and what one hears on the streets about AIDS. Most Americans should, by now, have a realistic impression of the AIDS crisis. However, no amount of education can really prepare one for the time the disease hits home.

Most persons confronting the AIDS crisis directly are members of the health care and social service systems or they are individuals whose personal lives have been hurt by the disease. I am a physician. I not only face AIDS in a professional context, the disease has also deeply affected my personal life. This chapter is intended to give my perspective, the personal perspective of a professional healer who has had his own spirit dramatically touched by AIDS.

I have worked in the field of public health and Addiction Medicine for 8 years. My discipline is now dealing with greater and greater public health challenges and AIDS is just one of them. I love being a physician, and I am always looking for ways to broaden my perspective on my work and to improve the quality of care I deliver.

I have a simplistic view of medicine's mission. Simply stated, medicine exists to alleviate pain and suffering and to save lives. In other words, the profession aims to preserve the quality of that which is most precious, human life. Disease is the enemy and my patients' well-being is my highest priority. Of

Anthony J. Puentes • Public Health and Addiction Medicine Specialist, San Francisco, California 94131.

Living and Dying with AIDS, edited by Paul I. Ahmed, Plenum Press, New York, 1992.

course, there is a strong element of intellectual curiosity and personal pursuit in how physicians perform their duties. Nevertheless, I entered medicine because of my belief in the mission and my innate sensitivity to other people's pain. It was not until the AIDS crisis became a personal reality for me that I experienced sensitivities to my own pain.

My personal experience with AIDS began in March of 1988. It was then that my lover, my dearest friend and partner, became sick with HIV disease. Rodger was his name. As with any other terminal disease, being told that you or someone close to you has AIDS or HIV disease is a chilling experience. Yes, chilled is the most appropriate word I can use to describe the way I felt when I learned Rodger had AIDS. Rodger died in March of 1989 at the age of 30.

There is now a growing number of helping professionals who have personally felt the pain of AIDS. I can't help thinking about how the whole experience of living with Rodger's illness has changed my life. Certainly, personal perspectives and accounts of the experience of AIDS must vary widely.

Being with my loved one who was living with dying from AIDS provided me a taste of reality that I was not taught in medical school. The experiences of having lived with AIDS and the effect they have on our lives are still very fresh in my mind, probably too fresh to be described totally objectively. Nevertheless, the lessons I learned are still valuable and can be shared.

My AIDS experience has affected me in a number of ways. My perspectives of medicine and the ways it is practiced are different now. I can see the profession from the viewpoint of the person in pain and needing help. I was feeling the pain of impending and actual loss of my loved one. The experience of grieving was something foreign to me. Thoughts of my own mortality and life after death are now a regular part of my life. Dealing with government systems proved to be very challenging. My relationships with my family and close friends have taken new and positive directions.

PERSPECTIVES ON MEDICINE

I love being a physician and I cannot imagine what I would do otherwise. In addition to my love for medicine, I have always maintained that my professional loyalty will always be to other physicians. After all, we have all been through the grueling experience of medical training together. Only another physician can truly understand what it is like to feel pressured by the ultimate responsibility for a patient's life. We share a common mission and passion for our work. During the last many months of living through Rodger's illness, I often wondered if my loyalty was wasted. That is, am I being loyal to a profession that

I now see as having so many serious flaws, especially in its inability to be sensitive to the pain of its patients?

As I have said before, the role of a physician is to fight disease. I often wonder if a physician can truly know disease if he has not experienced it? How can we, as physicians, understand what our patients are going through unless we have suffered the painful effects of illness ourselves? Lack of empathy for a patient's pain is a characteristic of many, if not most, physicians. Thus, as medical professionals, we have a serious handicap, an insensitivity to our patients' pain. A careless and cold medical environment often results.

I now see the health care system as having very little understanding of what it is like to be needy. Rodger's illness and death have given me the unfortunate opportunity to feel pain and a virtual helplessness that my profession so easily misunderstands. A couple of examples of what happened to us should illustrate my point.

In March of 1988, life seemed to be going on as usual. Work was busy as ever and life at home was fine. There was, however, a new problem. I was beginning to worry about Rodger. He had been looking very pale. As I am sure all doctors do at home, they often want to practice medicine on their loved ones, while at the same time becoming annoyed because they cannot get away from it. It's a matter of control. Doctors have to have control, and I was certainly no exception.

Over the next several days Rodger became more and more pale. He didn't seem to think that anything was wrong. As each day passed, I became more concerned about his health and I began asking questions. I am sure that my questions began to bother him. After all, if your own physician/lover gets worried, then something serious must be wrong. I began to insist that he see his own physician.

Rodger seemed very resistant to going to the doctor. It was obvious to me that he was getting sick, so why couldn't he see things my way? After all, I am a doctor. It never occurred to me that he was afraid, deathly afraid that he could have AIDS. I know now that he was worrying about AIDS well before I ever thought that it was even a possibility. After several days of pressuring him he finally agreed to see his family physician.

He consulted his physician on a Wednesday. After ordering a series of lab tests, she called him back to the office the next day to give him the results. He then called me that Thursday afternoon. It was a busy day for me. I had patients to see, charts to do, and a ton of paperwork to catch up on. Rodger called me at two o'clock. As soon as I heard his voice I knew it was bad news. His physician had told him that he was very sick and that she was sure it had something to do with AIDS. He had a hemoglobin level of 3.8 and low counts of every blood cell line you could think of. HIV antibody results were still pending but she was sure it had to be AIDS. Compounding the problem, she had no reservations about telling this distressing news to him alone in her office.

She immediately sent him to the hospital to have a bone marrow biopsy and several other diagnostic tests. He was scheduled to see an infectious disease specialist as well as a hematologist/oncologist as soon as possible. Rodger was being bombarded with all this bad news within a matter of minutes, and by this time he was getting very frightened.

My first reaction upon hearing all of this on the phone was, quite frankly, horror. The thought that Rodger could have AIDS terrified me. I then asked myself why would a physician suggest to someone they had AIDS without even an HIV antibody result? After all, he had no infections, no enlarged lymph nodes, nothing that was typical of HIV disease. Was she basing her diagnosis solely on a hunch? I thought that there had to be more to the story than that. Why wasn't she more understanding of Rodger's fear? Since she knew of our relationship, couldn't she wait until I was with him so that we could be told together?

I felt scared, and I felt like crying. I vividly remember feeling chilled— almost shocked. I couldn't do any more work that day. I wondered if I should explain to anyone at work what was happening. Most people at work didn't even know about my relationship with Rodger. I doubted that they would understand. I had no one to talk to and console me.

My next reaction was to call his physician and get the story firsthand. Maybe there was something she was not telling him. She was not in when I called. I called Rodger back and arranged to meet him at his house after his bone marrow biopsy since it would take me at least 2 hours to get home.

I arrived at Rodger's house 2 hours later. He was tired, pale, and he looked frightened. He looked just like any other patient that had just gone through the mill. But this patient was not just a patient, he was the person I loved most. He was a precious part of my life.

He began telling me about everything all over again. I tried calling his physician again. This time she was in. I would never have believed a physician could be so insensitive as she was until it happened to me personally. Since she knew I was an M.D., she began giving me all the test results and her impressions. Even though she admitted her diagnosis was not confirmed, she was certain it was AIDS.

I couldn't help but feel even more scared. I just sat there listening to this doctor tell me things that felt so shocking. I had never been in a position of receiving bad medical news. I had always been the one to deliver the bad news. I guess she was doing what any other doctor might do, but it felt so cold and matter-of-fact. "And by the way" she said, "is there a chance you could be exposed too?" When I told her that there probably was, she replied, "then you should see a doctor yourself as soon as possible because we have medicines now that can maybe help you live a long time or at least as long as possible."

And so there it all was—all that news in just 2 minutes. I guess that's just the way doctors do it. Present the case and move on to the next one quickly. Of course, she probably felt that since I was a physician I would want the news, good or bad, in clear, concise terms with no waste of time. Never mind that she was telling me that my lover may be dying and that it may be happening to me as well.

I remember feeling that I wanted her to slow down and tell me things step by step. I needed her to ask me how I felt about what I was going through. I wanted some sign of caring.

The next 12 months were difficult for both Rodger and me. It was doctor after doctor and opinion after opinion. Fortunately for us, it quickly focused down to a new primary physician who gave us some consistency in the messages we were getting. Rodger's original physician did, however, do some more damage.

About 2 weeks after the original work up, she phoned Rodger to tell him that his HIV antibody results were positive. Again, he was alone and of course he was scared. The bad news was difficult for him to take. I could not believe she had again done something so crude and insensitive. Physicians are taught to never give HIV results over the phone, *especially* those that are positive. This was lesson number one for me—physicians are not always the honorable people I thought they were. It turned out that her original diagnosis was wrong, and Rodger did not develop AIDS until 9 months later. Despite her original clinical instincts guiding her in the right direction, she needed to be slower and more sensitive in dropping the bomb on us.

I remember feeling like everything was happening to us, like we had no control over what we were being told and how it was being told to us. Rodger was especially frightened because it was all happening to him. He had no medical background, so very little made sense to him. I kept getting frustrated trying to explain things because I either did not understand them myself or did not want to know.

Rodger and I eventually developed a good rapport with the hematologist who became his primary caretaker. This relationship, however, also had its difficulties. On doctor's visits, when I was with Rodger, his hematologist would come into the exam room and talk to me about Rodger's granulocytes, reticulocytes, platelets, and other assorted blood and immune products. In essence, the doctor was talking to me, not to his patient. Poor Rodger would look at me after the doctor left the room and ask "what was he talking about?" There I was trying to explain things in terms that his own doctor should have done.

We asked his doctor to explain things to Rodger in simple terms. He did for a while, but then he resumed explaining things to me only. I guess the doctor felt more comfortable talking to me in technical language. Perhaps he figured I could pass the information to Rodger and then I could deal with Rodger's reactions and emotions. Most likely the doctor was avoiding an uncomfortable situation.

Several months before Rodger's death, I found myself getting more involved in helping him deal with the medical system. I began to feel more like a patient and less like a physician myself. The medical profession began to seem so different to me. I felt more like one of the system's victims and less like part of the system itself. Both Rodger and I felt like we were being tossed from lab to lab, clinic to clinic, and pharmacy to pharmacy.

I remember wishing several times for Rodger's health care providers to just slow down and take more time to talk with us and ask how we were dealing with his illness. Only a few times did anyone ask questions like, "How are you guys doing emotionally?" or "How are things otherwise?" When those questions were asked they were usually asked more out of courtesy than out of true concern. I am not sure if the persons asking really wanted to hear all about how bad things really were. After all, the last thing a busy physician or nurse wants is a patient who needs a lot of emotional support right there in the office. It takes too much time and energy to deal with all the emotional issues a patient might bring up. I know that is the case because I often feel the same way in my own practice.

I guess the lesson here for me is that in my own practice I always need to remind myself what it is like to deal with the system from the other side. Humility taught this physician that patients are people just like me. More importantly, I learned I am just as vulnerable as my patients. I hope that other physicians can learn the same lesson.

THE GRIEVING EXPERIENCE

Until my experience with Rodger's death, I never really understood the meaning of the word *grief*. I never had to. I had never grieved before. I had felt depressed, and I have had my ego bruised, but that wasn't grief.

After Rodger's death I began experiencing an intense series of emotions and physical reactions. First, I remember feeling strong relief immediately after his death, relief that he was no longer in pain. I now hoped that life for me could resume with some normalcy. I was also relieved that Rodger was in some greater place now.

I was soon overcome by strong feelings of abandonment. This was quickly followed by an overwhelming sense of incredible loneliness. I felt as if Rodger had been invited to a very special party and that I could not come along. It was as if he had refused the invitation several times before because he wanted to stay here with me, but this time he accepted and was going without me. He was now leaving me alone when he had never wanted to before, and there was nothing I could do about it. He had abandoned me.

I found it difficult to concentrate on work and I was always moody. Physical exhaustion became a fact of life and lasted for months.

Everyone kept telling me that I was feeling grief. That word kept coming up and I decided to look it up in the dictionary. Webster's defines it as "intense emotional suffering caused by loss, disaster, or misfortune; acute sorrow; deep sadness." I especially identified with the "deep sadness" part. The definition is perfect; that is exactly how I felt.

So, what is grief? For me, the process of grieving has been dynamic and complex. Over the 2 years since Rodger's death my own emotions have run the gamut from relief to sadness, loneliness to anger, and anxiety to peacefulness. Other feelings have included regret, guilt, confusion, and at times, real optimism. Grief often feels like a waxing and waning series of emotions. These emotions can come simultaneously or in cycles.

After Rodger's death, friends often asked me what they could do to help me during my grief. My best response was telling them what not to do. What bothered me most after Rodger's death was how people would just avoid bringing up his name in discussion. There must be a myth that the grieving do not want to talk about their loss. Some friends of mine would put pictures of Rodger and me away because they actually thought that I would not want to look at them. That could not be further from the truth. Talking about Rodger was exactly what I wanted to do. People sometimes acted like nothing had happened. I suspect they were afraid to bring up his name out of fear I might start crying or get depressed. I was already depressed, it couldn't get any worse.

Perhaps my friends were fearful of thinking about their own mortality or even thinking about the death of someone close to them. After all, since death can be scary to most people, perhaps we all needed to talk more with each other about all of our fears.

So, I would advise anyone wanting to help or care for a grieving person to please talk about the dead person if that person is, in fact, on their mind. The best way to get through grief is to experience it and express it. With AIDS it is especially important to talk about feelings of grief with one's closest friends and family. Family and friends may be the only persons who truly sympathize and understand because most people in society still have a very hard time facing the disease.

After Rodger's death, friends called me less often than before his death. It was as if they thought I wanted to be left alone. Quite the contrary, it was after his death that I needed human contact the most.

Even though 2 years have passed since Rodger's death, I still feel like I am being hit with waves of grief from time to time. The holidays are now approaching and I find myself thinking about his death more and more each day. It is an up-

and-down process, there are the highs and the lows and you do not know when your feelings are going to change suddenly. I have never experienced such a wide range of both physical and emotional sensations.

Grief has forced me to get in touch with feelings inside me that I have not known before. For example, feeling intense loneliness despite being surrounded by loving friends and family is a unique burden to me. The loneliness is uncontrollable. My emotional and artistic nature seems to be more expressed than ever before. Suddenly, I am renewing my interest in older more classical music and art to a degree I never have before. I feel more in touch with my feelings and less afraid to reveal my vulnerability to others. I also take my own health more seriously. My priorities are shifting; I want to be more at peace with what I already have instead of striving to get what I do not have and probably do not want. I have a greater appreciation for the process of life and its experiences rather than their results and outcomes. In short, I believe I have a stronger sense of love about me than ever before. It is like waking up to parts of me that had yet to be expressed.

Grief has also allowed me to discover just how much inner strength I really have. Before Rodger's illness I had always feared that I would not handle death well. When he became ill, I was afraid I might eventually run away from him and his illness out of fear. Fortunately, that did not happen. In fact, as his illness grew worse, I found myself truly wanting to help him even more and be there to support him. Frankly, I was surprised and proud of how I stood up to the crisis in my life.

Grief has been enriching and powerful as well as painful and exhausting. I have told my closest friends that, in an unusual way, Rodger's death process and that which followed has not only been the most painful experience of my life, it has been the most fertile and growing opportunity for me.

Shortly after Rodger's death I joined a 12-week bereavement group of surviving partners of persons who have died of AIDS. Participation in this group allowed me to talk about my ordeal with others who had been through the same crisis. Talking with others about the pain of losing Rodger became necessary so that I could express my grief. Others in the group could understand exactly how I felt because they too had felt the pain of loss. We shared a special bond and we needed each other's company. Besides sharing experiences, we provided each other with support. Joining the bereavement group was probably the most beneficial thing I could have done to help my grieving. Even though the group no longer meets, we have remained in close contact.

By no means is the grief process over for me. It is too soon to have experienced all that grief involves, but I understand it more and more as time passes.

I now also have a deeper appreciation for the word "faith." Since faith is what gets me through a crisis, I surely needed all that I could muster to help me through my own crisis of living with Rodger's illness and death. My faith is founded in a true belief in myself. I am confident that who I am and how I live my life is right and good. My faith is strong and it has helped me live through grief. It has helped make grief a healthy experience.

THOUGHTS ON DEATH AND DYING

The ordeal of watching close friends and peers die has usually been reserved for the elderly. The AIDS crisis has forced the realities of death and dying upon a new generation of young and productive people. Besides the Vietnam War there has probably been no other crisis in recent American history that has taken so many youthful lives.

Rodger and I had often talked and joked about growing old together. Just picture it, two old men on the porch in their rocking chairs. That prospect always created laughter amongst our friends. We had often hoped to spend the rest of our lives together as a couple. Who would have expected that one of us would get AIDS and die?

Since Rodger's illness never progressed to dementia, we were able to spend the last few weeks of his life really communicating, about ourselves, our fears around his illness, and most importantly, our feelings about each other. Like most relationships we too had our problems, but we certainly never stopped loving each other. I only hope that other gay couples, when faced with imminent death, have the time and strength to communicate their true love for one another. Hopefully, the realities of honest sharing will leave the surviving partner with a lasting sense of peace.

For Rodger and I, most of the last 3 months of his life were spent either visiting his doctors, being in the hospital, or at my home trying to deal with the realities of dying as best we could. We did a lot of talking about why we used to fight and argue. The reasons for the arguments seemed legitimate, but our angry reactions to each other now seemed wasteful. We apologized to each other several times. Only when Rodger's death seemed near were we able to go long stretches of time without our usual arguments.

Ironically, we had one of our nicest evenings together the night he informed me that his illness had progressed to AIDS. We dined at one of our favorite restaurants. I guess the reason the dinner went so well was that having Rodger with me seemed so precious now. He looked well that night but I knew he would probably die. I had known his lab results for sometime, and my clinical instincts told me that it was only a matter of time, very little time, before he would die. Moments with Rodger that night were precious. He managed to keep me smiling despite all the bad news.

Rodger and I also shared our fears about death during his last few weeks. Rodger had always feared dying alone. When he felt assured I would not leave him he began to focus his concerns on me. He feared that I would be alone after his death and that no one would be around to look after me. Rodger was always one to worry that I was not eating right or taking care of myself. He was always trying to get me not to work so hard. So, in his usual co-dependent manner, he was still worrying about his lover even when he was the one dying.

I did all I could to assure him that I would survive his death and that despite any pain, I would take care of myself. In fact, Rodger made me promise that I would never forget the lessons he taught me on how to stay well.

The most difficult issue for us to discuss was legalities. Rodger had always felt uncomfortable talking about issues like his last will and testament, living will, power of attorney, and life insurance. I guess those things made the prospect of death seem so real. One never thinks of the legal considerations as being urgent until one has very little time left. In fact, toward the end, one of the attorneys had to come out to the house to execute some of the documents. Despite his fears, Rodger dealt bravely with the lawyers and he was able to put most things in order.

Dealing with Rodger's family was also difficult. His family had always rejected his lifestyle and now they were afraid of his illness. For a time they even denied his diagnosis and impending death. His family has never accepted our relationship and their rejection made Rodger's dying even more difficult for both of us. We had only my family to look to for real support.

Despite my own acceptance of Rodger's certain death, I do not think he really appreciated the fact that he was going to die as soon as he did. He knew he was very ill, but he was not expecting things to fall apart so quickly.

Many couples faced with death certainly have to deal with some of the same issues that Rodger and I had to face. However, why did it have to happen so early in our life together? A day does not go by that I do not think of Rodger and the things we used to do together. The memories of the last few days of his life are the most painful. It hurts to remember how weak and in pain he was and how scared I felt seeing him deteriorate so quickly. This once energetic person was dying before me, and there was nothing I could do to prevent it from happening. My biggest fear was that one morning he would wake up and not know who I was. That never happened. In fact, Rodger never became confused. Though very weak, he was lucid and speaking to me right up to minutes before his death.

Besides thinking about Rodger everyday, I now think of my own mortality. What would death be like for me? It seems that from the moment of Rodger's death, my own death is not frightening at all. I used to feel like I had no real reason to die. I had always thought that the life beyond had very little to offer me. In a way I now look forward to death. Death now means my first opportunity to see Rodger again. That bright light that people say we walk into at death means that Rodger will be there waiting for me. It is like flying to a strange city and being afraid because you do not know anyone there and you do not know what to expect. It is easy to be frightened when you are alone and destined for a very strange place that you know nothing about. It sure makes things a lot easier if you could have a loved one waiting for you at the gate when you arrive. So, now, if I die, I will not be headed for a frightening unknown. I shall have someone waiting there for me; Rodger will be there for me. I did not have that assurance before. I cannot believe that he would not be there.

Of course, I do not want to or plan to die soon. It is just that if I am to die, so be it. I am not afraid anymore. If death comes soon then I welcome it because at this time in my life I am at peace with myself and my family. When Rodger died it was not goodbye. It was I'll see you later, somewhere, somehow. I truly believe he and I will be together again.

DEALING WITH BUREAUCRACY

As a physician, I work within the traditional health care delivery system. I believe the system, even though teeming with problems, does work. Unfortunately, it does not work all the time and it does not work for everyone. The system is so large now that it lacks the sensitivity so desperately needed by the people we are devoted to helping. The medical bureaucracy has become cold to the very people it serves. For the most part, it is the mechanism that is cold and not the people who work within it. When faced with a rigid and heartless system, patients are made to feel helpless and hopeless, judged, and even rejected. I know this to be true because it happened to Rodger and me.

From the first doctor visits, to the trips to the laboratory, to dealings with social service agencies, there was always some obstacle to overcome. Even the physical environment created its own barriers. One does not realize how long hallways are until one tries to help someone who can barely walk the distance. You never think about how a parking lot is filled with exhaust fumes until your lover cannot even breathe. I have never known a stairway to be insurmountable until Rodger tried to climb one.

In the hospital, I never realized how annoying it is to have to answer the same questions over and over again when giving one's medical history. Hospital admissions staff would often interview Rodger and me right out in the open. Complete strangers could hear and know why we were there. It's not that we had anything to be ashamed of, it is just that we felt we deserved privacy like anyone else.

In the laboratory waiting rooms, the take-a-number system means just that. You take a number no matter how uncomfortable or ill you are. So there we would sit, with Rodger weak and ill, waiting our turn while others who were obviously in no distress would go before him. You would think that a system could be developed so that sicker people would not have to wait as long. Simple considerations like this become so paramount when you are sick and dying.

Dealing with the government bureaucracies was always the worst obstacle. I had no idea how disorganized and insensitive the State Disability System was until I tried to deal with Rodger's disability claim. I sign disability forms all the time in my medical practice and they seem systematic and simple. However, being on the other side of the process is not so simple.

By the time Rodger was too ill to work, he was of course too weak to go downtown to file a claim. Naturally, we attempted to deal with questions and concerns by mail and telephone. When complicated matters about the claim came up, I knew I would have to go downtown and resolve the issue in person. Since I had Rodger's power of attorney I figured it would be an easy matter. No way!

I spent a good portion of my time downtown explaining why Rodger did not come in himself. People were always asking why I was given his power of attorney since I was not his next of kin and I was "just a friend." Society didn't validate my relationship with Rodger since we were not blood related or "married." I had to impress upon the bureaucrats that I was not trying to run a scam and take Rodger's money for myself. After being convinced that I was legally authorized to be handling Rodger's affairs, they would always require me to complete forms, and more forms. Filling out forms, of course, takes considerable time. It took at least three separate visits downtown to clear matters. It was exhausting, but things eventually got worked out and Rodger's check finally arrived.

Since I deal with bureaucracy all the time in my profession, I was able to catch on to the process fairly quickly. But what about people who are not familiar with the system and need things explained to them? What if I was not around for Rodger? Since he was too weak to deal with the business issues the last 2–3 months of his life, who would have deciphered the letters? Who would have contacted the disability office for him? How would things have gotten resolved if I had not gone downtown or I had not been authorized to handle his affairs? Since the system had no apparent way of allowing for and accommodating his weakened state and his inability to respond to requests for more information, what would have happened?

Rodger was fortunate that I was able to adjust my work schedule to find the time to help him. What about all those people with AIDS who do not have someone with them who knows the system and who knows how to cut through red tape? Even for me it was frustrating dealing with "downtown." I can only imagine how it would be for someone who is alone dying with AIDS.

Another frustrating time was when I had to talk with the Social Security office over the phone. Even though I knew I was speaking to a person on the other end, I felt like I was talking to a machine. The man did not seem to understand why I did not have the right documents and why I could not just put Rodger on the phone. Again, I was always being asked why I was handling things since I was not family or next of kin. As Rodger grew weaker, I was hoping for more sympathy and understanding from everyone I came in contact with. I didn't think that expecting kind words of understanding from people in a system that is designed to help those in need was unrealistic. It was certainly unrealistic here.

A nice relief came one day when I called Visiting Nurses and Hospice. Toward the end, as Rodger's illness worsened, I knew that caring for Rodger was draining my energies and that I needed help. On the suggestion of his physician I called for visiting nurse and home-attendant services.

What was difficult about this particular call to Hospice was that I was not accustomed to asking for help. I have always been the one to offer help and now I was asking for it. I guess that, as a physician, I find being needed and being the one to offer help a comfortable place to be. I don't like to show my vulnerabilities. Now I was very vulnerable, and I needed help.

I first spoke to an intake nurse who asked me a few questions about Rodger and me and inquired about how I was coping with things. She then asked what kind of help I needed in caring for Rodger. Finally I was talking to someone who seemed to care. I remember starting to cry over the phone when the nurse seemed so eager to help. I am not sure why I cried, but it just seemed such a relief to be able to tell someone that I felt desperate and needed help. Help eventually came. The home-attendant provided respite for me, and I was reminded that there are elements of the system that do work and are effective in providing quality care that is sensitive and warm.

I quickly learned from experiences like these that dealing with government agencies is difficult and frustrating. In contrast, my experiences with Hospice and some of Rodger's nurses in the hospital were quite positive. Just having some of the hospital nurses remember Rodger's name and show some true concern made all the difference in the world. Don't expect compassion from the government. I know, I tried.

LOVE AND MY FAMILY AND FRIENDS

The entire experience of having lived through Rodger's disease and his death created some realizations in my life. As I have mentioned before I have a greater appreciation for life's simple experiences and I am not so dependent on the future. Enjoying my friends and family seems more important now than expectations of wealth and security. I have had to adopt what feels healing to me and what connects me to the people I love.

My relations with my family and close friends have grown stronger and deeper ever since Rodger's death and I have a renewed optimism toward life. I now better understand how sometimes even strangers can be very caring. A recent experience in San Francisco reminded me of how much love there still is in the world and how I need to just let myself experience it. This new experience of love happened at a most unexpected time, the 1989 Gay Freedom Day Parade.

Since Rodger moved to San Francisco in 1986, we had made it a special point to go downtown and watch the Gay Freedom Day Parade together. The weather always managed to be nice and we usually were able to assemble a small group of our closest friends to make the trek downtown. If we got there early enough we were able to get a spot with a full view of the parade. If there was ever a day for Rodger and I to feel proud of what we had and how we felt about each other and our relationship, this was the day. During the parade it seemed as if the world had to accept gay people for what we were, just people like everyone else. Both straight and gay people alike would join in the celebration. The parade was an affirmation of our acceptance of one another. Hatred and prejudices had no place here.

In 1989 the parade was different. For one thing Rodger was not with me— it had been almost 3 months since his death. Also, I was not just watching but actually marching in the parade. I, along with about 50 other people, was marching as part of a newly formed contingent, Surviving Partners of Persons with AIDS. For the first time, a group had been formed of persons who had lived through the death of their partners. We felt the need to show people who we were and demonstrate publicly our pride in ourselves and in our partners. We knew we deserved recognition and support on this special day.

Our group marched just behind two other groups, Persons with AIDS and Parents of Persons with AIDS. These two groups had specifically invited us to march with them and share the honors of being at the front of this, the largest gay freedom parade in the world.

If you had told me just a few years ago that I would be marching I probably would not have believed you. Most likely I would have been afraid to acknowledge my homosexuality in public. Now times are different and I have a purpose. Rodger would have been proud.

The parade began and we all marched along the 3-mile route. The experience of marching as part of the Surviving Partner contingent proved to be enlightening. At first, I did not know what to expect. In fact, I do not think any of us knew what the crowd's reaction to our group would be. From the beginning and all along the route we were greeted with roaring cheers and applause. We were tossed thousands and thousands of greetings of "Love" in the universal sign language. It was as if the crowd was truly acknowledging the pain we had experienced and our strength to endure. I remember one man, in particular, who shouted out "life goes on." I immediately thought, "He's telling me?"

There were tears from the crowd and I saw several persons, men and women, crying and then being consoled by their friends as we passed by. I assumed that these people had also lost close friends and partners to AIDS and watching our contingent march by brought some of the pain back again. We had several people join us along the route and still others preferred to support us from the sides.

It felt like we were being blessed with love and warmth from all directions. We could hear the cheers and see the hand signals of love being sent from everywhere. It was an exhausting march but it was worth every second. By the time we reached the end I felt energized. I felt like a new person who had been given a special gift from all those thousands of people.

That special gift was an enveloping feeling of love and a reminder that there is still some hope and kindness from strangers. I am reminded of the words of the Maharishi Maheshi Yogi who, in his book *Love and God,* says "What a miracle God has created in Love." My experience during the parade was indeed a miracle.

I vividly remember feeling a natural high for several days after the march. It must have been obvious in my behavior because several of my friends commented on my heightened spirit. I look forward to marching in next year's parade.

That large dose of optimism during the parade began to overflow into other areas of my life. My relations with my family grew deeper and more enriched. My mother and I talk more about our feelings toward each other and about our fears concerning death. We seem to better understand each other and we have a greater appreciation for one another's way of living and thinking. We spend more time together just enjoying each other's company.

My father and I, two persons who rarely shared deep feelings with one another, now have begun talking about our personal lives in a way we had not before. We are beginning a new friendship and brotherhood with each other. My brothers and I are now enjoying a closer, more meaningful relationship.

As far as friendships go, I find myself being a lot more selective about who I spend time with. I have devoted more time to developing some closer ties with my serious and longtime friends, and I am spending less time on those friendships that provide me with very little benefit. I like my new selectivity.

I am not sure what specifically brought about all these positive changes in my relationships. I suppose they are a result of dealing in the last 3 years with the personal realities of human illness and mortality.

Certainly, faith has played a major role in my life. I have taken on new and positive changes. Confidence in myself and my acceptance of the love of my closest family and friends has proven to be one of my most treasured assets. The power of faith in getting me through my own AIDS crisis cannot be underestimated.

It is comforting to think that since Rodger has died he might, in some supernatural or spiritual way, be helping me put the pieces of my life together.

He was always wanting me to get closer to my family. Perhaps Rodger is somewhere giving me courage to face challenges. He could be influencing my behavior in ways that I cannot understand until I too have died. Maybe he is watching me as I write this chapter. Possibly he is with me as I relate to my parents; or maybe he is with me when I am renewing relations with my closest friends. Perhaps he is around me all the time. It is peaceful to think that he is still, in some healthy way, watching over me.

CLOSING

To truly appreciate the personal side of a family living and dying with AIDS one must personally live through the process. My own accounts reveal only what happened to Rodger and me but perhaps others can identify with what I have described. Watching Rodger die has certainly been a very spiritual and challenging experience for me. I now realize that no combination of written words will completely convey how I feel and what it is really like to be in a family with AIDS.

This chapter is not intended to give a complete and comprehensive picture of what it is like to actually live with the AIDS crisis at home. It is intended to simply illustrate the experiences of one man, a professional healer who is now himself a wounded healer. Being wounded has given me both pain and ultimate hope. Perhaps other healers can learn from my experiences.

A few closing comments may serve a purpose. Even though AIDS is still commonly associated with homosexual men, the disease represents the tragedy of illness and death no matter what the cause or who the victim. Since people of all colors and sexualities get sick and die, shouldn't we all have something to offer each other? Just like the thousands of people cheering me at the parade, we all have plenty of extra love to share; we just need to express that love.

Rodger and I often felt that we had to defend or justify our relationship to others so that we would not be judged. When one has AIDS, one might expect that people will be quick to judge. People do react negatively to AIDS patients all the time. Whether it is out of hatred, homophobia, or just plain fear, these negative reactions do no good. They help no one. Shame and fear about sexual secrets or sexual identity have no place in today's society and should never be the worry of a person seriously ill or dying from any disease. Rodger and I were honest about our love for each other. We did nothing wrong and we had every reason to expect the same love and respect from our caretakers that anyone else deserves.

It will be years before persons with AIDS will be welcomed into the mainstream medical care system as people who deserve love, kindness, and caring just like anyone else and not just because they represent an interesting research case or a clinical challenge. The medical establishment must realize that it is one of the professions that can lead society into a healthier acceptance and understanding of people with AIDS. We should help those with the disease regardless of who they are or how they got infected. I still have confidence in my profession, and I hope that responsible change is forthcoming. I truly hope that my own medical practice is enriched and that I never forget the lessons that Rodger's dying and death have taught me.

Personally, my experiences are still too fresh for me to be clearly objective in my comments. In fact, a number of unanswered questions persist in my mind. I am not sure if I will ever understand why the AIDS phenomenon struck Rodger and me and not our other friends. We did nothing wrong, so why us? Why does a disease like AIDS create such a horror in the community? Why do parents of AIDS patients often turn against their children? Is homophobia so strong that it splits up families at a time when they need to be together the most? Why do families of persons who have died of AIDS sometimes turn against the surviving partner? Why do churches, famous movie stars, and celebrities care so much about helping the cause against AIDS when they will not publicly accept or even acknowledge homosexuality? I guess only time will provide answers.

Why now have I chosen to be so honest and tell my story in such a public way? I guess it is because my own time for expression has come and I am very proud of my loving relationship with Rodger. We dealt well with the blow that fate struck upon us. We fought the AIDS battle together and I am now proud to be a surviving partner. I will continue the battle against AIDS with the help and love of my friends and family. Most of all, I feel proud of who I am.

AIDS and Special Groups

Coping with HIV Disease in the Army

ANN E. NORWOOD, JAMES R. RUNDELL,
MARIA E. ESPOSITO, LARRY H. INGRAHAM,
and HARRY C. HOLLOWAY

This chapter discusses challenges inherent in helping soldiers cope with HIV infection. We describe the history of HIV disease in the military and the development of a special HIV ward at the Walter Reed Army Medical Center. Ways in which we assist soldiers to adapt to the constraints of HIV infection are explored.

HISTORY OF HIV IN THE MILITARY

Coinciding with civilian efforts to ensure the safety of the nation's blood supply, the military began screening blood donations for the HIV antibody in July 1985. In August 1985, the Department of Defense instituted mandatory

The information presented here reflects the thoughts and opinions of the authors. It does not necessarily reflect the opinions of the Department of Defense, the Department of the Army, the Uniformed Services University of the Health Sciences, the Walter Reed Army Medical Center, the Walter Reed Army Institute of Research, the Walter Reed Retrovirus Research Group, or the Henry M. Jackson Foundation for the Advancement of Military Medicine.

ANN E. NORWOOD, JAMES R. RUNDELL, MARIA E. ESPOSITO, and HARRY C. HOLLOWAY • Department of Psychiatry, Uniformed Services University of the Health Sciences, Bethesda, Maryland 20814-4799.   LARRY H. INGRAHAM • Department of Military Psychiatry, Walter Reed Army Institute of Research, Washington, D.C. 20307-5100.

Living and Dying with AIDS, edited by Paul I. Ahmed, Plenum Press, New York, 1992.

blood testing for all individuals applying for induction. Expansion of mandatory screening was prompted by a recruit, later found to be HIV seropositive, who nearly died after receiving the standard smallpox immunization during basic training. On October 24, 1985, the Department of Defense expanded mandatory screening to cover all servicepersons already on active duty (Herbold, 1986).

The decision to institute universal testing was based on concerns unique to the military. The near fatality of the recruit raised the specter of endangering potentially immunocompromised service members with live virus immunizations, which are routinely administered to military personnel. Because service members are deployed to areas where infectious diseases are endemic and medical facilities sparse, protection of immunocompromised individuals from further risk was necessary. In addition, it was important to ensure the safety of the "buddy" blood supply system; under battlefield conditions and occasionally during disasters in peacetime, it has been found necessary to transfuse blood directly from soldier to soldier.

SCOPE OF THE PROBLEM

By November 1989, screening had identified approximately 1,800 HIV-seropositive soldiers (Brundage, personal communication, November 1989). Of this group, approximately 880 remained on active duty and 82 had died (Brundage, personal communication, November 1989). Upon reviewing HIV seroconversion rates from 1985–1989, McNeil et al. demonstrated a downward trend, estimating that approximately 220 soldiers were infected with HIV during 1989 and 1990 (McNeil et al., 1991).

Clinical goals of the army's medical program are early detection, treatment, and prevention. Research efforts are under way in all of the uniformed services to better characterize the natural history of the infection, to develop a vaccine against the virus, to prevent transmission, and to improve patient care. Walter Reed Army Medical Center (WRAMC) has developed an HIV ward to further these goals.

Initial Diagnosis

In April 1988, the army implemented an HIV regulation (AR 600-110). Soldiers are screened for HIV at least every other year, and commanders must provide at least 4 hours of unit-level education about HIV/AIDS annually. This education, consisting of a movie, followed by a question-and-answer session facilitated by a community health nurse, constitutes the pretest counseling for soldiers.

Blood is screened for HIV using the ELISA technique, which is sensitive but not specific. If the blood tests positive, it is retested using the same method. After a second positive test, an aliquot of the specimen is forwarded for confirmation testing using the Western Blot, an immunoelectrophoresis technique that is highly specific.

Individuals confirmed HIV seropositive are notified individually by a physician. The soldier's unit commander is informed of the positive test result in advance and accompanies the soldier to receive the news. Additionally, each army post is required to identify a support network of individuals trained to provide assistance to HIV-seropositive soldiers. This network generally consists of mental health professionals, preventive medicine physicians and nurses, internists, and chaplains. Commanders and physicians often elect to have a mental health professional or chaplain from this team available to provide additional support, as indicated.

In breaking the news to the soldier, the physician informs the individual that he or she has had a positive Western Blot, which may signify infection with HIV. This is carefully phrased to include the possibility that, while unlikely, there may have been an error and that further evaluation is necessary. The soldier is counseled on behaviors that transmit the virus and common myths are discussed. The individual is instructed to refrain from known transmission behaviors pending definitive evaluation at a medical center.

After physician counseling, the soldier's commander is required to formally counsel the soldier. Counseling includes a direct order to inform partners of the infection prior to engaging in intimate sexual behaviors. A direct order is also given to refrain from unprotected sexual relations with persons other than their spouses and not to donate blood, tissues, sperm, or body organs. Soldiers, who disobey this order, are subject to disciplinary action.

Notification of seropositivity produces varied responses including anxiety, denial, sadness, shock, and fear. Physicians and commanders working with newly identified seropositive soldiers are instructed to observe the individuals closely for behavioral changes that might indicate suicidal ideation. If suicidal ideation is suspected, the soldier is referred to a mental health professional for evaluation.

While the reactions to initial notification may be profound, soldiers rarely require psychiatric hospitalization. More commonly, supportive outpatient treatment is indicated to help the individual manage anxiety generated by the presumptive diagnosis of HIV infection. Soldiers are sent rapidly to the post's designated medical center to shorten the time they must cope with uncertainty.

Evaluation at the Medical Center

Shortly after initial notification, the soldiers go to one of six army medical centers for medical evaluation. The progression of disease is assessed using the

STAGE	HTLV III ANTIBODY AND/OR VIRUS ISOLATION	CHRONIC LYMPHADEN-OPATHY	T HELPER CELLS/mm3	DHS	THRUSH	O.I.
WR 0	−	−	>400	NL	−	−
WR 1	+	−	>400	NL	−	−
WR 2	+	+	>400	NL	−	−
WR 3	+	+/−	<400	NL	−	−
WR 4	+	+/−	<400	P	−	−
WR 5	+	+/−	<400	C and/or +		−
WR 6	+	+/−	<400	PC	+/−	+

FIGURE 1. The Walter Reed staging classification for HTLV-III/LAV infection. DHS denotes delayed hypersensitivity; NL, normal; P, partial cutaneous anergy, which is defined as an intact cutaneous response to only one of the four test antigens; C, complete anergy to the four test antigens; and O.I., opportunistic infection. (From "The Walter Reed Staging Classification for HTLV-III/LAV Infection," by R. R. Redfield, D. C. Wright, & E. C. Tramont, 1986, The New England Journal of Medicine, 314, 131–132.)

Walter Reed classification system (see Figure 1). Soldiers are returned to duty or medically retired, based on the severity of these findings. Soldiers who are Walter Reed stages 1–2 (T4 > 400) are returned to active duty, and soldiers who are Walter Reed stages 3–6 (T4 < 400) are medically retired.

HISTORY OF AN HIV WARD

The history of Ward P-8 illustrates problems that soldiers encountered in the early days of the testing program and the actions that were taken to address them.

The evolution of the ward has paralleled society's maturation in dealing with this new disease. Its scope has expanded from its original clinical and administrative focus to one that includes research. The ward will be referred to by a pseudonym, Ward P-8.

Just as universal testing for all potential inductees was prompted by a vaccine-related tragedy, Ward P-8's inception was catalyzed by a death. In January 1986, one of the original group of inductees found to be HIV seropositive committed suicide in the barracks. This initial group of inductees was not well established, with little in common other than seropositivity. They could not provide effective support for one another. Housed in the barracks while awaiting administrative actions, their HIV status was soon discovered by the other, nonHIV patients, who were also housed there. The HIV patients were subsequently subjected to harassment ("queer-baiting" and unsolicited sexual advances) and even physical assaults. Attending infectious disease physicians and psychiatrists working with these patients accurately assessed the need for a safe holding environment for the patients. Plans were still in the review process when the suicide occurred. Within a matter of days, Ward P-8, a ward that previously had been dedicated to housing ambulatory care patients, was rededicated to the support of HIV-seropositive patients (Rothberg *et al.*, 1990).

These events occurred during the same period of time in which civilian AIDS patients were also subjected to threatening behaviors based on people's fear and ignorance. In some settings, even health care providers reinforced the stigma, donning protective clothing more suitable to space exploration than to patient care. It was against this backdrop that Ward P-8 was developed.

Ward Milieu

Ward P-8 is an administrative hybrid. While the operation of the ward falls under the auspices of internal medicine, there is a strong psychiatric presence. Technically speaking, it is probably incorrect to describe the ward as a "therapeutic milieu." However, milieu principles gleaned from psychiatry play a prominent role in the treatment design. Gunderson (1978) has described the five functions of therapeutic milieus: containment, support, structure, involvement, and validation.

Containment "acts to prevent assaults, homicides, and suicides, and to minimize the chances of physical deterioration or of dangerous accidents in those who lack judgment" (Gunderson, 1978, p. 329). This function of milieu therapy is not a prominent part of Ward P-8. Patients who manifest psychotic processes or active homicidal/suicidal ideation are transferred to the psychiatric ward.

In contrast, support plays a prominent role. Gunderson (1978, p. 329) describes support as "conscious efforts by the social network to make patients feel better and to enhance their self-esteem." The ways in which the ward provides support will be discussed later in the chapter.

Ward P-8's structure provides a framework to organize the patients' varied medical appointments and activities. Most patients are presented with a daily schedule of activities, such as support group discussions, relaxation techniques, and art therapy. Certain activities are voluntary while others are mandatory.

Patient involvement is a cornerstone of the ward. The ward affords HIV-seropositive patients the opportunity to meet others encountering similar problems. Patients can share experiences about helpful ways of dealing with family members' and co-workers' reactions to their diagnosis. Because patients of all stages are frequently on the ward, they have a wealth of experience to discuss.

Validation refers to "the ward processes which affect a patient's individuality" (Gunderson, 1978, p. 331). This includes all aspects of the ward that support the individual's efforts to master loss, tolerate uncertainty, and accept change.

These five functions and the degree to which some of them predominate at different times help to conceptualize ward operations. While not fundamentally changing these functions, the military aspect of the ward influences the ways in which they are manifested.

Military discipline pervades the ward's functions. Initially, active duty soldiers and retirees are addressed by their rank. "Hello, Sgt. Jones" is a common greeting. Often the therapeutic limits incorporate military courtesy and regulation; while it might be appropriate—and perhaps encouraged—to tell the medical ward officer to "go to hell" in the context of group therapy, this would not be condoned if it took place at the front desk.

Military staff members often act as ready targets for patients' displaced anger at "the army" and the conflicts it engenders in them. Officers helping HIV-infected soldiers deal with perceived injustices experience similar conflicts and feelings. Transference and countertransference issues have been helpful in understanding dilemmas created by HIV infection.

On the ward we seek to strike a balance between keeping the environment "military enough" to maintain the military identity of those soldiers returning to duty, yet not "too military" so as to impede the transition from soldier to civilian. An example of this is the ward policy on duty uniform, that is, whether patients should wear pajamas, street clothes, or uniforms. We weighed the potential impact of each choice of clothing on the milieu. Pajamas, we felt, might foster regression, reinforce the sick role, and frighten newly diagnosed patients. Uniforms, on the other hand, could accentuate differences in rank and exacerbate isolation. In the end, street clothes became the "uniform-of-the-day" for all patients except those confined to bed.

Curfews and other rules have been developed by staff, who also solicit patient participation in determining how the ward can best serve patient needs. As in psychiatric milieus, emphasis is placed on helping patients develop standards and social norms that promote mutual help and respect. Consistent with the coping and social supports literature, we have found peer support to be invaluable for helping individuals deal with HIV disease.

Ward Composition

The patient population comprises individuals in all stages of HIV disease, although there is a predominance of those in the earlier stages. During initial staging, soldiers are hospitalized on Ward P-8 and attend various classes. HIV-seropositive patients are followed on a quarterly, semi-annual, or annual basis depending on the severity of the illness. Most of the patients returning to Walter Reed for restaging elect to stay on the ward; others stay with friends or in motels. In addition, patients who are scheduled for reevaluation for disability purposes (Temporary Disabled Retirement List, TDRL) and those who are involved in research protocols are members of the milieu.

The ward is staffed to support a 40-bed moderate care medical ward. A medical officer (currently a family practitioner) is in charge of the ward and reports to the Chief of the Infectious Disease Service. The other military staff include the head nurse (a field grade officer) and the wardmaster (a noncommissioned officer). Civilian staff assigned to the ward include nurses (most of whom have medical/surgical backgrounds), practical nurses, a psychiatric clinical nurse specialist, and physician assistants. The staff is augmented by full- and part-time staff provided by other departments. Two social workers, one psychologist, and two psychiatrists support Ward P-8 exclusively. In addition, a recreation therapist, an art therapist, a chaplain, infectious control nurse specialists, and a drug and alcohol counselor provide part-time consultation to the ward.

Recently, the ward's capabilities have been expanded to provide care for more seriously ill patients. Thus the ward also houses HIV-seropositive patients with illnesses that do not require critical or intensive nursing care; patients with medical and psychiatric illnesses that do not require restraint or a locked ward environment can now be treated on P-8.

Ward Routine

Nurses complete assessments after patients arrive on the ward, and a physician's assistant performs a history and physical examination. All patients fill out a psychiatric screening sheet consisting of yes/no questions that assess past history of psychiatric illness and recent suicidal ideation and substance abuse. If the patient responds positively to any of these questions, or if the nurse or physician's assistant has concerns about the patient, he or she receives immediate psychiatric consultation. In most cases, however, the patient is not seen by a psychiatrist until the second or third hospital day.

A nurse orients patients admitted for initial staging to the ward and introduces them to other patients, who informally serve as sponsors. Patients sleep in 4- to 8-person bays. Private rooms are located nearest to the nursing station and are reserved for patients in need of closer nursing observation.

Before attending the various ward activities, patients have blood drawn for laboratory analysis and anergy panels applied. The results of these tests are then available when they see their infectious disease physicians later in the week.

WARD TREATMENT PROGRAM

Patients are placed in one of four program tracks depending on the purpose of their admission. Each track consists of mandatory and optional classes and groups. Patients undergoing initial staging enter track 1, the most intensive program with exposure to all ward activities. Patients coming back for follow-up visits, involved in research protocols, or awaiting medical retirement enter tracks 2–4, which emphasize voluntary participation except for activities specific to individual treatment goals.

Treatment Goals

The milieu provides an environment in which specific goals of hospitalization can be carried out. While the multidisciplinary team specifies individual goals for each patient, the ward's general goals as formulated by the staff in April 1989, are the following:

Goal 1: Medical evaluation. To provide HIV staging and evaluation, treatment intervention, and medical disposition for active duty service members and other eligible health care beneficiaries.

Goal 2: Research. To support the Walter Reed Retrovirus Research Group's efforts for further understanding of HIV infection, treatment, and care for health care beneficiaries.

Goal 3: Education. To provide education on health maintenance and transmissibility of HIV to enable patients to manage their health effectively and to diminish transmission of the virus.

Goal 4: Psychiatric/psychosocial support. To provide inpatient psychiatric/ psychosocial evaluation and treatment for military personnel and their health care beneficiaries infected with HIV, in order to enhance their quality of life and to promote responsible sexual behavior.

Group Activities

Numerous classes and small groups address the goals enumerated above. Education by groups and classes about HIV are supplemented by focusing on peer support, enhancement of coping skills, and health promotion. Peer support is a cornerstone of the entire program, and most therapeutic activities happen in a group setting. Helping patients to help each other is a major emphasis and promotes social norms and pressures supporting safe sex. The formal groups and classes include the following.

Socialization group. The recreation therapist facilitates patients getting to know one another and teaches numerous topics. Class content varies depending on needs of the current patient population. Topics and skills covered include communication, assertiveness training, problem solving and recognizing one's needs and how they change (e.g., how one can modify one's recreation to match constraints imposed by illness).

Sexuality group. This group is facilitated by a psychiatric clinical nurse specialist and a physician's assistant. Its goal is to explore beliefs and values about sexuality and ways in which these have been changed by HIV disease. The group assists patients in expanding their ideas about what constitutes sexuality and sensuality and seeks to reduce resistance to safe sex practices.

Medical evaluation board (MEB) group. This group is led by a social work noncommissioned officer. He educates soldiers being medically retired about their benefits and entitlements. He also keeps them apprised of the status of their boards as they proceed through administrative channels.

Recreation therapy and assessment group. Patients are asked to fill out forms that assess their current leisure activities and their satisfaction with them. These are then the subject of group discussion, with a goal of facilitating behaviors that are health promoting. In this context, education is provided about ways patients can spend enjoyable leisure time without drinking alcohol and/or smoking. Recreation therapy also sponsors outings in which patients become acquainted with activities that are fun and health promoting.

Art therapy. The weekly art therapy is mandatory. Patients draw or sculpt, and the group then discusses the work. Frequently, the artwork stimulates and facilitates the discussion of feelings by the patients. The artwork also provides staff with glimpses into the patients unconscious, especially helpful for patients who have difficulty expressing themselves verbally. In addition, patients use the studio in the evenings and during open art periods. Patient artwork displayed on the ward softens the institutional atmosphere. The art therapist has developed a moving audiovisual presentation of patient's artwork entitled "If I Could Tell You." This slideshow is an eloquent reminder of the human dimensions of this infection.

Support group. The group meets twice a week. Former patients are encouraged to continue to participate as outpatients. Two social workers in the group facilitate, and other staff attend as space permits. Patients cite the support group as the most helpful experience for them. Topics are generally introduced by the patients. Recurring themes include how and when to inform family members and friends about the HIV diagnosis, fears about illness and death, improving relationships, how to protect confidentiality, and the like.

Well springs. The chaplain meets with all interested persons to discuss spirituality. In an informal atmosphere patients talk about their thoughts and feelings on spirituality. This has been especially helpful for those patients estranged from their organized religions because of their sexual practices or drug use.

Stress reduction and imagery class. Organized and taught by the art therapist, this group teaches patients how to use meditation and relaxation techniques. Many patients find these techniques helpful for dealing with anxiety and stress-related symptoms.

Alcohol and substance abuse. This group is led by the drug and alcohol counselor. Patients' thoughts and comments about substances are elicited. Education about substance abuse and available treatment options are discussed. Times and places for AA and other 12-step meetings are provided. Usually there is at least one patient already involved in a recovery program who is willing to share his or her experiences.

Meeting with protocol nurses. Nurses involved with various research protocols inform patients about them. Patients also have the opportunity to ask questions and to schedule individual appointments to learn more about experimental treatments.

TRACK 1 WEEKLY SCHEDULE

HOUR	MONDAY	TUESDAY	WEDNESDAY	THURSDAY	FRIDAY
0800	orientation patient ...	morning ...	orientation assembly in ...	dayroom ...	(Mon-Fri)
0900					
1000	socialization group	HIV support group A (1000-1130)	stress reduction with imagery class (0930-1100)	infection control class	HIV support group B (1000-1130)
1100	MEB information group		health maintenance diet therapy (1100-1230)		
1200					
1300	sexuality group	rec. therapy intake and assessment	multi-D management	community outing	responsible sex
1400	art therapy for MEB (1400-1630)	well springs	alcohol & drug education		
1500		protocol group	class (cont.) (1430-1600)		
1600		introduction to art therapy (1600-1730)			
1700			meeting: while you are here		

FIGURE 2. Scheduled activities for an initial-staging patient enrolled in track 1.

Figure 2 shows the scheduled activities for an initial-staging patient enrolled in track 1.

Individualized Assessment and Treatment Plan

The first step in any rehabilitation strategy is patient assessment. On Ward P-8, staff members compare their impressions of the patients and identify problem areas for the multidisciplinary team. Treatment discussions occur weekly in the treatment planning conference (TPC); modifications can be made during the daily nursing reports.

Each patient is discussed at the TPC. The patient's strengths and weaknesses are outlined by the various disciplines. A plan is then developed to work on problems delineated at the TPC. If the patient has a substance abuse problem or significant psychiatric illness, a behavioral contract will be negotiated between the patient and staff. A person with a history of alcohol dependence, for example, might agree to attend the substance-use class and go to at least one AA meeting. A patient with major depression could agree to a contract in which he would gradually increase his involvement in the milieu and report for medications at the stated times.

Psychiatric diagnoses reported in the civilian community also occur in the military environment (Pace, Rundell, & Paolucci, 1990). Because suicide rates are high in AIDS patients (Marzuk, Tierney, & Tardiff, 1988) and following the notification of positive HIV test results (*Clinical Psychiatry News*), the program emphasizes assessment of suicide potential. Patients are especially vulnerable to suicidal ideation at times of disease progression. A psychiatrist assesses patients whose T4 helper cell count has dropped significantly. Actively suicidal patients are transferred for inpatient psychiatric care.

Substance abuse is another major focus of concern. Alcohol abuse has long been associated with suicide, poor judgment, impulsive behavior, auto accidents, and drowning (Holloway, Perdue, & Wegner, 1988.) Moreover, substance abuse has been implicated in increasing HIV transmission via high-risk behaviors (Stall, McKusick, Wiley, Coates, & Ostrow, 1986.) The military offers both residential and outpatient treatment for alcohol problems. Drug rehabilitation is more limited in the military; generally, retirees are referred to civilian programs for drug problems that require residential treatment.

Severe psychiatric disorders are grounds for medical retirement. In many cases, however, soldiers return to duty when their illnesses resolve. For example, soldiers have returned to duty when their major depressive disorders have ameliorated in response to therapy. They then receive follow-up psychiatric care at their home posts.

DISCHARGE PLANNING IN THE ARMY: ADVANTAGES AND DISADVANTAGES

Soldiers and retirees come to WRAMC from all over the world. This presents problems in arranging follow-up care. Social workers take responsibility for coordinating discharge planning and aftercare. While there are constraints associated with being an HIV-positive soldier, the army holds many benefits, as well.

The importance of material resources (implicit in the relationship noted among economic status, stress, and adaptation) is rarely addressed in the literature (Cohen & Lazarus, 1984.) Yet, WRAMC patients describe the monies and medical care provided by the army as being an important source of support. Eligible family members and retirees have access to conventional and experimental treatments through military and Veterans Administration medical facilities. They also have the option of seeking medical care through civilian facilities with partial reimbursement (usually 75%) provided by the CHAMPUS (Civilian Health and Medical Program of the Uniformed Services) program. Because of these resources, then, discharge plans for retirees may well contain more options than found in many segments of the civilian community. Soldiers returning to duty present a different set of challenges for health care providers. The military constraints involved in treating HIV-positive soldiers affect treatment and disposition.

CONSTRAINTS AND CHALLENGES UNIQUE TO THE MILITARY

While there are similarities between military and civilian treatment of HIV-infected persons, there are also differences. All known modes of HIV transmission have been identified in the military: sexual behaviors, intravenous drug use, blood transfusions, and perinatal transmission. Homosexual acts and illicit substance abuse are illegal under the Uniform Code of Military Justice (UCMJ). Moreover, confidentiality is not guaranteed in the military physician–patient relationship (Auster, 1985). One of the major challenges for the ward, then, has been to create an environment in which soldiers can talk safely and candidly about themselves and their partners; the ability to assess and treat patients is compromised when patients do not feel safe in doing so.

The limits of confidentiality remain ambiguous. In October 1986, Congress passed a law stating that information disclosed during epidemiological assessment could not be used in ways that are contrary to the patient's interests, notably involuntary separation or adverse personnel actions (Howe, 1988). It is less clear whether information obtained during other portions of medical evaluation is given similar safeguards. For the present, military physicians must reach decisions individually as to how they will address these ethical dilemmas.

While confidentiality remains a focus of concern for physicians, Auster (1985) notes "that whatever the regulation, no physician in any of the services is known to have been disciplined for failing to report homosexuality, alcoholism or cannabis use in his patients." It appears that patient perceptions of the practitioner's comfort in talking about sex and substance abuse and a nonjudgmental stance affect rapport more than whether or not the provider wears a uniform. Regardless, some patients remain circumspect when dealing with staff, leaving the question to what degree they would experience similar difficulties with trust in the civilian sector.

"Fitness for duty" evaluation is also unique to the military. This function of the ward can also complicate assessment and treatment. Immunosuppressed soldiers must be medically retired. For soldiers who are not medically boarded, the physician must document any limitations that would affect the soldier's duty performance. In addition to documenting physical limitations, consideration must be given to psychiatric conditions that could hamper a soldier's ability to perform his duties. By regulation (AR 635-200), most major psychiatric disorders render the soldier unfit for duty and lead to medical retirement. Soldiers who fail substance abuse rehabilitation, however, are administratively separated; that is, they are ineligible for continued military benefits but qualify for medical care at Veterans Administration hospitals.

Concerns about disposition prompt soldiers to downplay or to exaggerate psychological complaints based on hopes of returning to duty or medically retiring. Soldiers who meet retention standards based on HIV disease (stages 1 and 2) sometimes explore the possibility of receiving medical retirement based on psychiatric grounds. For most psychiatrists, psychiatric diagnosis and its impact on patient disposition can pose a greater dilemma than does confidentiality.

Many patients experience the diagnosis of HIV infection as a traumatic event. While most military HIV-infected patients do not develop psychiatric disorders following this news, high levels of psychological distress are common (Rundell et al., 1989). Some soldiers have adjustment disorders, but because these disorders are self-limiting, they are not conditions leading to disability separation. The treatment team must then assist the soldiers in preparing emotionally for the return to duty. Sometimes highly motivated soldiers will experience signs and symptoms of depression but will prefer to "suffer in silence" rather than risk not being allowed to go back to work. These soldiers also present the milieu with special challenges.

Duty limitations imposed by AR 600-110 engender strong feelings in the patients that must be addressed by the treatment team. Soldiers frequently voice concerns that their careers are effectively over after learning the specifics of the regulation. The limitations include exclusion from overseas assignments, disqualification for jump (parachute) status, ineligibility for recruiting and drill instructor assignments, mandatory stabilization at current duty assignments, and significant restrictions on further schooling. Motivated soldiers sometimes become demoralized due to these restrictions. Moreover, as discussed later, commanders at some posts have developed local policies that further restrict HIV-seropositive soldiers.

It is counterproductive to defend army policy in the face of patient disappointment and anger. Rather, the treatment team tries to validate their feelings (when appropriate) and encourage patients to channel these feelings in a constructive fashion. In the past, HIV policymakers have been invited to the ward to meet with patients, and this has proved to be a good learning experience for both. Also, while soldiers fear that HIV disease will prevent them from being promoted, a review of personnel files on matched controls found that there was no statistically significant difference between seropositive soldiers and their contemporaries (Prier, McNeil, & Burge, 1990). However, these findings must be interpreted cautiously as it is too early to judge the long-term consequences of HIV-related restrictions on career progression.

RETURN TO DUTY

The soldier's unit is a potential source of significant support. HIV-seropositive individuals commonly fear rejection and harassment should others become aware of their diagnosis. Informed, compassionate commanders and supervisors have been of tremendous benefit to the soldiers. Our patients describe good leaders as exhibiting care and concern, yet also conveying their expectations that the soldier will continue to "drive on," performing to the best of his or her ability.

Soldiers who find that they can still function effectively in their occupational roles after diagnosis are reassured. For soldiers from dysfunctional families, being a member of "the army family" is often the closest they come to feeling a sense of belonging and respect. These soldiers are particularly vulnerable to rejection by members of their unit or other elements of the army.

Ward P-8 staff attempt primary prevention of psychiatric morbidity by educating commanders about HIV infection. This process enables commanders to address their own anxieties concerning HIV and its attendant issues. Work is under way to develop a handbook for commanders that will provide practical guidance; it draws heavily on the experiences of commanders who have worked well with HIV soldiers.

Command decisions at higher levels also impact on the daily life of soldiers. Generally, we are unsuccessful in influencing these decisions and therefore focus on helping soldiers adapt. The experience at Fort Hood, Texas, is an example of such a situation. It also illustrates the dilemma commanders must face; namely, that while concern for individual soldiers is very important, the mission comes first.

In April 1988, after receiving authority from higher headquarters, the commanding general of III Corps, Fort Hood, reassigned HIV-positive soldiers en masse to the post's headquarters company, a decision reportedly affecting 65 soldiers. The rationale used to support this move was mission support; soldiers with HIV are nondeployable to overseas assignments and hence were occupying positions that could be filled by soldiers without duty limitations. Soldiers affected by this move complained that it compromised their confidentiality and created the appearance of a "leper colony." Moreover, it meant the loss of their parent units, a potentially traumatic event in itself.

Some HIV-positive soldiers affected by this decision asked the Inspector General to investigate the situation. The *Army Times* (Roth, 1989) quoted from a copy of the Inspector General's report that had not been officially released. They quoted the report as saying that Fort Hood policy was "more restrictive than current army policy allows" (p. 15). The Inspector General reportedly found no evidence of antipathy toward the soldiers and felt that the "policy apparently was prompted by a genuine concern for unit readiness, an issue of primary importance to deployable units" (Roth, 1989, p. 15). The potential conflict between the needs of the HIV-infected soldier and the mission continues to be a focus of concern and research.

SUMMARY

As reflected in this chapter, army efforts to support HIV-positive soldiers have been based heavily on clinical intuition and experience. As our research efforts mature, we hope to be able to present quantitative, as well as qualitative, data about the natural history of HIV infection and its impact on soldiers' coping and adaptation. In the meantime, we continue to assist HIV-positive soldiers to be all they can be within the constraints of HIV infection and army policy.

ACKNOWLEDGMENT.   The authors gratefully acknowledge Charlene Lewis, Wendy Weigert, and Helena Poole for their assistance.

REFERENCES

Auster, S. L. (1985). Confidentiality in military medicine. *Military Medicine, 150*, 341–346.
Cohen, J., & Lazarus, R. S. (1984). The concept of coping. In R. S. Lazarus & S. Folkman (Eds.) *Stress, appraisal, and coping* (pp. 117–140). New York: Springer.

Gunderson, J. G. (1978). Defining the therapeutic processes in psychiatric milieus. *Psychiatry, 41,* 327–335.

Herbold, J. R. (1986). AIDS policy development within the Department of Defense. *Military Medicine, 151,* 623–627.

Holloway, H. C., Dixon, M. S., & Wegner S. A. (1988). The active alcoholic in the medical and surgical inpatient environment. *Physical Medicine and Rehabilitation: State of the Art Review, 2*(2), 121–138.

Howe, E. G. (1988). Ethical aspects of military physicians treating patients with HIV/Part I-III. *Military Medicine, 153,* 7–9, 72–76, 140–142.

Marzuk, P. M., Tierney, H., & Tardiff, M., *et al.* (1988). Increased risk of suicide in persons with AIDS. *Journal of the American Medical Association, 259,* 1333–1337.

McNeil, J. G., Brundage, J. F., Gardner, L. I., *et al.* (1991). Trends of HIV seroconversion among young adults in the US Army. *Journal of the American Medical Association, 265,* 1709–1714.

Pace, J., Brown, G., Rundell, J., *et al.* (1990). Prevalence of Psychiatric Disorders in a Mandatory Screening Program for Infection with Human Immunodeficiency Virus: A Pilot Study. *Military Medicine, 155,* 76–80.

Prier, R. E., McNeil, J. G., & Burge, J. R. (1991). HIV infection: Military occaptional sequelae. *Military Medicine, 156,* 108–113.

Redfield, R. R., Wright, D. C., & Tramont, E. C. (1986). The Walter Reed staging classification for HTLV-III/LAV infection. *The New England Journal of Medicine, 314,* 131–132.

Roth, M. (1989). The Army wrestles with AIDS. *Army Times,* August 28, pp. 14–16.

Rothberg, J. M., Bain, M. W., Boggiano, W., Cline, W. R., Grace, W. C., Holloway, H. C., & Rock, N. L. (1990). Dealing with the stress of an HIV-positive diagnosis at an Army medical center. *Military Medicine, 155,* 1–27.

Stall, R., McKusick, L., Wiley, J., Coates, T. J., & Ostrow, D. G. (1986). Alcohol and drug use during sexual activity and compliance with safe sex guidelines for AIDS: The AIDS Behavioral Research Project. *Health Education Quarterly, 13,* 359–371.

"Underscore urgency of HIV counseling: several suicides follow positive tests," (1987, November). *Clinical Psychiatry News,* p. 1.

13

The Impact of HIV on Minority Populations

IRENE JILLSON-BOOSTROM

This chapter describes the extent to which minority populations in the United States have been affected by the HIV epidemic, and the degree to which services are available for them to cope with the social and psychological burdens of the disease.

RACIAL/ETHNIC DISTRIBUTION OF HIV AND AIDS CASES

More than 171,876 cases of AIDS had been reported in the United States through March 1991 (Centers for Disease Control, 1991), and an estimated 1 to 1.5 million Americans are currently infected with HIV (Centers for Disease Control, 1991). African Americans and Hispanic Americans have been disproportionately affected by HIV, as is demonstrated in both HIV seroprevalence and in the numbers of reported cases of AIDS. For example, 28% of total cumulative U.S. adult cases thus far have been among African Americans and 16% among Hispanics. This compares with their proportional representation in the U.S. population: African Americans comprised 12% and Hispanics 8%, of the total population in the United States in 1988 (Bureau of Census, 1991). The remainder of this chapter presents data concerning seroprevalence, diagnosed cases, and case fatality; discusses prevention and treatment among minority populations; and addresses such issues as access to psychological care and cost of treatment.

IRENE JILLSON-BOOSTROM • Policy Research, Inc., Clarksville, Maryland 21029.

Living and Dying with AIDS, edited by Paul I. Ahmed, Plenum Press, New York, 1992.

HIV Seroprevalence

The Centers for Disease Control (CDC) has estimated that between 1 and 1.5 million Americans are currently infected with the virus (Centers for Disease Control, 1990b). No national HIV seroprevalence studies have been conducted in the United States, but the results of several population studies of seroprevalence suggest significant differences in racial/ethnic distribution of HIV positivity. Between October 1985 and December 1990, nearly 2.5 million military recruits were tested for HIV. The cumulative seroprevalence rate was 0.06% for white recruits, 0.35% for African Americans, and 0.19% for Hispanics (Centers for Disease Control, 1990a).

An indicator for unsafe sex practices (e.g., nonmonogamous sex or anal intercourse without use of condoms), and thus an indicator for HIV seroprevalence, is the prevalence of syphilis. Rates of syphilis have decreased for white males since the onset of AIDS prevention programs but have increased for African American males, according to a number of studies; in some studies the increase has been significant (Landrum, Beck-Sangue, & Kraus, 1988; Mays & Cochran, 1988b). One of these studies, conducted in Georgia, also found differences by income group, with low-income individuals showing an increase in syphilis. National data for increases in primary and secondary syphilis for the years 1986–1987 also show significant increases for African Americans and Hispanics, as compared with whites. For example, the rate per 100,000 persons aged 15–64 increased 36% for African American males (106.2 to 144.9/100,000) and 43% for African American females (55.5 to 79.4/100,000). The CDC reported that for Hispanics, the increases were 22% for males (2.2 to 2.6/100,000) and 24% for females (17.8 to 22.0/100,000). The rate for white males actually decreased in the same time period (6.4 to 5.7/100,000), while it increased for white females, although not as much as for African Americans and Hispanics (7%, from 2.2 to 2.6/100,000) (Centers for Disease Control, 1988b).

In a national study of HIV prevalence among prostitutes in seven geographic areas in the United States, African American and Hispanic prostitutes had higher seroprevalence rates than did whites. Of the 280 African American or Hispanic prostitutes tested, 15.4% were HIV positive, versus 6.7% of the 284 white prostitutes tested. Acknowledged IV drug use may have been a factor in the disparate rates among the racial/ethnic groups, although the African American prostitutes were twice as likely to be HIV positive: 25% of the African American or Hispanic IV drug user prostitutes were HIV positive, versus 10.2% of white prostitutes who acknowledged IV drug use (Cohen & Wofsy, 1987).

HIV-antibody screening data for Job Corps applicants is perhaps the most useful available data to estimate HIV prevalence among economically disadvantaged youth. Applicants, all of whom are economically disadvantaged, are aged 16–21, and are predominantly racial and ethnic minorities; they include both inner-city and rural poor. Between 1987 and 1989, 60,000 Job Corps entrants were screened for HIV. The overall seroprevalence for these disadvantaged youth from 16 to 21 years of age was 0.36%. The rate for African American entrants was five times that of white entrants, and the rate for Hispanic entrants was twice that of white entrants (Centers for Disease Control, 1990b).

In calculating the relative risk of AIDS by race, ethnic group, age, risk behavior, and geographic area, researchers have found that the risk of AIDS in African American and Hispanic men was almost 3 times as great as that in white men. More significantly, they found that African American women and children had 13.2 and 11.6 times the risk of AIDS, respectively, compared to their white counterparts.

The reader is cautioned that epidemiological estimates regarding HIV and AIDS are considered by many to be low and that projections of seroprevalence and cases range considerably. This is true because assumptions underlying these epidemiological estimates and projections are necessarily based on information that is not verifiable (e.g., homosexual/bisexual activity, extent of prostitution and practices of prostitutes, and intravenous drug use). Epidemiological data and information are particularly difficult to obtain for minority and low-income populations, in view of the fact that household surveys and other commonly used forms of data collection underrepresent those populations. This is even more true for minorities who are intravenous drug abusers, a population of increasing concern in the HIV epidemic.

Diagnosed AIDS Cases

More than one-quarter (28%) of the total cumulative U.S. adult cases through March 1991 have been among African Americans and 16% have been among Hispanic Americans. In addition, 52% of all female cases of AIDS were among African American women and 21% were among Hispanic women (Centers for Disease Control, 1991). For cumulative cases from 1981 to 1988, the rate per 100,000 population has been 84/100,000 among African Americans, 73/100,000 among Hispanics, and 26/100,000 among whites. The rates are substantially lower for Asian and Pacific Islanders (14/100,000) and American Indian/Alaskan Natives (6/100,000) (Centers for Disease Control, 1989).

Pediatric and adolescent cases of AIDS are increasing dramatically; for example, the number of newly diagnosed pediatric cases (children under 13 years of age) increased from 50 in 1985 to 605 in 1989, a twelve-fold increase and the number of newly diagnosed cases for youths 13–19 increased from 29 in 1985 to 89 in 1989, a three-fold increase (National Center for Health Statistics, 1991). African American and Hispanic American youth are significantly overrepresented in both pediatric and adolescent cases. Half (52%) of the 2963 pediatric AIDS cases diagnosed as of March 1991 are among African Americans, and 25% are among Hispanics. As of March 1991, there had been 670 diagnosed cases among adolescents 13–19 years of age (38% of whom were African American, 42%, white and 18% Hispanic) (Centers for Disease Control, 1991).

Between 1982 and 1987, there was no significant change in the percentage of reported cases by race or ethnicity. For those years, an average of 60% of cases were white, 26% were African American, and 13% were Hispanic (National Center for Health Statistics, 1988). However, by 1990 there had been a substantial increase in the proportion of minority members diagnosed over those diagnosed in 1985: 31% of the newly reported cases in 1990 were African American, 17% were Hispanic, and 52% were white, versus 26%, 14%, and 60%, respectively, for 1985. (Centers for Disease Control, 1991; National Center for Health Statistics, 1991). Figure 1 shows the difference in distribution of newly diagnosed cases in 1985 and 1990.

Table 1 shows the distribution of reported cases by transmission category, sex, and year (through 1988, with provisional data for both 1989 and 1990) for whites, African Americans, and Hispanics. Although some of the differences are undoubtedly explained by the variation by racial and ethnic group of differential probabilities of sharing needles, becoming ill (with AIDS-related or other illnesses), and using emergency rooms, these findings support others that seem to

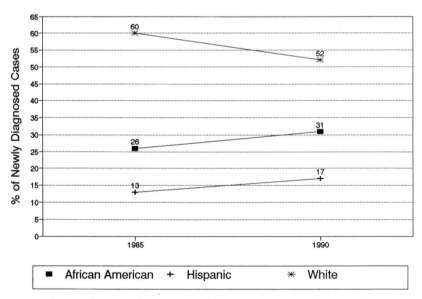

FIGURE 1. Distribution of AIDS cases by race/ethnicity, 1985 and 1990. Compiled by Policy Research Incorporated using data from the National Center for Health Statistics and Centers for Disease Control.

indicate an overrepresentation of African Americans and Hispanics among IV drug abusers. For example, recent National Institute for Drug Abuse (NIDA) data for drug-related deaths show that 30% of these whose deaths were reported from 27 metropolitan areas for 1988 were African American, and 13% were Hispanic. This excludes deaths in which AIDS was reported. Notably, these are the same percentage breakdowns as AIDS cases for 1988. For all drug-related deaths in 1987, the mortality–race ratio was 2.2 for African American and white deaths (National Center for Health Statistics, 1989).

Minorities are overrepresented in the transmission categories related to IV drug use. Of the 32,329 cumulative AIDS cases among IV drug abusers as of December 1989, 44% were African American and 25% were Hispanic. Moreover, 51% of the 2871 adult heterosexual cases involving sexual contact with an IV drug user have been among African Americans and 26% of such cases have been among Hispanics.

Minority males are significantly overrepresented in this transmission category. Of the 24,212 cases attributed to IV drug use with no homosexual/bisexual contact, 50% were African American and 29% Hispanic, compared with 20% white. When IV drug users with homosexual/bisexual contact are added, the differences are reduced somewhat: 44%, 25%, and 30% for African American, Hispanic, and white, respectively.

For minority women, the differences are even more striking; as of the end of 1989, 58% of all AIDS cases among African women are in this transmission category (IV drug use); 52% of all Hispanic female AIDS cases; and 41% of white female AIDS cases. When women who have had sex with an IV drug user (but who are not themselves IV drug users) are added to this category, the differences are more prominent: 76% and 83% of all African American and Hispanic women, respectively, as compared with 55% of white women, have contracted HIV because of IV drug abuse (their own or their sexual partner's). The findings of Peterson and Bakeman (1988) suggest that minority status and IV drug use may interact to create an extremely high risk of exposure to HIV. According to their analysis of CDC data as of April 1987:

- The numbers of cases among African American and Latin IV drug using men were 22.6 and 21.4 times the rate of white male IV drug users.
- The numbers of cases among African American and Latin IV drug using women were 17.9 and 11.2 times the rate of white female IV drug users (Peterson & Bakeman, 1988).

Nearly 20 years ago, Ball and Chambers, among others, found that minorities were overrepresented among IV drug abusers (Ball & Chambers, 1970). Recent data show that this phenomenon has not changed. For example, according to emergency room data reported to NIDA in 1988, 41% of heroin/morphine addiction diagnoses were among African Americans and 13% were among Hispanics

TABLE 1

AIDS Cases, According to Race/Ethnicity, Sex, and Transmission Category for Persons 13 Years and over: United States, 1984–1990[a,b,c]

	Number of cases, by year of report								Percent distribution			
	Cumulative[d,e]	1984	1985	1986	1987	1988	1989[e]	1990[e]	Cumulative[d,e]	1984	1989[e]	1990[e]
Total[f]	145,056	4,386	8,053	12,938	20,793	30,281	33,105	32,649	100.0	100.0	100.0	100.0
Male homosexual/bisexual	88,367	2,863	5,416	8,500	13,552	17,901	19,604	18,748	60.9	65.3	59.2	57.4
Intravenous drug use	29,695	774	1,395	2,240	3,537	6,872	7,186	7,179	20.5	17.6	21.7	22.0
Male homosexual/bisexual and intravenous drug use	9,639	408	587	986	1,533	2,001	2,109	1,747	6.6	9.3	6.4	5.4
Hemophilia/coagulation disorder	1,306	36	74	123	211	294	284	266	0.9	0.8	0.9	0.8
Born in Caribbean/African countries	1,968	112	139	218	267	367	383	348	1.4	2.6	1.2	1.1
Heterosexual contact[g]	5,430	56	139	338	632	1,169	1,464	1,603	3.7	1.3	4.4	4.9
Sex with intravenous drug user	3,790	42	106	237	433	844	1,036	1,069	2.6	1.0	3.1	3.3
Transfusion	3,399	50	166	302	624	825	732	670	2.3	1.1	2.2	2.1
Undetermined[h]	5,252	87	137	231	437	852	1,343	2,088	3.6	2.0	4.1	6.4
White, not Hispanic	83,266	2,680	4,930	7,778	12,880	17,011	18,523	17,834	100.0	100.0	100.0	100.0
Male homosexual/bisexual	63,640	2,156	4,035	6,196	10,023	12,834	13,835	13,262	76.4	80.4	74.7	74.4
Intravenous drug use	6,536	145	251	406	817	1,487	1,703	1,621	7.8	5.4	9.2	9.1
Male homosexual/bisexual and intravenous drug use	5,845	264	375	646	990	1,160	1,261	996	7.0	9.9	6.8	5.6
Hemophilia/coagulation disorder	1,106	26	63	113	183	241	237	226	1.3	1.0	1.3	1.3
Born in Caribbean/African countries	6	1	1	1	1	1	—	2	0.0	0.0	—	0.0
Heterosexual contact[g]	1,645	17	33	96	205	366	444	480	2.0	0.6	2.4	2.7
Sex with intravenous drug user	908	10	19	48	102	207	259	262	1.1	0.4	1.4	1.5
Transfusion	2,480	37	129	233	472	607	541	436	3.0	1.4	2.9	2.4
Undetermined[h]	2,008	34	44	87	189	315	502	811	2.4	1.3	2.7	4.5
Black, not Hispanic	41,362	1,091	1,996	3,286	5,218	8,807	9,978	10,198	100.0	100.0	100.0	100.0
Male homosexual/bisexual	15,024	402	794	1,323	2,116	3,079	3,580	3,441	36.3	36.8	35.9	33.7
Intravenous drug use	16,172	404	751	1,206	1,882	3,711	3,978	3,989	39.1	37.0	39.9	39.1
Male homosexual/bisexual and intravenous drug use	2,712	97	142	238	384	596	630	559	6.6	8.9	6.3	5.5

Exposure category	No.	No.	No.	No.	No.	No.	No.	No.	%	%	%	%
Hemophilia/coagulation disorder	87	5	4	4	11	27	17	19	0.2	0.5	0.2	0.2
Born in Caribbean/African countries	1,941	111	139	216	263	361	376	342	4.7	10.2	3.8	3.4
Heterosexual contact[g]	2,768	22	80	161	317	563	767	846	6.7	2.0	7.7	8.3
Sex with intravenous drug user	2,081	17	64	120	245	442	579	604	5.0	1.6	5.8	5.9
Transfusion	589	10	26	45	93	142	124	147	1.4	0.9	1.2	1.4
Undetermined[h]	2,069	40	60	93	152	328	506	855	5.0	3.7	5.1	8.4
Hispanic	18,944	593	1,066	1,750	2,485	4,165	4,208	4,256	100.0	100.0	100.0	100.0
Male homosexual/bisexual	8,720	289	543	892	1,260	1,781	1,946	1,819	46.0	48.7	46.2	42.7
Intravenous drug use	6,832	224	385	615	828	1,640	1,456	1,532	36.1	37.8	34.6	36.0
Male homosexual/bisexual and intravenous drug use	1,024	46	68	98	147	239	201	177	5.4	7.8	4.8	4.2
Hemophilia/coagulation disorder	86	4	7	5	10	22	20	17	0.5	0.7	0.5	0.4
Born in Caribbean/African countries	11	—	—	—	3	3	2	2	0.1	—	0.0	0.0
Heterosexual contact[g]	965	17	26	78	107	225	231	268	5.1	2.9	5.5	6.3
Sex with intravenous drug user	771	15	23	69	85	186	184	197	4.1	2.5	4.4	4.6
Transfusion	252	2	6	18	41	59	55	69	1.3	0.3	1.3	1.6
Undetermined[h]	1,054	11	31	44	89	196	297	372	5.6	1.9	7.1	8.7
Male	131,390	4,110	7,530	11,967	19,114	27,234	29,728	29,050	100.0	100.0	100.0	100.0
Homosexual/bisexual	88,367	2,863	5,416	8,500	13,552	17,901	19,604	18,748	67.3	69.7	65.9	64.5
Intravenous drug use	22,728	604	1,112	1,759	2,701	5,257	5,441	5,452	17.3	14.7	18.3	18.8
Homosexual/bisexual and intravenous drug use	9,639	408	587	986	1,533	2,001	2,109	1,747	7.3	9.9	7.1	6.0
Hemophilia/coagulation disorder	1,272	34	71	119	206	290	277	257	1.0	0.8	0.9	0.9
Born in Caribbean/African countries	1,436	95	109	162	192	262	251	252	1.1	2.3	0.8	0.9
Heterosexual contact[g]	1,602	10	27	66	158	332	481	526	1.2	0.2	1.6	1.8
Sex with intravenous drug user	1,118	9	25	47	113	233	358	332	0.9	0.2	1.2	1.1
Transfusion	2,099	29	107	197	410	496	452	391	1.6	0.7	1.5	1.3
Undetermined[h]	4,247	67	101	178	362	695	1,113	1,677	3.2	1.6	3.7	5.8

(continued)

TABLE 1
(Continued)

	Number of cases, by year of report								Percent distribution			
	Cumulative[d,e]	1984	1985	1986	1987	1988	1989[e]	1990[e]	Cumulative[d,e]	1984	1989[e]	1990[e]
Female	13,666	276	523	971	1,679	3,047	3,377	3,599	100.0	100.0	100.0	100.0
Intravenous drug use	6,967	170	283	481	836	1,615	1,745	1,727	51.0	61.6	51.7	48.0
Hemophilia/coagulation disorder	34	2	3	4	5	4	7	9	0.2	0.7	0.2	0.3
Born in Caribbean/African countries	532	17	30	56	75	106	132	96	3.9	6.2	3.9	2.7
Heterosexual contact[g]	3,828	46	112	272	474	837	983	1,077	28.0	16.7	29.1	29.9
Sex with intravenous drug user	2,672	33	81	190	320	611	678	737	19.6	12.0	20.1	20.5
Transfusion	1,300	21	59	105	214	329	280	279	9.5	7.6	8.3	7.8
Undetermined[h]	1,005	20	36	53	75	157	230	411	7.4	7.2	6.8	11.4

[a] Data are based on reporting by state health departments.
[b] The AIDS case definition was changed in September 1987 to allow for the presumptive diagnosis of AIDS-associated diseases and conditions and to expand the spectrum of HIV-associated diseases reportable as AIDS. Excludes residents of U.S. territories.
[c] Source: National Center for Health Statistics. (1991). *Health, United States, 1990.* Hyattsville, MD: Public Health Service.
[d] Includes cases prior to 1984.
[e] Data are as of September 30, 1990, and reflect reporting delays.
[f] Includes all other races not shown separately.
[g] Includes persons who have had heterosexual contact with a person with human immunodeficiency virus (HIV) infection or at risk of HIV infection.
[h] Includes persons for whom risk information is incomplete (because of death, refusal to be interviewed, or loss to followup), persons still under investigation, men reported ony to have had heterosexual contact with prostitutes, and interviewed persons for whom no specific risk is identified.

(National Institute on Drug Abuse, 1989). Peterson and Marin (1988) and Mays and Cochran (1988a) have pointed out important differences in attitudes and beliefs, information sources and access, lack of social networks, high-risk sexual behavior, and sharing of IV needles (for illicit drug use as well as for medications and vitamins) among African Americans and Hispanics. These differences have important implications for transmission as well as for prevention programs.

As of October 1989, 415 adolescents had been diagnosed with AIDS (44% of whom were white, 35% African American, and 18% Hispanic). Six Asian Pacific Islander adolescents have been diagnosed, as have four American Indians/ Alaskan Natives.

RACIAL/ETHNIC DIFFERENCES IN MORTALITY RATES

There appears to be no significant racial/ethnic differences in the death rate from HIV infection through 1990. Overall, of the 45,466 cumulative diagnosed cases among African Americans as of the end of 1990, 63% had died; of the 25,649 cumulative cases among Hispanics, 62% had died. Similarly, 63% of the total 88,342 reported white cases had died during the same period (Centers for Disease Control, 1991). Table 2 shows the distribution of deaths by race, sex, and exposure category through December, 1990. However, two other measures indicate differences in mortality: rank of AIDS in causes of death and life expectancy after diagnosis. For African American and Hispanic males, HIV infection was the 6th leading cause of death in 1988; for white males in the same year it was the 10th leading cause of death (National Center for Health Statistics, 1991). The mean survival time after diagnosis for African Americans is eight months, versus 18–24 months for whites (National Center for Health Statistics, 1990b).

A number of reasons have been proposed for these differences in life expectancy after diagnosis; these include:

- The higher percentage of African American and Hispanic cases who are IV drug users, with a generally poorer health status
- Delay in diagnosis among minority and low-income populations (the latter of whom are overrepresented among African Americans and Hispanics)
- Longer mean survival times among those whose initial AIDS-related diagnosis is KS (Friedman *et al.*, 1987) (African Americans and Hispanics are less likely to have a diagnosis of KS than are whites)

AIDS PREVENTION AMONG MINORITY POPULATIONS

Although African American and Hispanic populations are disproportionately at risk for HIV and AIDS, their level of risk is largely dependent upon the

TABLE 2
Number of Deaths from AIDS by Category, United States, 1981–1990[a]

Characteristic	Number	Percent
Total	100,777	100.0
HIV exposure group		
Homosexual/bisexual men	59,586	59.1
Intravenous-drug users		
Women and heterosexual men	21,126	21.0
Homosexual/bisexual men	6,894	6.8
Persons with hemophilia		
Adult/adolescent	945	0.9
Child	74	0.1
Transfusion recipient		
Adult/adolescent	2,793	2.8
Child	150	0.1
Heterosexual contact	3,587	3.6
Persons born in countries where HIV infection occurs primarily through heterosexual contact	1,160	1.2
Perinatal	1,186	1.2
No identified risk	3,276	3.3
Race/ethnicity		
White, non-Hispanic	55,494	55.1
Black, non-Hispanic	28,575	28.4
Hispanic	15,805	15.7
Asian/Pacific Islander	608	0.6
American Indian/Alaskan Native	138	0.1
Unspecified	157	0.2
Age at death (yr)		
<5	1,141	1.1
5–14	308	0.3
15–24	3,266	3.2
25–34	36,418	36.1
35–44	37,634	37.3
45–54	14,256	14.1
≥55	7,405	7.3
Unspecified	349	0.3
Sex		
Male	90,715	90.0
Female	10,056	10.0
Unspecified	6	<0.1

[a] Source: Centers for Disease Control. (1991, January 25). *Morbidity and Mortality Weekly Report, 40*(3).

degree to which individual members of these racial/ethnic groups engage in risk-related behaviors. Thus, an individual's general knowledge about HIV and its transmission and his or her ability to make health-protective decisions are critical in risk reduction. Information is becoming available that points to racial/ethnic group differences in knowledge and attitudes regarding HIV and AIDS.

For example, according to a report of results of the National Health Interview Survey (NHIS) conducted in November 1987, 22% of white adults stated that they knew a lot about AIDS, compared to 14% of African American adults (Dawson & Thornberry, 1988). The proportion of white adults responding to the same survey who indicated that they knew nothing about AIDS was 9%, compared to a startling 26% of African American adult respondents (Dawson & Thornberry, 1988). When the same survey was conducted in mid-1990, only 19% of whites, 17% of African Americans, and 18% of Hispanics reported that they knew a lot about AIDS. This is a startling finding, given the extent of dissemination of information to the general public and the expressed concern for prevention on the part of the public and private sectors. Importantly, 9% of white respondents, 17% of African Americans, and 18% of Hispanics reported that they knew nothing about AIDS (Fitti & Cynamon, 1990).

Importantly, in terms of prevention, African American and Hispanic adult respondents to the 1990 survey were consistently less knowledgeable about prevention methods in terms of sexual transmission than white adults. For example, when asked about the effectiveness of condoms in preventing AIDS, only 2% of white adults responded "Don't know method" compared to 4% of African American and 6% of Hispanic respondents. These results have implications for family planning as well as for prevention of transmission of HIV and other sexually transmitted diseases. In contrast, all groups were about equally likely to have received no AIDS information in the past month (10% of white and African American respondents and 12% of Hispanic respondents). White respondents were far more likely to have received information about AIDS in the previous month from a newspaper than were African American or Hispanic respondents (59% versus 47% and 42%, respectively). In contrast, African Americans were more likely to have read a health department brochure (26% versus 17% of white and 18% of Hispanic respondents).

In a study of AIDS knowledge and attitudes among 628 adolescents in San Francisco high schools, DiClemente *et al.* found substantial differences based on racial/ethnic group. While nearly 72% of white youth reported that they were aware that using condoms would decrease the risk of transmission of HIV, only 60% of African American youth and 58% of Hispanic youth were so aware (DiClemente, Boyer, & Morales, 1988). The previously referenced report of syphilis rates in Atlanta is also indicative of racial/ethnic differences in effectiveness of AIDS prevention campaigns, in view of the fact that the Atlanta area had been the target of broad-based AIDS prevention programs. In another recent study of AIDS knowledge among 250 adolescent girls (81% of whom were African Americans residing in urban areas), while 90% knew that unprotected sexual intercourse placed them at risk for AIDS, only 38% of them had used a condom when they had most recently had sex, and 72% did not know that use of a spermicide can reduce the risk of HIV infection (Fishein, 1988).

Some public health officials are seeing IV drug abusers, prostitutes, and the sexual partners of both of these populations as the groups of increasing concern in terms of relative risk. This is true in part because, from the beginning of the epidemic, many of the known successful prevention programs have been initiated by community-based gay organizations that, for the most part, have been sought out by white males. Although prevention activities directed at both the general public and at other target populations (including racial/ethnic minorities and IV drug abusers) have increased substantially since 1988, there is as yet little evidence of success with these prevention programs. In fact, there is some evidence that AIDS prevention programs have been relatively unsuccessful in minority, low-income communities (Fullilove, 1988; Communication Technologies, 1990).

While there were calls early on in the epidemic for targeted prevention programs, these needs have only recently been addressed. At the community level, most grassroots programs were developed by the gay community in the early 1980s. In 1987, however, prevention activities began to expand into minority communities, including among local and national organizations (e.g., the Southern Christian Leadership Conference, Black Coalition on AIDS, and local churches) (Friedman et al., 1987). At the federal level, the CDC, the National Institute on Drug Abuse, the Office of Minority Health, the Health Resources and Services Administration, and other agencies have begun to fund research and demonstration projects directed toward minority populations.

Resource allocations do not reflect the relative seriousness of the problem in minority groups. For example, while CDC expenditures for HIV prevention have expanded considerably from $136 million in fiscal year 1987 to an estimated $400 million for fiscal year 1989 (Centers for Disease Control, 1988a), less than 10% of those funds were targeted to the minority population. In fact, of the $3.1 billion estimated by the Presidential Commission on the Human Immunodeficiency Virus Epidemic as needed to carry out its recommendations, less than 10% ($300 million) was allocated to prevention (Watkins, 1988).

AIDS TREATMENT AMONG MINORITY POPULATIONS

An important factor in the way in which persons with AIDS can cope with the disease is the degree to which treatment services are available, and the economic impact of such services.

Most AIDS patients in the United States are treated in hospitals. Treatment is provided for the illnesses (or infections) that the patient has contracted as a result of AIDS (for the pneumonia, or Kaposi's sarcoma), and where available, AZT is provided in an attempt to slow the progression of the disease. Some large urban hospitals also have hospices and home health care arrangements; group homes operated by private voluntary groups (primarily gay organizations) are also available in some urban areas.

Estimates of the cost of AIDS treatment vary considerably, depending on the assumptions made about life expectancy, utilization of hospital-based versus home health or voluntary care, and geographic location. The average estimated lifetime cost (i.e., an average per month of postdiagnosis remaining lifetime) for treating an AIDS patient following diagnosis in this country ranges from approximately $7000 per month for inpatient care alone in San Francisco (Scitovsky, Cline, & Lee, 1986), to $7000 per month for both inpatient and outpatient care in Boston (Seage *et al.,* 1986). The average lifetime costs of treating AIDS (i.e., from diagnosis to death) ranges from $40,000 to $75,000 according to recent published estimates (Green & Arno, 1990).

The Presidential Commission on HIV reported that the average cost of home health care for HIV infection is $15,000 per year, and the average cost of nursing home care is $24,000 to $60,000 (Watkins, 1988). A study of home-based hospice care in San Francisco showed monthly costs of $2820. However, the Presidential Commission also noted that few nursing homes in the United States accept "patients with advanced HIV illness" (Watkins, 1988, p. 18).

Given the high cost of AIDS treatment in the United States, to what degree is the economic impact differentially felt among minority and low-income populations? Nationally, the percentage of persons under 65 years of age who are covered by private health insurance decreased since 1980 from 78.8% to 75.9% in 1986 (National Center for Health Statistics, 1990a). African Americans (who are at much higher risk for AIDS) are much less likely to have private health insurance; for example, 57% of African Americans were covered in 1986 versus 79.1% of whites. Similarly, only 31.3% of those earning less than $10,000 had private health care coverage, and only 58.1% of those earning between $10,000 and $14,999 were so covered (as compared with 88.3% of those earning between $20,000 and $34,999) (National Center for Health Statistics, 1990a). Importantly, 22.6% of African Americans, and 37% of those earning less than $10,000 were not covered by any type of health insurance (National Center for Health Statistics, 1990a).

Krieger has noted that, while the overall cost of AIDS remains low in comparison to the major causes of morbidity and mortality (e.g., accidents, violence, cancer, and cardiovascular disease), the fiscal impact of AIDS is hardest on those geographic areas most severely hit by the disease, which are also areas in which large percentages of the population are minorities and low income (Krieger,

1988). For example, in New York City, AIDS was the leading cause of death among men 30 to 49 and women 20 to 39 in 1989 (Smith et al., 1991). Between April 1990 and March 1991, there were 6674 newly reported cases of AIDS (Centers for Disease Control, 1991). In terms of health-services utilization, the NYC Department of Health has estimated that there were 70,000 New York City residents with ARC in 1986 (Weinberg & Murray, 1987). Most of the patients in New York City are low-income minorities, and the financial burden of their care falls heavily on the public health system and on voluntary groups in New York. In 1985, for example, 20% of New York City's AIDS patients were not covered by any type of health insurance (Krieger, 1988).

It is important to note that the concept of "low income" has to be reconsidered when discussing AIDS. According to the Presidential Commission on HIV:

> Overall, the provision of health care services to African Americans and Hispanics has been hampered by the large number of uninsured persons, i.e., persons with neither public nor private health insurance, including significant numbers who are employed (Watkins, 1988, p. 15).

The socioeconomic impact of the disease has, in fact, created a new, large group of medically indigent individuals, including:

- Those who were covered by private health insurance through their employers and who have been terminated from employment because of their disease
- Those who remain covered by private health insurance companies, but who must pay out-of-pocket for diagnostic tests and treatment procedures determined to be related to experimental treatment and thus not covered through the medical insurance
- Those not previously privately insured (e.g., self-employed individuals) who have had to "spend down" to become eligible for Medicaid

Examining the percent distribution of AIDS deaths by family income in 1986 (the latest available data) indicates that 43% had incomes less than $11,000 (Kapantais & Powell-Griner, 1989). In 1986, this would have been below the poverty line. When the percent distribution of AIDS deaths was examined by assets at death, the largest group, 38%, had no assets at death, and 28% had assets below $5000. Only 23% had assets of $25,000 or more (Kapantais & Powell-Griner, 1989).

Further, while all states' Medicaid agencies provide coverage to eligible individuals and their families, the covered services and eligibility criteria vary considerably by state. The Presidential Commission noted that "the great variability in Medicaid coverage by states creates totally different service pictures in states such as Texas, Florida, Mississippi, and Alabama as compared to New York or California" (Watkins, 1988, p. 15).

Medicare, the only other major public program subsidizing disability medical services, has not yet been a factor in AIDS-treatment financing. Although AIDS is considered a disability, the two-year waiting period for medical coverage under Medicare, and the 18-month average life expectancy of AIDS patients, results in *de facto* restrictions on coverage through that federal program. As of May 1991, there were no plans to waive the two-year waiting period for Medicare coverage (Health Care Financing Administration, 1991). Another gap in the financing of health care arises from restrictions on coverage of nontraditional therapies. Even in cases in which "modern medicine" has a cure for an illness, increasingly in the past 20 years or so, Americans have turned to alternative forms of care for a variety of health problems. With AIDS, for which there is no known cure, the seeking of alternative therapies, particularly among those who are educated, middle class patients aware of such alternatives, is relatively common. Such treatments have included, for example, acupuncture, biofeedback, and homeopathy (Moffatt, Spiegel, Parrish, & Helquist, 1987). Few health insurance programs cover these treatment alternatives.

Coverage through private-sector insurance is variable, and many companies have attempted to limit their risk by screening out applicants who may be "at risk," limiting coverage for preexisting conditions that may be related to HIV/AIDS, and limiting coverage for treatment related to "experimental therapies" (which necessarily includes most AIDS treatment procedures). In an effort to ensure that private insurance companies maintain equitable coverage related to HIV/AIDS, most states have developed and implemented some form of policy designed to protect the benefits of HIV/AIDS patients. However, at least two states (Alabama and Wyoming) have no such policies (Pascal, Cvitanic, Bennett, Gorman, & Serrato, 1989).

ACCESS TO PSYCHOLOGICAL COUNSELING

A still largely neglected area has been psychological counseling for those who are at risk for AIDS (e.g., homosexual or bisexual males and IV drug users), those who are HIV positive, and those who have the disease. Although the National Institute of Mental Health began to fund research into psychological needs and appropriate treatment of these groups in 1986, there is still relatively little psychological support available for the AIDS patient, and most of the research has focused on homosexual or bisexual males. There are few psychological counseling programs directed toward minorities. The problems that have made psychological counseling for minorities difficult under any circumstances (e.g., cultural appropriateness of diagnostic and treatment regimes, use and interpretation of language) pertain with regard to counseling to those who are HIV positive, and are compounded by the issues of sexuality (including homosexuality/bisexuality and having a sexual partner who is homosexual/bisexual) and/or illicit drug use. However, the psychological needs of minority and low-income individuals at risk and those with AIDS or ARC should not be underestimated. According to one researcher:

> The diagnosis of AIDS can precipitate a psychosocial crisis. Concerns about loss of career, social isolation and stigmatization, loss of independence and autonomy because of physical symptoms, about future uncontrolled pain, and fears of death and dying are frequent sources of distress (Wolcott, 1986, pp. 95, 96).

In addition, the loss of physical and sexual contact and the not infrequent abandonment by friends and loved ones places extraordinary stress on the person infected with HIV, at any stage of infection, including those who are asymptomatic and those with confirmed cases of AIDS. Those who currently engage (or in the past engaged) in high-risk behaviors (such as gay or bisexual men or IV drug users) can be under stress, even though they have not yet been tested; for them, the decision to test is itself stressful, particularly given the fact that no *cure* yet exists (although AZT does seem to prolong life in most recipients of the drug).

Not surprisingly, although statistics are difficult to obtain, "clinical experience indicates that suicidal crises are relatively common in newly diagnosed AIDS patients" (Wolcott, 1986, p. 97). According to a study done in 1988, using data from 1985, the rate of suicide for men aged 20–59 years diagnosed with AIDS was 680 deaths for 100,000 person years of life with AIDS. This represents a relative risk for that population 36 times that of men in this age group in the general population. The rate for males and females older than 10 years diagnosed with AIDS was 614 deaths per 100,000 person years of life with AIDS, which yields a relative risk 66 times that of the general population (Marzuk *et al.,* 1988).

In his 1986 article, Wolcott presented a list of psychosocial concepts important to the care of AIDS patients; that list follows:

- Past psychosocial history. Interpersonal relationships, education, and career, psychologic symptoms, nonprescribed drug and alcohol use, psychiatric care, community organizations
- Stress/distress and crisis. Level of anxiety, fear, and behavioral disorganization, specific losses and threats the patient is experiencing, duration, intensity, and precipitants of the crisis
- Coping. Previous patterns of understanding problems and methods of problem resolution; what approaches have been successful in the past; what approaches are currently being tried
- Social support. Sources of support: family, lover, friends, other social network, size and number of trusted friends, social identity (both cultural

and subcultural), types of support needs and satisfaction, e.g., practical assistance, social interaction, emotional support

- Life-cycle phase. Goals, resources, skills related to age and social roles
- Psychosocial illness phase. Existential plight, accomodation and mitigation, recurrence and relapse, deterioration and decline.
- Individual identity, uniqueness, and future orientation. Sources of self-esteem, valued achievements, future goals, and their relationship to the personal meaning of the illness
- Loss and grief. What losses the individual has experienced or anticipates as a result of the illness, the person's previous experiences with loss and grief, and current grief.

Psychological counseling for loved ones, family members and friends is extraordinarily important in this disease. This is true because there is so much that is not known, because it raises issues that are very difficult for us to confront as individuals, and because, in the case of homosexual and bisexual men, family and friends may have been estranged from the patient, or may have been unaware of his sexual preference. The onset of AIDS is a sudden, horrific way for the family to learn of this preference, for both the patient and his family. Women who are HIV positive or who have AIDS as a result of sexual contact with men who are IV drug users or bisexual may have particular anger toward the individual through whom they contracted the virus, in particular when they have not been aware of their sexual partner's risk behavior. Men, women, and children who have contracted the disease through blood transfusions may have anger toward the health care system from which they received the blood transfusion, and even toward the risk groups from which the contaminated blood was received.

Unfortunately, in spite of the obvious and extensive need for counseling services for these populations, such services are not widely available. In the report of the President's Commission, scant attention was paid to coping services. For example, in the section on expanding the provider base, no mention was made of the need for counseling services. In the section on "Therapists' Role in Prevention," no mention is made of the need for coping services linked with counseling related to prevention. In a special issue on AIDS, the journal of the American Psychological Association focuses on prevention and on psychoimmunology (American Psychologist, 1988).

Since 1986, the National Institute of Mental Health has funded a total of 21 contracts (primarily to universities) to develop and implement training programs for those involved with the HIV epidemic. These contracts have included training with regard to psychological support for both patients and health care providers. While the projects have produced training materials and other documents, they are not widely disseminated, and no published evaluation report is available that could be used by community-based and other organizations to determine which strategies for coping services are most effective, in particular with minority and low-income populations that are increasingly the victims of the epidemic.

TOWARD A HUMANE CARE SYSTEM FOR MINORITY POPULATIONS

HIV infection is a disease for which there is no known cure and only very limited (and expensive) experimental treatment (such as azidothymidine, or AZT). There is no vaccine to prevent contracting the virus or developing the illness, and experts now predict that one is not likely to be available for non-experimental use for 10 years or more. Because of its disproportionate impact on the minority and low-income populations in the U.S., prevention of HIV infection among those populations, as well as the provision of coping services, must continue to be a high priority in the public and private sectors.

REFERENCES

American Psychologist. (1988, November). Special Issue: Psychology and AIDS, *American Psychologist, 43*(11).

Ball, J. C., & Chambers, C. D. (1970). *The epidemiology of opiate addiction in the United States.* Springfield, IL: Charles C. Thomas.

Centers for Disease Control. (1988a, August). Preventing HIV infection and AIDS in racial and ethnic minorities. Presented at: National Conference on the Prevention of HIV Infection and AIDS among Racial and Ethnic Minorities in the United States, Washington, DC.

Centers for Disease Control. (1988b, August). Syphilis and congenital syphilis—United States, 1985–1988. *Morbidity and Mortality Weekly Report, 37*(32), 486–490.

Centers for Disease Control. (1989, May 12). AIDS and human immunodeficiency virus infection in the United States: 1988 update. *Morbidity and Mortality Weekly Report, 38*(Suppl. S-4), 1–38.

Centers for Disease Control. (1990a). National HIV seroprevalence surveys: Summary of results. HIV/CID/9-90/006.

Centers for Disease Control. (1990b, November 30). HIV prevalence estimates and AIDS case projections for the U.S.: Report based upon a workshop. *Morbidity and Mortality Weekly Report, 39*(RR-16), 1.

Centers for Disease Control. (1991, April). HIV/AIDS Surveillance. U.S. AIDS cases reported through March 1991.

Cohen, J., & Wofsy, C. (1987, March 27). *Antibody to human immunodeficiency virus in female prostitutes.* Atlanta, GA: Centers for Disease Control, U.S. Public Health Service, Department of Health and Human Services.

Communication Technologies. (1990). HIV-related knowledge, attitudes, and behaviors among San Francisco gay and bisexual men: Results from the fifth population-based survey. San Francisco: Communication Technologies.

Dawson, D. A. (1989, August). *AIDS knowledge and attitudes for January–March, 1989* (National Center for Health Statistics, Advance Data from Vital Health Statistics, No. 176. DHHS Pub. No. PHS 89-1250). Hyattsville, MD: U.S. Government Printing Office.

Dawson, D. A., & Thornberry, O. T. (1988, March). *AIDS knowledge and attitudes for November, 1987* (National Center for Health Statistics, Advance Data from Vital Health Statistics, No. 151. DHHS Pub. No. PHS 88-1250). Hyattsville, MD: U.S. Government Printing Office.

DiClemente, R. J., Boyer, C. B., & Morales, E. (1988, January). Minorities and AIDS: Knowledge, attitudes and misconceptions among Black and Latino adolescents. *American Journal of Public Health, 78*(1), 55–57.

Fishein, J. (1988, December). Teenage girls know about AIDS, but don't act accordingly. In: *The Nation's Health*. Washington, DC: American Public Health Association.

Fitti, J. E. & Cynamon, J. (1990, December). *AIDS knowledge and attitudes for April–June 1990* (National Center for Health Statistics, Advance Data from Vital and Health Statistics, No. 195, December 18, 1990, Table I). Hyattsville, MD: U.S. Government Printing Office.

Friedman, S. R., Sotheran, J. L., Abdul-Quader, A., Primm, B. J., Des Jarlais, D. C., Kleinman, P., Mauge, C., Goldsmith, D. S., El-Sadr, W., & Maslansky, R. (1987). The AIDS epidemic among Blacks and Hispanics. *The Milbank Quarterly, 65*(Suppl. 2), 455–499.

Fullilove, R. E. (1988, Winter). Minorities and AIDS: A review of recent publications. *Multicultural Inquiry and Research AIDS, 2*(1), 3–5.

Green, J., & Arno, P. (1990, September). The medicaidization of AIDS. Trends in the financing of HIV-related medical care. *Journal of the American Medical Association, 264*(10), 1261.

Health Care Financing Administration. (1991, May). Personal communication.

Kapantais, G., & Powell-Griner, E. (1989). *Characteristics of persons dying from AIDS: Preliminary data from the 1986 National Mortality Followback Survey* (National Center for Health Statistics, Advance Data from Vital and Health Statistics, No. 173. DHHS Pub. No. PHS 89-1250). Hyattsville, MD: U.S. Government Printing Office.

Krieger, N. (1988). AIDS funding: Competing needs and the politics of priorities. *International Journal of Health Services, 18*(4), 521–541.

Landrum, S., Beck-Sangue, C., & Kraus, S. (1988). Racial trends in syphilis among men with same-sex partners in Atlanta, Georgia. *American Journal of Public Health, 78,* 66–67.

Marzuk, P. M., Tierney, H., Tardiff, K., Gross, E. M., Morgan, E. B., Hsu, M., & Mann, J. J. (1988, March). Increased risk of suicide in persons with AIDS. *Journal of the American Medical Association, 259*(9), 1333–1337.

Mays, V., & Cochran, S. D. (1988a, November). Issues in the perception of AIDS risk and risk reduction activities by Black and Hispanic women. *American Psychologist, 43*(11), 949–957.

Mays, V., & Cochran, S. D. (1988b, December). Black gay and bisexual men coping with more than just a disease. *Focus: A Guide to AIDS Research, 4*(1), 1–3.

Moffatt, B. C., Spiegel, J., Parish, S., & Helquist, M. (1987). *AIDS: A self-care manual.* Santa Monica, CA: IBS Press.

National Center for Health Statistics. (1988). *Health United States, 1987* (DHHS Pub. No. PHS 88-1232). Hyattsville, MD: U.S. Government Printing Office.

National Center for Health Statistics. (1989). Advance Report of Final Mortality Statistics, 1987. *Monthly Vital Statistics Report, 38*(5 Supplement) (DHHS Pub. No. PHS 89-120). Hyattsville, MD: U.S. Government Printing Office.

National Center for Health Statistics. (1990a). *Health United States, 1989* (DHHS Pub. No. PHS 90-1232). Hyattsville, MD: U.S. Government Printing Office.

National Center for Health Statistics. (1990b). Advance Report of Final Mortality Statistics, 1988. *Monthly Vital Statistics, 39*(7 Supplement) (DHHS Pub. No. PHS 91-1120). Hyattsville, MD: U.S. Government Printing Office.

National Center for Health Statistics. (1991). *Health United States, 1990.* (DHHS Pub. No. PHS 91-1232). Hyattsville, MD: U.S. Government Printing Office.

National Institute on Drug Abuse. (1989). *Data from the Drug Abuse Warning Network (DAWN)* (Series 1, No. 7). Washington, DC: DHHS Public Health Service Alcohol, Drug Abuse and Mental Health Administration.

Pascal, A., Cvitanic, M., Bennett, C., Gorman, M., & Serrato, C. A. (1989, Fall). State policies and the financing of acquired immunodeficiency syndrome care. *Health Care Financing Review, 11*(1), 91–104.

Peterson, J., & Bakeman, R. (1988, Winter). The epidemiology of adult minority AIDS. MIRA newsletter, *Multicultural Inquiry and Research on AIDS, 2*(1), 1–2.

Peterson, J. L., & Marin, G. (1988, Nov). Issues in the prevention of AIDS among Black and Hispanic men. *American Psychologist, 43*(11), 871–877.

Scitovsky, A., Cline, M., & Lee, P. (1986, December 12). Medical care costs of patients with AIDS in San Francisco. *Journal of the American Medical Association, 256*(22), 3101–3106.

Seage, G. R., Landers, S., Barry, M. A., Groopman, J., Lamb, G. A., & Epstein, A. M. (1986, December). Medical care cost of AIDS in Massachusetts. *Journal of the American Medical Association, 256*(22), 3107–3109.

Smith, P. F., Mikl, J., Hyde, S., & Morse, D. L. (1991, May). The AIDS epidemic in New York State. *American Journal of Public Health, 81*(Supplement), 54–60.

Watkins, J. D. (1988). *Report of the Presidential Commission on the Human Immunodeficiency Virus Epidemic.* Washington, DC: U.S. Government Printing Office.

Weinberg, D. S., & Murray, H. W. (1987, December). Coping with AIDS: The special problems of New York City. *New England Journal of Medicine, 317*(23), 1469–1472.

Wolcott, D. L. (1986, August). Psychosocial aspects of acquired immune deficiency syndrome and the primary care physician. *Annals of Allergy, 57,* 95–96.

14

Coping with AIDS in Hemophilia

BRIAN M. WICKLUND and MARY ANNE JACKSON

INTRODUCTION

Hemophilia is a lifelong, chronic disease caused by a deficiency of a clotting factor in the blood. The bleeding episodes caused by that deficiency, especially hemorrhages into the joints, have been the source of pain, suffering, and death to the people who inherited it, from ancient times until just the last half of this century.

Background of Hemophilia Treatment

Initial attempts to treat the bleeding in hemophiliacs depended on the use of human plasma infusions, and were usually unsuccessful because a large volume of plasma had to be infused to control even a minor bleeding episode. Development of cryoprecipitation, to concentrate the missing clotting factor in a smaller volume, allowed the first practical replacement infusions to treat episodes of bleeding (Hershgold, Pool, & Pappenhagen, 1966). However, the need to store cryoprecipitate in blood bank freezers forced patients to come to a hospital for treatment. In the mid- to late 1960s, the techniques were developed to further extract the missing clotting factors from pooled human plasma. Each lot of clotting factor concentrate is made from the pooled plasma donations of several thousand donors. Lyophilization (drying) of the clotting factor concentrates reduced the handling and storage difficulties by putting the factor in a powdered form that could be stored without freezing. It reconstituted to a significantly smaller volume of material than cryoprecipitate to treat a bleeding episode

---

BRIAN M. WICKLUND and MARY ANNE JACKSON • University of Missouri, Kansas City, Children's Mercy Hospital, Kansas City, Missouri 64108.

Living and Dying with AIDS, edited by Paul I. Ahmed, Plenum Press, New York, 1992.

(Johnson, Newman, Howell, & Puszkin, 1967). Factor concentrates allowed the next major improvement in the treatment of hemophilia, the development of home factor infusion programs.

Beginning of an Improved Lifestyle

Self-infusion with lyophilized factor concentrate permitted the hemophiliac to treat his bleeding episodes when they happened, without going to a hospital or medical facility. Comprehensive care programs started in the 1970s, and provided a yearly assessment of the patient by a full team of medical specialists to provide coordinated care for all of the hemophiliac's problems (Levine & Britten, 1973). With these systems in place, hemophiliacs began to have the chance for a more normal, productive life.

Advantages of Home Infusion

One study looked at the experience of patients at a comprehensive center during the first 5 years of a home infusion program. It showed an increase in life expectancy, an increase in the number of men in professional and semi-professional jobs, a significant reduction in the use of pain medications for hemophilic joint disease, an increase in the number of 18- to 35-year-olds who were in school full time, and a decrease in the number of adult patients on unemployment. The authors also noted that the hemophiliac population was beginning to look more like the general population with respect to the age at marriage, time in school, and job performance (Hernandez, Gray, & Lineberger, 1989). Studies from the National Hemophilia Foundation report a 74% reduction in unemployment, a 73% reduction in days lost from school, an 83% reduction in hospitalization, and a 74% reduction in the costs of medical care since the introduction of home therapy (National Hemophilia Foundation, 1988).

Complications: Hepatitis and AIDS

The success of the hemophilia treatment programs also brought with it major problems with infections due to viruses transmitted in the clotting factor concentrates and cryoprecipitate.

Hepatitis. Hepatitis B and C infection has been a frequent complication in patients treated with commercial factor concentrates (Gerety & Barker, 1976; Seeff & Hoofnagle, 1976). Although the majority of patients are asymptomatic, cases of chronic active hepatitis and cirrhosis have been documented (Kasper & Kipres, 1972). Liver disease was the second leading cause of death in hemophiliacs, after bleeding, in the pre-AIDS era (Aledort, 1989).

AIDS. Among the first evidence that AIDS was transmitted by blood products was the report of three patients with hemophilia A who developed *Pneumocystis carinii* pneumonia (Centers for Disease Control, 1982). Since then, seroprevalence studies have shown that between 33% and 92% of hemophilia A (factor VIII deficient) patients and 14% to 52% of hemophilia B (factor IX deficient) patients have been infected by the HIV virus (Gjerset *et al.*, 1985; Goedert *et al.*, 1985; Jason *et al.*, 1986; Kreiss *et al.*, 1986; Stehr-Green, Holman, Jason, & Evatt, 1988; Waskin, Smith, Simon, Gribble, & Mertz, 1986).

AIDS IN HEMOPHILIA

Overall Impact on the Hemophilia Community

As of January 1, 1991, 1617 cases of AIDS in hemophiliacs and patients with related bleeding disorders had been reported to the Centers for Disease Control. This represents 1% of all adult AIDS cases in the United States (Centers for Disease Control, 1991). Since there are estimated to be only 20,000 hemophiliacs in the United States, this means that almost 1 out of every 12 hemophiliacs has already been diagnosed with AIDS. The experience of other nations has been just as bad, as the French report that out of 3500 hemophiliacs, 1500 have antibodies against HIV, 200 have developed AIDS, and 80 have died (Coles, 1989).

At our center in Kansas City, we follow 105 patients with hemophilia, of whom 65 have agreed to testing for HIV infection. Of the individuals tested, 45 (69%) were seropositive. Of that group, 14 (31% of all HIV seropositives) have died, 12 with the diagnosis of AIDS. There are 4 patients who have AIDS and are still alive, and 27 (60% of the HIV positives) who are still asymptomatic. This means that at our center, 1 out of every 7 patients has or has died of AIDS. The distribution of patients at our center is skewed toward the moderate and severe hemophiliacs who are more likely to require the transfusion of blood products, and we have relatively few mild patients who rarely or never require an infusion.

Impact on the Hemophiliac: The Individual and the Family

"Victim"

Many hemophiliacs view themselves as the "innocent victims" of AIDS, and identification or confusion with other high-risk groups such as homosexuals, prostitutes, and IV drug abusers causes extreme anger and emotional distress (Ross, 1989). They and their families report a period of very strong anger after their HIV infection is diagnosed. The anger is often directed at the "unknown" people who donated the contaminated plasma.

Rejection and Isolation

Fears of rejection and ostracism are shared by hemophiliacs with all other HIV-positive individuals. Yet hemophilia is the only situation where the individual must declare himself to authorities as a member of a high-risk group for the protection of his own health. The best example is the informing of school administrators about a child's hemophilia when he is enrolled, to insure that provision is made for treatment of bleeding episodes while at school. Others at the same school may be members of risk groups for HIV infection due to blood transfusions or drug abuse, but nothing will immediately identify them to the authorities. The potential this provides for selection and punitive action is frightening, and it is something that the individual and family is powerless to do anything about.

Social Isolation

Hemophilia is a relatively rare disease. One male in every 7500 has hemophilia, thus it is estimated that there are 20,000 affected individuals in the United States (National Hemophilia Foundation, 1988). Beyond the immediate family, there is often little chance of finding others with the same problems to talk to. Outside major cities, provision of adequate care is difficult, and establishment of support groups for hemophiliacs and their families involves overcoming geographic isolation. Some families travel as much as 60 to 100 miles to attend meetings at our center. For patients and families trying to deal with HIV infection, self-help and support groups organized through local hemophilia centers or National Hemophilia Foundation chapters have been instrumental in working through the anxieties, guilt, and grief caused by what has happened within their families.

Stigma and Discrimination

Two of the most notable examples in the popular media of discrimination against people with AIDS come from within the hemophilia community. The television movie "The Ryan White Story" dramatized the experience of a boy with hemophilia and AIDS who was expelled from school and whose family had to sue to have him reinstated. The story of the three Ray brothers, all HIV-positive hemophiliacs, received extensive national media attention. They had also been removed from school, and when their parents pursued legal action to have them reinstated, the family's house was burned by an arsonist. Discrimination against the hemophiliac extends to the entire family, including the non-affected family members. Although the association between hemophilia and AIDS may not be as closely linked in the public's perception as the hemophilia community might think (Ross, 1989), issues of discrimination continue to be reported by almost every affected individual.

Distrust of the Medical Profession

Because the hemophiliac contracted HIV infection through infusion of a physician-prescribed product that was necessary for treatment of their bleeding, anger and distrust of the medical community must often be dealt with. Despite the development of more-purified factor concentrates that are free of HIV (Lusher, 1989), hemophiliacs experience a continued fear of using any blood product. Adolescent hemophiliacs reported that 42% did not believe that heat-treated factor was free of virus, and 27% were self-restricting their use of factor concentrate for known or suspected bleeding (Overby, Lo, & Litt, 1989). In a survey of all age ranges of hemophiliacs, 33% postponed treating bleeds and 36% used less factor in an attempt to lessen the probability of HIV exposure (Wilson & Wasserman, 1989).

The new methods of purification have not only increased the purity and safety of the factor concentrates, they have also increased the cost of a unit of factor concentrate and reduced the number of units that can be recovered from a given amount of donor plasma. Shortages of factor concentrate from 1987 to 1989 resulted in the delay of elective surgery, reduction in treatment of some bleeding episodes, and significant restrictions of home care supplies by up to 25% (Aledort, 1989). This has been a great problem for younger hemophiliacs, where the goal of previous treatment programs was to allow as normal a lifestyle as possible.

Financial Impact

A significant financial impact of HIV was felt by all hemophiliacs in the cost of factor concentrate. As mentioned above, both the supply of factor dropped after 1987, and the price increased. The cheapest factor concentrate in 1987 cost $0.06 to $0.07 per unit of factor VIII activity. Factor concentrates that had been heat-treated to inactivate viruses cost from $0.09 to $0.13 per unit of factor VIII activity. One year later, the much purer monoclonally purified factor concentrates that have had either heat treatment or a solvent-detergent treatment to inactivate viruses cost between $0.43 and $0.65 per unit of factor VIII activity (National Hemophilia Foundation, 1988). This represents between a 617% to 829% increase in the cost of factor within 2 years. Since the average severe adult hemophiliac uses between 80,000–100,000 units of factor per year (Aledort, 1989), the bill for just the factor cost for a year increased from $5,000–10,000 per year to as high as $70,000–100,000 per year (Augustyniak, personal communication, December, 1989).

Insurance. Many families get assistance from some state programs in meeting the costs of factor concentrate, but most of the burden falls on the insurance coverage the person or family has, or on Medicaid or Social Security benefits. Insurance companies are moving to reduce their losses in this area, as hemophiliacs are excluded from group coverage. The father of one family at our center has worked for the same small company for many years, and his son's hemophilia costs were covered through their group health insurance. When health care providers for the company changed, no other insurer would provide group coverage the small company could afford that included the son with hemophilia. Reliance on state programs is necessary but often unsatisfactory for these families. State officials also have reason to be wary about costs, as the increases in the cost of factor concentrate could bankrupt an entire state's funding for the handicapped (Aledort, 1989).

Insurance is a great concern for the adolescent who is about to leave the parent's insurance coverage and go out to work on his own. Many hemophiliacs, both HIV negative and positive, are finding great difficulty in obtaining insurance coverage of any type, and are again being forced back on public programs. Others are finding a secondary insurance program necessary to cover waiting periods in employers policies. Finally, lifetime major medical caps are in place in most policies, limiting the lifetime benefits to one million dollars, or about $43,000 per year (Aledort, 1989; Tetrick, 1989). Between the costs of factor, routine medical care, and the costs of HIV therapy such as AZT, these benefits are often being exhausted by early adulthood.

Jobs. Concerns about the ability to hold a job and the stress associated with it are significant. There can be outright discrimination in the workplace, with refusal to hire or termination when a person's HIV-positive status is discovered by the employer. Also, a more insidious discrimination occurs, as the HIV-positive individual is not given assignments or promotions at the same pace as his co-workers. The management's concern is that he may not always be counted on to be at work in the future. This concern is also a significant one for the employee, as absences due to opportunistic infections mean that work will be shifted onto co-workers, adding to their loads and generating hostility (Ross, 1989). A Canadian study of families with an HIV-positive hemophiliac within the household found higher rates of unemployment (33% vs. 5%), a lower average annual income ($17,600 vs. $27,700), a higher rate of separation and divorce (11% vs. 0%), and described more stress and other difficulties at work and school than in hemophilia families without an HIV-positive individual (Mindell, O'Neill, & French, 1989). Forty-five percent of the respondents felt that they had been refused employment or lost job opportunities due to health concerns. One-quarter of the families with an HIV-positive individual even experienced a decrease in the family's income. This figure included the impact on caregiving spouses or parents of lost wages while providing care for the affected hemophiliacs (Mindell *et al.,* 1989).

Sexuality

Adults often feel an upsurge in their need for affection and feelings of attachment when they learn about their HIV-positive status (Weiss, 1988). Yet surveys show that sexual activity is markedly reduced in the newly seropositive group and that a minority of men (16%) ended all sexual relationships (Wilson & Wasserman, 1989).

In the past, a hemophiliac was the equal of all other men, in that he could have children. All his sons would be normal, and while his daughters would be carriers of the disease, they would not be directly affected. Now, if this man is seropositive, he faces the risk that he may infect his wife through unprotected intercourse. If she becomes infected, then the child also has a 20% to 50% chance of infection (Johnson *et al.,* 1989). Even in the face of these risks, and advice from the Public Health Service and the National Hemophilia Foundation that HIV-positive hemophiliacs use condoms in combination with nonoxynol 9 (spermicide) and forgo having children, multiple couples have elected to go on with pregnancies, and HIV-infected infants have been born.

Our center has tested 17 sexual partners of HIV-positive hemophiliacs and found 5 to be HIV positive (29%). One sexual partner has died of AIDS, and there is 1 proven seropositive infant born to a hemophiliac and his wife. Seventy nine cases of AIDS have been reported nationally in sexual contacts of hemophiliacs and 9 children of HIV-infected hemophiliacs have developed AIDS (Centers for Disease Control, 1991). There have been 11 studies published reporting HIV seropositivity rates of from 0% to 21% in the sexual partners of hemophiliacs (Lawrence, Jason, Holmen, & Murphy, 1989). The federal government has made the prevention of infections in the spouses and sexual partners of HIV-positive hemophiliacs one of the leading goals of the federally funded HIV risk reduction programs in the comprehensive centers (Barrett, 1989).

People with established relationships. With the concerns about increasing HIV infection rates among sexual partners of hemophiliacs, it is distressing to find that less than half of the couples with a known HIV-infected partner use the risk reduction measures promoted by hemophilia treatment centers on a regular basis (Ragni *et al.,* 1988). Only 18% of women questioned in a different study used condoms "nearly always," and only 12% followed the recommended strategy of avoidance of oral/genital sex, together with the use of condoms (Lawrence *et al.,* 1989).

Several issues are felt to underlie this lack of compliance. First, the women are usually healthy and only have limited contact with the hemophilia center personnel. Second, issues of confidentiality with "their" patient (the hemophiliac) inhibit some hemophilia center workers from directly addressing HIV issues with a spouse or sexual partner. Third, the women may avoid discussion of HIV issues with their local physicians due to fear of community reaction, and finally, the hemophiliac may not inform his partner of his status for fear of losing her or in an attempt to protect her (Ragni *et al.,* 1989). The toll taken by the threat of HIV infection was brought home to the authors of one study when they began to investigate why women did not participate in a follow-up study. There were "poignant descriptions of estrangements, divorces, embitterment at the medical profession, and grief" (Lawrence *et al.,* 1989).

People without established relationships. For the hemophiliac without an intimate partner, avoidance of relationships seems to be a frequent coping method. In a previously cited study, 32% of single hemophiliacs stated that they had postponed having an intimate relationship. Twenty-one percent felt that the AIDS threat made earlier dating problems worse, and were unwilling to pursue further intimate relationships with anyone (Wilson & Wasserman, 1989). A young professional with hemophilia and HIV infection described his situation as "a life in limbo" (Boyer, 1989).

Adolescents. Self-esteem and self-image are very serious concerns for the child or adolescent with hemophilia and have significantly expanded importance when HIV problems are added. Hemophiliacs are unable to participate in many of the sports activities that adolescent males use to define themselves. Then HIV positivity adds the question about a sexual identity and if he will be able to look toward having a sexual life and feelings.

If the adolescent does start to date, many ethical questions are raised. Should the girl be told about his HIV status, and if so, when? If the adolescent hemophiliac has sex with his date without telling her about his HIV status, what are the medicolegal ramifications for the adolescent and his parents. Can an adolescent girl make an informed decision about as critical an issue as the risk that might be posed to her by intercourse with an HIV-positive adolescent boy? There are no answers to the above questions, but from experience with adolescents, the issues may be more than they can deal with.

Teenagers often handle problems by ignoring them. When this is combined with feelings of "invulnerability" and that something bad only happens to other people, the possibility for a disaster looms. At several centers, the policy is to ask the teenage hemophiliac if he has thought about how he would feel if a girlfriend became infected and got AIDS because of something he did. It is hoped that this type of approach will have more success, as direct factual knowledge about AIDS was not found to be "predictive of behavior with regard to safe sexual practices" in adolescent hemophiliacs (Overby *et al.,* 1989).

Encephalopathy

For one of the authors a first encounter with an AIDS patient came in 1985, when a 12-year-old hemophiliac with a 9-month history of increasing learning and behavior problems was brought in by his mother. He had been an advanced student, who would write short stories for enjoyment. During the preceding spring, the quality of his school work dropped off and he stopped writing stories. Then, over the summer, while his local pediatrician investigated him for hypothyroidism, he continued to lose intellectual milestones and became unable to even write a sentence. When he finally presented to the hemophilia center, his appearance was that of a 90-year-old man in the body of a child, with a slack expression, the inability to hold a conversation, and the echoing back of the last two or three words of the question asked to him. We were unable to find any other cause for the cerebral atrophy that was present on his CT scan, and we had nothing to slow the progressive worsening of his dementia. His mother dropped out of nursing school to care for him over the next half year until he died. At the time of his death, he had AIDS-related complex, as the revision of the definition of AIDS to include retroviral encephalopathy did not take place until 1987.

Many hemophiliacs have the same fear as other HIV-positive individuals regarding the development of dementia. A hemophiliac with a very responsible professional job now questions himself any time he forgets something. His fear of intellectual deterioration has made him wary of taking on new jobs or responsibilities. A family whose son died of AIDS took comfort from the fact that his terminal event was rapid—overwhelming liver failure, and not encephalopathy. He had been able to attend the National Hemophilia Foundation annual meeting and appear on a television talk show discussing AIDS in adolescents just weeks before his death. He and his family were familiar with another hemophiliac who died with encephalopathy, and had been blind and demented for a significant period of time. The boy's parents confided that this had been his worst nightmare, and they were glad that both he and they had not had to "go through it." Estimates are that eventually two-thirds of patients with AIDS will have a clinically overt dementia, and one-quarter of the patients will have a subclinical AIDS dementia complex (Price *et al.,* 1988).

Impact on Families of Hemophiliacs

In assessing the impact of HIV infection, AIDS, and hemophilia, all problems must be viewed as affecting a family, not just one individual. While one-third of boys with hemophilia represent a new genetic deletion, and happen in families that have not had a previously affected individual, the majority of children come from families where the gene has been present for many generations.

Multiple Generations Affected

Many times, when an extended family has several generations of hemophiliacs, they may also have several generations with multiple HIV-positive individuals. A mother may be faced with both her father's and uncles', as well as her sons', illnesses with AIDS. The emotional toll on the uninfected, as well as the asymptomatic HIV infected, leads to a survivorlike mentality.

Guilt and Blame

The parents of hemophiliacs with HIV infection have an additional concern due to the genetic pattern of transmission of the disease. Considerable guilt is often felt by the mothers of affected children, and in-laws have sometimes added to this by placing the "blame" for the child's problems on the mother and her genes. The parents of children who were on home transfusion programs also have to come to terms with the fact that they unknowingly infused the contaminated factor concentrate that caused their child's infection.

Overprotection

Overprotection of boys with hemophilia has been a long-standing problem (Mattsson and Gross, 1966) which had been helped by the introduction of home infusion programs. Now that HIV infection has added to the complexity of medical management, and medications like AZT require adherence to strict medication schedules, parental overprotection has again become an issue (Agle, Gluck, & Pierce, 1987; Ross, 1989). The capabilities of the HIV-infected adolescent vary with time and illness, and it is difficult for parents to give back to the adolescent the independence that is necessary for the development of his sense of identity. Adolescence is also the time of risk-taking behavior, which may be of extreme concern to the parent who is trying to balance the need for their child to be independent with the desire to control risks involving either sexual behavior, lack of attention to self-care, or drug abuse.

Discussion of HIV- and AIDS-related issues with children can be extremely difficult for parents. The scope of this discussion is intensive and includes talk of the child's possible death, illness, an explanation of how he became infected, and other mechanisms of transmitting HIV infection. These discussions are extremely important, as the child's understanding of these issues may be incomplete or wrong. The information must be straightforward and given in a manner that will be comprehensible for the child or adolescent. If the information is misunderstood, potentially damaging consequences may result. An example of this is the situation in which a child with hemophilia is accused of being a homosexual by schoolmates who have not understood what has been in the media (Ross, 1989).

Infected and Noninfected Children

The fears and anxieties of the parents may so overwhelm them that they are unable to deal with their child's fears and needs. Parents may still be in the denial phase and may try to maintain the "HIV" secret both within and outside of the family. They may try to protect the child from information they feel he "does not yet need to know" and want the child to remain "untainted" by the knowledge of HIV infection. Knowledge of the HIV status may be kept secret from some family members, but not others, and from friends and relatives. This serves to generate an unmentionable topic for the family and the additional stress of remembering who is on the "informed list" and who isn't. For small children, a special problem of feeling that there is something dirty about themselves that cannot be discussed with others leads to diminished feelings of self-worth. Reactions of children whose parents or loved ones have HIV include isolation, fear, anger, loss, shame, and a need to hide (Sinclair, 1989).

As children grow older, the age of consent becomes a problem. Issues about who determines if the child should be told about his HIV status can cause significant battles between parents and medical caregivers. Many times children and young adolescents will often ask for this information from their parents, who are unwilling or unable to provide answers. Medical staff may attempt to provide this information, such as a discussion of HIV status or information about safer sexual practices, if the child and parents request.

OUTLOOK FOR THE FUTURE

Safe Factor Concentrates

With the development of monoclonal antibody-based purification systems for the isolation of clotting factor concentrates free of viral contamination, safe factor concentrates are now available (Addiego et al., 1989). The introduction of recombinant DNA-produced human clotting factor from cell cultures is presently in clinical trials, and promises to provide clotting factor concentrate that is totally free of any viral contamination, as well as concentrate supplies that are free of the dependence on donations of plasma (Kingdon et al., 1989).

AIDS as a Chronic Disease

Clinical data from trials with zidovudine (AZT) show that it may prolong life and relieve severe AIDS symptoms in children and adults. Also, patients suffering from serious or life-threatening AIDS-related conditions for which there are no satisfactory treatments have the opportunity to obtain promising experimental drugs that have already undergone initial testing to determine that they are safe. Although opinions differ regarding the likelihood that researchers will develop an AIDS vaccine within the next 5 years, promising data from the study of an AIDS-like monkey virus vaccine are encouraging.

Recombinant Gene Technology to Cure Hemophilia

The possibility to "cure" hemophilia exists if the missing or defective DNA could be replaced in the hemophiliac's cells by fresh DNA that properly coded for the missing clotting factor. Experiments have been done using a rat model, where cells containing the gene for human factor IX were implanted under the rat's skin. These cells secreted sufficient levels of human factor IX into the rat's blood so that a human with hemophilia B would have been changed from a severe to a mild hemophiliac (Palmer, Thompson, & Miller, 1988). If this can be adapted to the much larger factor VIII gene, a potential cure for hemophilia exists, and further problems due to contamination of factor concentrates can be avoided.

REFERENCES

Addiego, J., Gomperts, E., Gill, J., Hilgartner, M., Abildgaard, C., Parmley, R., Shapiro, A., Andes, A., Krill, C., Werner, E., Aznar, J., Courter, S., & Kingdon, H. (1989, October, 14). Lack of viral transmission in previously untreated hemophiliacs using a monoclonal ab purified, organic solvent/detergent treated plasma derived from factor VIIIc concentrate. In abstracts from the *41st Conference of the National Hemophilia Foundation* (p. 1), Chicago, IL.

Agle, D. P. (1975). Psychological factors in hemophilia—the concept of self-care. *Annals of the New York Academy of Science, 240,* 221–225.

Agle, D., Gluck, H., & Pierce, G. F. (1987). The risk of AIDS: Psychologic impact on the hemophilic population. *General Hospital Psychiatry, 9,* 11–17.

Aledort, L. M. (1989). Concentrates: meeting the demand. *Life Paths, 1*(2), 6–7.

Barret, S. (1989, January). Presentation to *HIV Risk Reduction within the Hemophilia Community Conference,* Las Vegas, NV.

Boyer, P. B. (1989, April 1). A life in limbo. *The New York Times Magazine,* p. 48.

Centers for Disease Control. (1982). Pneumocystis carinii pneumonia among persons with hemophilia A. *Morbidity and Mortality Weekly Report, 31,* 507.

Centers for Disease Control. (1991, May 8). *HIV/AIDS surveillance report,* pp. 1–10.

Coles, P. (1989). French haemophiliacs awarded damages. *Nature, 340,* 253.

Gerety, R. J., & Barker, L. F. (1976). Viral antigens and antibodies in hemophiliacs. In *National Heart, Lung, and Blood Institute: Unsolved Therapeutic Problems in Hemophilia* (pp. 51–56). Washington, DC: U.S. Government Printing Office.

Gjerset, G. F., McGrady, G., Counts, R. B., Martin, P. J., Jason, J., Kennedy, S., Evatt, B., & Hansen, J. A. (1985). Lymphadenopathy-associated virus antibodies and T cells in hemophiliacs treated with cryoprecipitate or concentrate. *Blood, 66,* 718–720.

Goedert, J. J., Sarngadharan, M. G., Eyster, M. E., Weiss, S. H., Bodner, A. J., Gallo, R. C., & Blattner, W. A. (1985). Antibodies reactive with human T cell leukemia viruses in the serum of hemophiliacs receiving factor VIII concentrate. *Blood, 65,* 492–495.

Hernandez, J., Gray, D., & Lineberger, H. P. (1989). Social and economic indicators of well-being among hemophiliacs over a 5-year period. *General Hospital Psychiatry, 11,* 241–247.

Hershgold, E. J., Pool, J. G., & Pappenhagen, A. R. (1966). The potent antihemophilic globulin concentrate derived from a cold insoluble fraction of human plasma: characterization and further data on preparation and clinical trial. *Journal of Laboratory and Clinical Medicine, 67,* 23–32.

Jason, J., Holman, R. C., Dixon, G., Lawrence, D. N., Bozeman, L. H., Chorba, T. L., Tregillus, L., & Evatt, B. L. (1986). Effects of exposure to factor concentrates containing donations from identified AIDS patients. A matched cohort study. *Journal of the American Medical Association, 256,* 1758–1762.

Johnson, A. J., Newman, J., Howell, M. B., & Puszkin, S. (1967). Purification of antihemophilic factor (AHF) for clinical and experimental use. *Thrombosis, Diathesis, and Haemorrhage,* 377–381.

Johnson, J. P., Nair, P., Hines, S. E., Seiden, S. W., Alger, L., Revie, D. R., O'Neil, K. M., & Hebel, R. (1989). Natural history and serologic diagnosis of infants born to human immunodeficiency virus-infected women. *American Journal of Diseases of Children, 143,* 1147–53.

Kasper, C. K., & Kipnis, S. A. (1972). Hepatitis and clotting factor concentrates. *Journal of the American Medical Association, 221,* 510.

Kingdon, H. S., Liu, S. L., Bagby, B., Cox, D., Gracien, M., Lee, M., & Courter, S. (1989, October 14). Preliminary result of recombinate™ clinical safety and efficacy. In abstracts from the *41st Conference of the National Hemophilia Foundation* (p. 6), Chicago, IL.

Kreiss, J. K., Kitchen, L. W., Prince, H. E., Kasper, C. K., Goldstein, A. L., Naylor, P. H., Preble, O., Stewart, J. A., & Essex, M. (1986). Human T cell leukemia virus type III antibody, lymphadenopathy, and acquired immune deficiency syndrome in hemophiliac subjects. Results of a prospective study. *American Journal of Medicine, 80,* 345–350.

Lawrence, D. N., Jason, J. M., Holman, R. C., Heine, P., Evatt, B. L., & the Hemophilia Study Group. (1989). Sex practice correlates of human immunodeficiency virus transmission and acquired immunodeficiency syndrome incidence in heterosexual partners and offspring of U.S. hemophilic men. *American Journal of Hematology, 30,* 68–76.

Lawrence, D. N., Jason, J. J., Holman, R. C., Murphy, J. J. (1989, February). Human immunodeficiency virus transmission from hemophilic men to their heterosexual partners. In *Proceedings of the CONRAD 2nd International Workshop,* Norfolk, VA.

Levine, P. H., & Britten, A. F. H. (1973). Supervised patient-management of hemophilia. A study of 45 patients with hemophilia A and B. *Annals of Internal Medicine, 78,* 195–201.

Lusher, J. M. (1989, October 14). Update on safety of clotting factor concentrates. In abstracts from the *41st Conference of the National Hemophilia Foundation* (p. 26). Chicago, IL.

Mattsson, A., & Gross, S. (1966). Adaptational and defensive behavior in young hemophiliacs and their parents. *American Journal of Psychiatry, 122,* 1349–1356.

Mindell, W., O'Neill, R., & French, S. (1989). The social and economic impact of HIV on Canadians with hemophilia. Presented at *The Vth International Conference on AIDS,* Montreal, Canada.

National Hemophilia Foundation (1988). *What you should know about hemophilia.* New York: National Hemophilia Foundation.

National Hemophilia Foundation (1989, November 22). MASAC policy on access to AIDS clinical trials. *Hemophilia Information Exchange, 97,* 1–2.

Overby, K. J., Lo, B., & Litt, I. F. (1989). Knowledge and concerns about acquired immunodeficiency syndrome and their relationship to behavior among adolescents with hemophilia. *Pediatrics, 83,* 204–210.

Palmer, T. D., Thompson, A. R., & Miller, A. D. (1988, October 15). Recombinant human factor IX in rodents produced by gene transfer. In abstracts from the *40th Conference of the National Hemophilia Foundation* (p. 12), Anaheim, CA.

Price, R. W., Brew, B., Sidtis, J., Rosenblum, M., Scheck, A. C., & Cleary, P. (1988). The brain in AIDS: central nervous system HIV-1 infection and AIDS dementia complex. *Science, 239,* 586–592.

Ragni, M. V., Gupta, P., Rinaldo, C. R., Kingsley, L. A., Spero, J. A., & Lewis, J. H. (1988). HIV transmission to female sexual partners of HIV antibody-positive hemophiliacs. *Public Health Report, 103,* 54–58.

Ragni, M. V., & Nimorwicz, P. (1989). Human immunodeficiency virus transmission and hemophilia. *Archives of Internal Medicine, 149,* 1379–1380.

Ross, J. (1989). People with hemophilia and HIV. *Life Paths, 1,* 7–9.

Seeff, L. B., & Hoofnagle, J. (1976). Acute and chronic liver disease in hemophilia. In *National Heart, Lung, and Blood Institute: Unsolved therapeutic problems in hemophilia* (pp. 61–72). Washington, DC: U.S. Government Printing Office.

Sinclair, R. (1989). The impact on children whose parents or loved ones have HIV disease. Presented at *The Vth International Conference on AIDS,* Montreal, Canada.

Stehr-Green, J. K., Holman, R. C., Jason, J. M., & Evatt, B. L. (1988). Hemophilia-associated AIDS in the United States, 1981 to September, 1987. *American Journal of Public Health, 78,* 439–442.

Tetrick, A. P. (1989). *Medical insurance policy scrutiny. Guidelines for families with chronic disease.* Worcester, MA: New England Hemophilia Center.

Waskin, H., Smith, K. J., Simon, T. L., Gribble, T. J., & Mertz, G. J. (1986). Prevalence of HTLV-III antibody among New Mexico residents with hemophilia. *Western Journal of Medicine, 145,* 477–480.

Weiss, R. S. (1988). The experience of AIDS: Hypotheses based on pilot study interviews. *Journal of Palliative Care, 4,* 15–25.

Wilson, P. A., & Wasserman, K. (1989). Psychosocial responses to the threat of HIV exposure among people with bleeding disorders. *Health and Social Work, 14,* 176–183.

Index